TRANSESOPHAGEAL ECHOCARDIOGRAPHY OF CONGENITAL HEART DISEASES

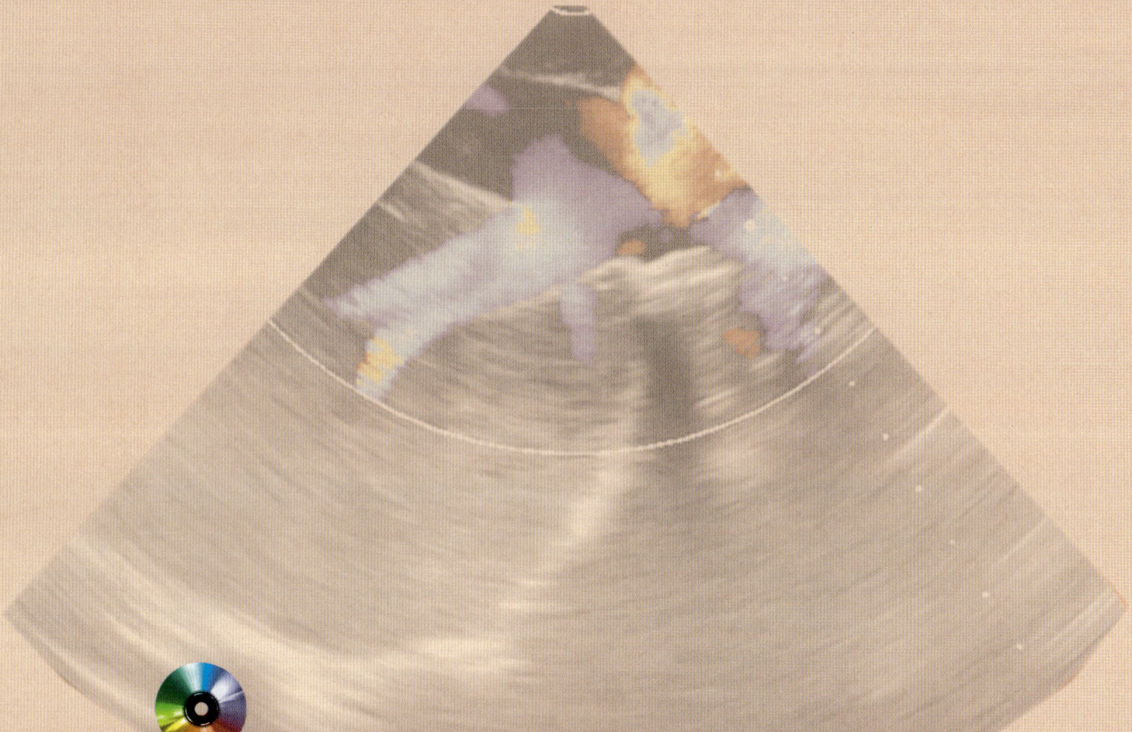

System requirement:

- Operating System—Windows Vista or above
- Web Browser—Google Chrome, Mozilla Firefox, Internet Explorer 9 and above
- Essential plugins—Java and Flash Player
  - Facing problems in viewing content—it may be, your system does not have Java enabled.
  - If videos do not show up—it may be the system requires Flash Player or need to manage Flash setting. To learn more about Flash setting click on the link in the help section.
  - You can test Java and Flash by using the links from the help section of the **CD/DVD**.

Accompanying DVD-ROM is playable only in Computer and not in DVD player.

CD/DVD has autorun function—it may take few seconds to load on your computer. If it does not work for you, then follow the steps below to access the contents manually:

- Click on my computer.
- Select the **CD/DVD** drive and click open/explore—this will show list of files in the **CD/DVD**.
- Find and double click file—"launch.html".

For more information about troubleshoot of autorun click on:
http://support.microsoft.com/kb/330135

TRANSESOPHAGEAL ECHOCARDIOGRAPHY OF CONGENITAL HEART DISEASES

Editors

Poonam Malhotra Kapoor

MD DNB MNAMS FIACTA FTEE FISCU

Professor
Department of Cardiac Anesthesia
Cardio-Neuro Center (CNC)
All India Institute of Medical Sciences, New Delhi, India
Secretary
Society of Cardiac Anesthesia
Delhi and NCR Branch
Coordinator
Indian Association of Cardiovascular Thoracic Anesthesiologists (IACTA)
Education and Research Cell
Co-editor
Annals of Cardiac Anesthesia

Sarvesh Pal Singh

MD DM FIACTA FTEE

Senior Resident
Department of Cardiac Anesthesia
Cardio-Neuro Center (CNC)
All India Institute of Medical Sciences
New Delhi, India

Forewords

MC Misra, Navin C Nanda, Balram Airan
Usha Kiran, Yatin Mehta

Under the Aegis of SCA—Delhi and NCR

JAYPEE

JAYPEE BROTHERS MEDICAL PUBLISHERS (P) LTD

New Delhi • London • Philadelphia • Panama

Jaypee Brothers Medical Publishers (P) Ltd.

Headquarters
Jaypee Brothers Medical Publishers (P) Ltd.
4838/24, Ansari Road, Daryaganj
New Delhi 110 002, India
Phone: +91-11-43574357
Fax: +91-11-43574314
E-mail: jaypee@jaypeebrothers.com

Overseas Offices

J.P. Medical Ltd.
83, Victoria Street, London
SW1H 0HW (UK)
Phone: +44-2031708910
Fax: +44(0)2030086180
E-mail: info@jpmedpub.com

Jaypee-Highlights Medical Publishers Inc.
City of Knowledge, Bld. 237, Clayton
Panama City, Panama
Phone: +1 507-301-0496
Fax: +1 507-301-0499
E-mail: cservice@jphmedical.com

Jaypee Medical Inc.
The Bourse
111, South Independence Mall East
Suite 835, Philadelphia, PA 19106, USA
Phone: +1 267-519-9789
E-mail: jpmed.us@gmail.com

Jaypee Brothers Medical Publishers (P) Ltd.
17/1-B, Babar Road, Block-B, Shaymali
Mohammadpur, Dhaka-1207
Bangladesh
Mobile: +08801912003485
E-mail: jaypeedhaka@gmail.com

Jaypee Brothers Medical Publishers (P) Ltd.
Bhotahity, Kathmandu, Nepal
Phone: +977-9741283608
E-mail: kathmandu@jaypeebrothers.com

Website: www.jaypeebrothers.com
Website: www.jaypeedigital.com

Inquiries for bulk sales may be solicited at: jaypee@jaypeebrothers.com

Transesophageal Echocardiography of Congenital Heart Diseases

First Edition: **2014**

ISBN: 978-93-5152-219-5

Printed at Replika Press Pvt. Ltd.

Dedicated to

My father and family

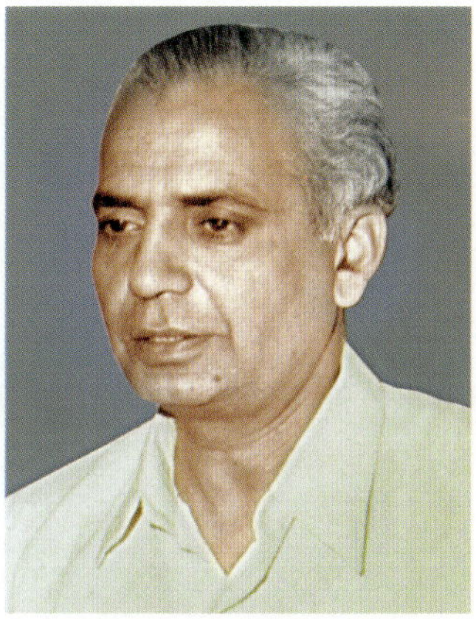

Dr KK Malhotra
(4.7.1929–4.1.2011)

My father is a never-ending song in my heart—of comfort, happiness and well-being. I may sometimes forget the words but I always remember the tune.

My mentor, guide and inspiration in life
An extraordinary physician and human being with boundless affection, witty, hardworking and godly qualities who three years after he's gone, still inspires me to read and write. He is my bridge and good luck charm.

—Poonam Malhotra Kapoor

Dedicated to

IACTA Education and Research Cell (IERC)

Contributors

Ajay Jha
Senior Resident
Department of Cardiac Anesthesia
Cardio-Neuro Center (CNC)
All India Institute of
Medical Sciences (AIIMS)
New Delhi, India

Arin Choudhury
Senior Resident
Department of Cardiac Anesthesia
Cardio-Neuro Center (CNC)
All India Institute of
Medical Sciences
New Delhi, India

Arindam Choudhury
Assistant Professor
Department of Cardiac Anesthesia
Cardio-Neuro Center (CNC)
All India Institute of
Medical Sciences
New Delhi, India

Arun Subramaniam
Senior Resident
Department of Cardiac Anesthesia
Cardio-Neuro Center (CNC)
All India Institute of
Medical Sciences
New Delhi, India

Balaswaroop Sahu
Senior Resident
Department of Cardiac Anesthesia
Cardio-Neuro Center (CNC)
All India Institute of
Medical Sciences
New Delhi, India

Dinesh Chandra
Senior Resident
Department of Cardio-Thoracic and
Vascular Surgery
Cardio-Neuro Center (CNC)
All India Institute of
Medical Sciences
New Delhi, India

Jitin Narula
Senior Resident
Department of Cardiac Anesthesia
Cardio-Neuro Center (CNC)
All India Institute of
Medical Sciences
New Delhi, India

Kalpana Irpachi
Senior Resident
Department of Cardiac Anesthesia
Cardio-Neuro Center (CNC)
All India Institute of
Medical Sciences
New Delhi, India

Kulbhushan Saini
Senior Resident
Department of Cardiac Anesthesia
Cardio-Neuro Center (CNC)
All India Institute of
Medical Sciences
New Delhi, India

Milind Hote
Additional Professor
Department of Cardio-Thoracic and
Vascular Surgery
Cardio-Neuro Center (CNC)
All India Institute of
Medical Sciences
New Delhi, India

Minati Choudhury
Additional Professor
Department of Cardiac Anesthesia
Cardio-Neuro Center (CNC)
All India Institute of
Medical Sciences
New Delhi, India

Neeti Makhija
Professor
Department of Cardiac Anesthesia
Cardio-Neuro Center (CNC)
All India Institute of
Medical Sciences
New Delhi, India

Pankaj Kumar
Senior Resident
Department of Cardiac Anesthesia
Cardio-Neuro Center (CNC)
All India Institute of
Medical Sciences
New Delhi, India

Parag Gharde
Additional Professor
Department of Cardiac Anesthesia
Cardio-Neuro Center (CNC)
All India Institute of
Medical Sciences
New Delhi, India

Pawan Jain
Senior Resident
Department of Cardiac Anesthesia
Cardio-Neuro Center (CNC)
All India Institute of
Medical Sciences
New Delhi, India

Poonam Malhotra Kapoor
Professor
Department of Cardiac Anesthesia
Cardio-Neuro Center (CNC)
All India Institute of Medical Sciences, New Delhi, India
Secretary
Society of Cardiac Anesthesia
Delhi and NCR Branch
Coordinator
Indian Association of Cardiovascular Thoracic Anesthesiologists (IACTA)
Education and Research Cell
Co-editor
Annals of Cardiac Anesthesia

Rajshekhar
Assistant Professor
Department of Cardio-Thoracic Vascular Surgery
Cardio-Neuro Center (CNC)
All India Institute of Medical Sciences
New Delhi, India

RS Rajput
Senior Resident
Department of Cardiac Anesthesia
Cardio-Neuro Center (CNC)
All India Institute of Medical Sciences
New Delhi, India

Sachin Talwar
Additional Professor
Department of Cardio-Thoracic Vascular Surgery
Cardio-Neuro Center (CNC)
All India Institute of Medical Sciences
New Delhi, India

Sameer Taneja
Senior Resident
Department of Cardiac Anesthesia
Cardio-Neuro Center (CNC)
All India Institute of Medical Sciences
New Delhi, India

Sandeep Chauhan
Professor
Department of Cardiac Anesthesia
Cardio-Neuro Center (CNC)
All India Institute of Medical Sciences
New Delhi, India

Sanjay Kumar
Senior Resident
Department of Cardiac Anesthesia
Cardio-Neuro Center (CNC)
All India Institute of Medical Sciences
New Delhi, India

Sarvesh Pal Singh
Senior Resident
Department of Cardiac Anesthesia
Cardio-Neuro Center (CNC)
All India Institute of Medical Sciences
New Delhi, India

SN Das
Additional Professor
Department of Cardiac Anesthesia
Cardio-Neuro Center (CNC)
All India Institute of Medical Sciences
New Delhi, India

Suruchi Ladha
Senior Resident
Department of Cardiac Anesthesia
Cardio-Neuro Center (CNC)
All India Institute of Medical Sciences
New Delhi, India

Suruchi Hasija
Assistant Professor
Department of Cardiac Anesthesia
Cardio-Neuro Center (CNC)
All India Institute of Medical Sciences
New Delhi, India

Ujjwal Chowdhury
Professor
Department of Cardio-Thoracic Vascular Surgery
Cardio-Neuro Center (CNC)
All India Institute of Medical Sciences
New Delhi
India

Umed Kumar
Senior Resident
Department of Cardiac Anesthesia
Cardio-Neuro Center (CNC)
All India Institute of Medical Sciences
New Delhi
India

Usha Kiran
Professor and Head
Department of Cardiac Anesthesia
Cardio-Neuro Center (CNC)
All India Institute of Medical Sciences
New Delhi
India

V Devagourou
Additional Professor
Department of Cardio-Thoracic Vascular Surgery
Cardio-Neuro Center (CNC)
All India Institute of Medical Sciences
New Delhi
India

Vishwas Malik
Additional Professor
Department of Cardiac Anesthesia
Cardio-Neuro Center (CNC)
All India Institute of Medical Sciences
New Delhi
India

अखिल भारतीय आयुर्विज्ञान संस्थान
अंसारी नगर, नई दिल्ली–110029

All India Institute of Medical Sciences
ANSARI NAGAR, NEW DELHI-110029

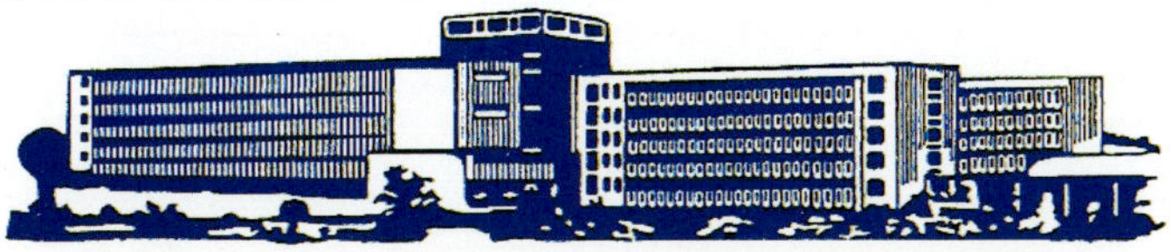

फैक्स सं०/Fax No.: 91-11-26588663, 26588641
दूरभाष/Phone: (का०/Offi) 26588000, 26594800, 25694805
Phones (नि०/Res.) +91-11-26594500
E-mail : director@aiims.ac.in, director.aiims@gmail.com

प्रो० महेश चन्द्र मिश्र
निदेशक

Prof. M. C. Misra
MS, FRCS, Hon. FRCS (Glasg.) FCLS, FAMS, FACS
DIRECTOR

संख्या/No...

दिनांक/Date 02nd May, 2014

Foreword

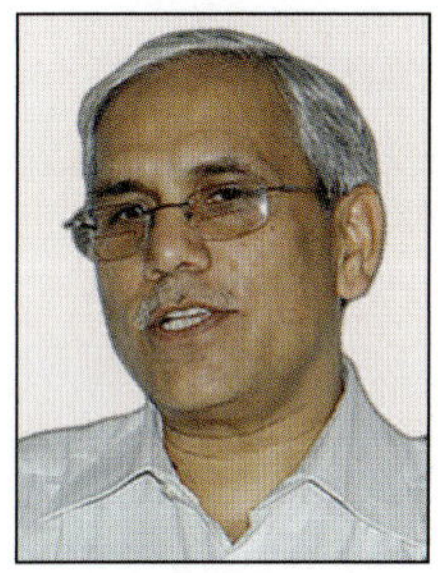

A precise and complete diagnosis of congenital heart disease has always been a very challenging problem. Cardiac catheterization had to be resorted to it in all cases prior to surgery especially in congenital heart disease. The access to echo-Doppler has enabled the echocardiographer to deliberate the pathoanatomy and pathophysiology of congenital heart disease with great ease and perfection, and a major chunk of this population is now submitted directly to surgery. The availability of perioperative transesophageal echocardiography (TEE) has paved the way for evaluation of all cases in a tertiary center like All India Institute of Medical Sciences (AIIMS), New Delhi, India, enabling good surgical outcomes in complex pediatric patients undergoing corrective cardiac surgery.

The intraoperative echocardiography and echocardiography during catheter interventions have also proved very gratifying. The key to success in congenital heart disease is to proceed in a much planned systemic way. *Transesophageal Echocardiography of Congenital Heart Diseases* by Dr Poonam Malhotra Kapoor and Dr Sarvesh Pal Singh is so elegantly edited and illustrated that it will automatically pave the way for a correct and complete diagnosis of congenital heart disease. I am confident that the contents of the book are original and the editors have exercised extreme caution while reproducing text, pictures and diagrams.

The book will continue to vibrate you from beginning-to-end and going through the book is a pleasure. The reading shows that the editors of the book are unmatched in their pediatric perioperative TEE skills and have excelled in their fields.

I am sure that the book will find a permanent place on the desk of all echocardiographers interested in congenital heart diseases. I compliment and congratulate Dr Poonam Malhotra Kapoor and her team for this wonderful endeavor, and wish the book and all of them a great success.

MC Misra
Director
All India Institute of Medical Sciences
New Delhi, India

Foreword

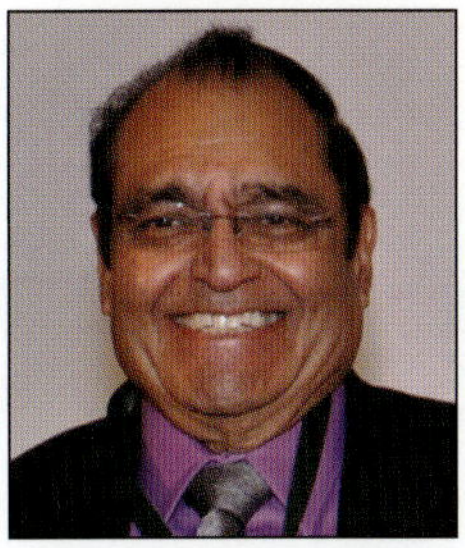

Traditionally, transesophageal echocardiography (TEE) provides a very clear picture in most cardiac congenital diseases, for diagnosing various pathologies and is a rapid diagnostic screening tool, though not universally available, because of its cost.

This book tries to present a very easy-to-use practical approach to TEE in complex and simple congenital heart diseases, which is not an easy subject in itself.

We are well aware, that three-dimensional (3D) TEE is now a potent visual medium which can be used by the novice or experienced echocardiographer and beautifully complements the traditional 2D and 3D imaging and it also permits visualization of any cardiac structure of interest from multiple perspectives.

Transesophageal Echocardiography of Congenital Heart Diseases represents a unique work, the only textbook of its kind that focuses specifically upon the applications of TEE in congenital heart disease (CHD). In each chapter, the contributors—highly regarded specialists and leaders in the field—provide practical and instructive information on many different aspects of CHD evaluation by TEE. The textbook is extensively supplemented with figures/illustrations and high quality videos (available online) and all from All India Institute of Medical Sciences (AIIMS), New Delhi, India. This reference will prove an invaluable resource for those who use TEE in the care of both children and adults with CHD, whether they be cardiologists, surgeons, anesthesiologists, intensivists, sonographers, or trainees wishing to obtain basic knowledge or advance their understanding of the field.

The details of each lesion on TEE are very beautifully illustrated with tables, figures and adequate videos which are self-explanatory.

The textbook will rekindle everyone's interest in the operating room especially amongst postgraduates, dealing with the subject to this powerful tool TEE.

The wealth of information provided in the book is truly awesome. Every clinician who sees patients with congenital lesions of the heart would want a copy of the book, close at hand. I wish the editors all success in their academic endeavor. It is with pleasure that I write a foreword to the book.

Navin C Nanda
Professor
Department of Medicine and Cardiovascular Disease
Director
Heart Station/Echocardiography Laboratories
University of Alabama
Birmingham, Alabama, USA

Foreword

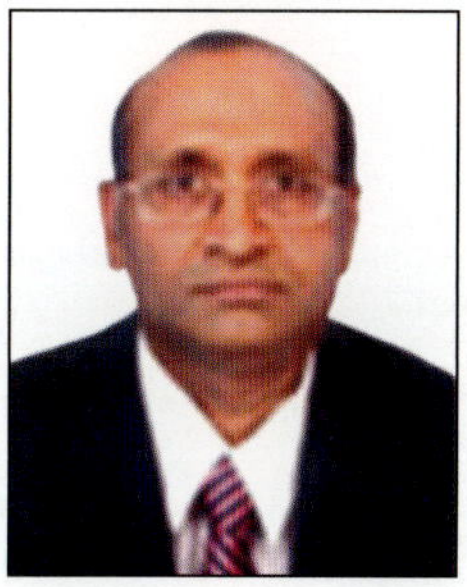

Transesophageal Echocardiography of Congenital Heart Diseases is an important and admirable book. It is thorough, lucid and extremely practical, and is a manual of all echocardiographers need to know about their proper role in the operative room and the intensive care unit (ICU), postoperative about the adequacy of surgery.

This is an excellent addition to the library of books on TEE. It is concise yet thorough, well-written with excellent illustrations, and tables that enhance the reading, and provides an outstanding review of the subject. I would highly recommend this to all cardiothoracic anesthesiologists/surgeons, especially fellows in training of the subject and taking examinations.

It is not only a practical guide to best practice in TEE of CHD, but also sets out the procedure which apply to reach the diagnosis of disease and clinical negligence cases. The text is expressed in clear and accessible terms, and also offers useful practical guidance on many of the difficult issues that arise in obtaining good views of this subject.

All-in-all, the *Transesophageal Echocardiography in Congenital Heart Diseases,* is a very important entry into what I would consider the "examination preparation" category of echocardiography textbooks for fellows and students in the subject. The chapters are well-illustrated, and most have an extensive number of topics that they may need to review in greater depth. With expert contributors and sound editing, the book would be a valuable addition to the library of anesthesiologists, surgeons and cardiologists interested in a text covering the breadth of topics related to transesophageal echocardiography in congenital heart disease.

The eyes do not see what the mind does not know is very true about TEE in congenital heart disease. As a result, a simple atrial septal defect (ASD) may be missed. There is a great need for a book of this type and editors' present work goes a long way in fulfilling this need.

I wish the editors all success in their venture.

Balram Airan
Professor and Head
Department of Cardiothoracic and Vascular Surgery (CTVS)
Chief
Cardiothoracic Center
All India Institute of Medical Sciences
New Delhi, India

Foreword

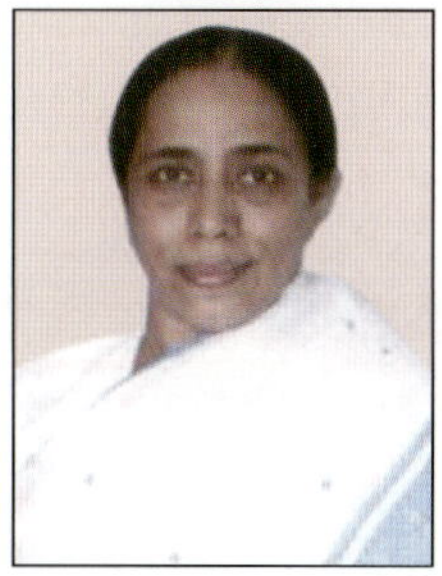

It has been my experience that transesophageal echocardiography (TEE) is highly essential tool for intraoperative monitoring and guiding surgical procedures. Advancement in non-invasive and invasive perioperative monitorings has grown by leaps and bounds in last two decades. Transesophageal echocardiography though invasive but evidence narrates almost negligible complications and is as safe as noninvasive technology in expert hands.

Any technology will be useful, if proper training skills are developed to make maximum use. Experience is substantiated by a nationwise survey and conducting various transesophageal echocardiography workshops and hand-on training programs. Faculty and resident doctors involved in cardiac anesthesia have shown a lot of interest in learning their skills.

Transesophageal Echocardiography of Congenital Heart Diseases is a practical guidance for those doctors who want to get benefit of advanced perioperative monitoring and are thoroughly involved in pediatric care.

Hoping that, this book will be highly useful for Cardiac Anesthesia Residency Training Program and for those, anesthesiologists involved in subspecialties like neurosurgery, orthopedic surgery especially those who are managing the patients with the higher risk of thromboembolic phenomenon.

May I thank the editors and Department of Cardiac Anesthesia as well as Department of Cardiothoracic Vascular Surgery of All India Institute of Medical Sciences (AIIMS), New Delhi, India, their staff and technical officers for consistent efforts in bringing out the book with illustrations and videos from patients who underwent successful surgery in cardiothoracic center at AIIMS.

Usha Kiran
Professor and Head
Department of Cardiac Anesthesia
Cardio-Neuro Center (CNC)
All India Institute of Medical Sciences
New Delhi, India

Foreword

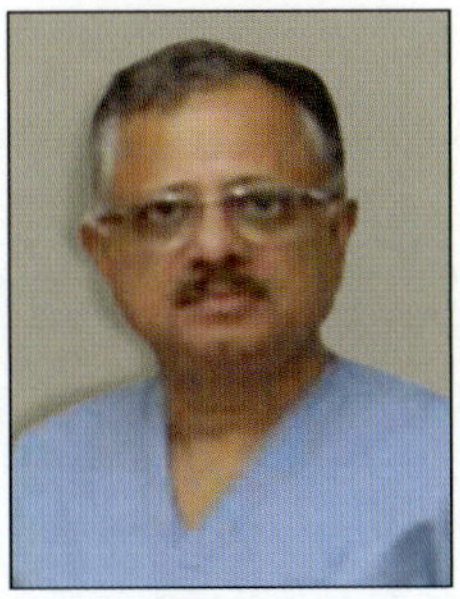

Transesophageal Echocardiography of Congenital Heart Diseases by Professor Poonam Malhotra Kapoor is another landmark book in a series of books from her. Each book gets better than the previous and all within a year!

It is a commendable effort, timely and highly recommended. This is a book for a quick read or for refreshing ones memory prior to a viva or examination! It is particularly useful for MD, DM, FIACTA or FNB examination going candidates for a quick revision prior to a presentation or examination or for a senior cardiac anesthesiologist like me who mostly does adult anesthesia and does not have time for a detailed time consuming reading! It has twenty-five chapters each with a few salient features of that particular pathology with pre- and postoperative TEE images of very good quality along with brief description of the ECGs and X-ray chest views for the same pathology as TEE.

It is a unique, easily readable book with just the right amount of information in right doses. M/s Jaypee Brothers Medical Publishers (P) Ltd, New Delhi, India, has done a very good job as usual, and printing and image quality is excellent. It is along with a DVD-ROM which is an additional attractive feature containing videos.

I would strongly recommend the book for everyone dealing with pediatric-cardiac patients, surgeons, anesthesiologists, cardiologists and intensivists.

Yatin Mehta
Chairman
Medanta Institute of Critical Care and Anesthesiology
Medanta—The Medicity
Gurgaon, Haryana, India

Preface

The purpose of *Transesophageal Echocardiography of Congenital Heart Diseases* is to provide the definitive advanced reference text on the diagnostic utility of echocardiography in clinical practice. Put simply, the book reflects our role as clinicians caring for patients with congenital heart disease. The clinical information in the book will be of value to all cardiovascular specialists, anesthetists and surgeons not just those focused on cardiovascular imaging. The book will also be of interest to cardiology fellows, cardiovascular anesthesiologists, and other healthcare providers using echocardiographic approaches in the clinical setting, including interventional cardiologists, electrophysiologists, emergency medicine physicians, and internists with an active interest in cardiovascular disease with congenital heart diseases and titling in the lacunae have done along with Dr Poonam Malhotra Kapoor, Dr Sarvesh Pal Singh for the videos and text, and Dr Jitin Narula for editing.

We have many people to thank for their efforts in producing the book. First, the contributors have done a superb job of producing authoritative chapters that synthesize vast amounts of scientific and clinical data to create state-of-the-art descriptions of medical disorders. In today's information rich, rapidly evolving environment, they have ensured that this information is current. Helpful suggestions and critical inputs have been provided by a number of colleagues; particularly notable was the advice and encouragement of Dr Usha Kiran. We are most grateful to all our colleagues in each of our chapters who have kept track of the operating rooms and helped us complete it directly or indirectly.

Why is this book necessary? Today echo facility is available in most operating rooms doing pediatric-cardiac surgery. Further, echo is reported by technicians and clinicians who are otherwise good but have less exposure to echo in congenital heart disease.

The book will also appeal to all examinees wanting to know about the echo which is simple, safe, cost-effective, and the excellent noninvasive diagnostic tool that is easily available and the videos can be used by them to have a perfect picture. We hope readers will be richly benefited by the book and do well in all examinations, such as DNB, DM, FIACTA, and perioperative TEE examinations.

Thank you all and happy reading.

Poonam Malhotra Kapoor
Sarvesh Pal Singh

Acknowledgments

At the outset we would like to thank the God Almighty for enabling us to put this book to print. It has been a proud privilege to work at All India Institute of Medical Sciences (AIIMS), New Delhi, India, for all these years. We would like to thank the whole staff of Cardiothoracic Center at AIIMS for the exceptional work, they have been doing for years. We thank Professor Balram Airan, Chief, Cardiothoracic Center for his exceptional leading capacity and unrelenting support. We extend our gratitude to Professor Usha Kiran, Head, Department of Cardiac Anesthesia and Professor Sandeep Chauhan for their constant encouragement and supervision and expert suggestions at all time. Our special thanks to the Faculty, Department of Cardiac Anesthesia and to Dr Sachin Talwar for his invaluable inputs regarding the aspects of different complex surgeries.

Thanks to Professor MC Mishra, The Director, AIIMS, for his amiable, communicative and for AIIMS in having a 'doer' director personality and one who is inspirational, encouraging and has unbridled enthusiasm, to go ahead and get things done. He is a true leader and we are lucky at AIIMS to be having him direct us, we thank him, and Dr Navin C Nanda, Professor Balram Airan and Professor Usha Kiran whole-heartedly for writing forewords in the book and encouraging us with expert suggestions.

Our heartfelt gratitude to Dr Yatin Mehta for his untiring effort and support for SCA—Delhi and NCR and his motivation for this book. A leader like him has made us put in all efforts in building up a strong academics society within 5 years time. He is an encouraging and inspirational senior. He is a true maestro and stalwart.

Our office team Mr Sandeep, Mr Manoj Mishra, Mr Pradeep, Mr Sachin Balyan, and Miss Poonam are to be especially thanked for their data and reference input and typing and preparation of the book in such a short time. We could not work without them!

We express our sincere gratitude to all contributors of the individual chapters, faculty and senior residents at Department of Cardiac Anesthesia, Cardio-Neuro Center (CNC), AIIMS. Without their hard work and dedication, this textbook could not have been completed.

We are heartily thankful to Shri Jitendar P Vij (Group Chairman), Mr Ankit Vij (Group President), Mr Tarun Duneja (Director-Publishing), Mr Sunil Kumar Dogra (Production Executive), Mr Neelambar Pant (Production Coordinator), Mr Chandra Dutt (Typesetter), Mr Gurnam Singh (Senior Proofreader), Mr Binay Kumar (Proofreader) Mr Manoj Pahuja (Graphic Designer-Head) of M/s Jaypee Brothers Medical Publishers (P) Ltd., New Delhi, India, and also like to acknowledge the professionalism and talent of Shri Jitendar P Vij and his publishing team for a speedy and professional academic venture for the fourth time, within a year. Thanks to their editorial efforts to improve the book overall.

Special thanks to DSS, CAE viamedix team of Mr Kandhari, Mr Praveen and Mr Manish Bansal for their "simulation" inputs in the chapter of "TEE views". A heartfelt thank also goes to Dr Varun Kapoor, for always looking at the bright side of life, Mr Pranav Kapoor, for making us realize what is really important in life and our family members who are our moral and emotional supporters at all adverse moments, we thank Almighty for his utmost blessings on us, AIIMS and SCA—Delhi and NCR. Thank you God for everything.

Poonam Malhotra Kapoor
Sarvesh Pal Singh

Contents

DVD Contents

Chapter 3
TEE VIEWS IN CONGENITAL HEART DISEASE

S. No. Video Name

1. *Video 1:* Midesophageal four chamber view for identification of four chambers, IAS, IVS, MV and TV.
2. *Video 2:* Midesophageal two chamber view to show the LV and LA and also provide detailed evaluation of the mitral valve and regional assessment of the LV anterior and inferior walls.
3. *Video 3:* Midesophageal bicommissural view for a detailed view of LA, LV and MV leaflets and their scallops.
4. *Video 4:* Midesophageal long-axis view for LV function, MV disease, AV and aortic root disease to view the aortic over-ride and IVS in detail.
5. *Video 5:* Midesophageal aortic valve long-axis view showing the aortic and mitral valves and regional assessment of LV, also excellent for aortic annulus and AML length.
6. *Video 6:* Midesophageal aortic valve short-axis view the 3 cusps of AV, calcification in the 3 cusps, presence and quantification of AS and AR.
7. *Video 7:* Midesophageal bicaval view outline and video to see the IAS.
8. *Video 8:* Midesophageal descending thoracic aorta long-axis view showing the descending thoracic aorta in the center.
9. *Video 9:* Midesophageal descending thoracic aorta short-axis view showing the descending thoracic aorta. Ideal for IABP placement evaluation and see left pleural effusion.
10. *Video 10:* Midesophageal ascending aorta long-axis view showing the relation of the RPA and aorta.
11. *Video 11:* Midesophageal ascending aorta short-axis view showing the ascending aorta, superior vena cava (short-axis), main pulmonary artery, right pulmonary artery, left pulmonary artery (turn probe tip to left), pulmonic valve.
12. *Video 12:* Midesophageal left atrial appendage view showing left atrial appendage and left upper pulmonary valve.
13. *Video 13:* Midesophageal modified bicaval view showing right atrial appendage and superior vena cava.
14. *Video 14:* Midesophageal right pulmonary vein view to show the position between aorta, superior vena cava and the right pulmonary artery, seen to the right side in figure B.
15. *Video 15:* Midesophageal right ventricle inflow-outflow view showing the right ventricle and atrium, left atrium, right atrium tricuspid valve, aortic valve, right ventricle outflow tract, pulmonic valve and main pulmonary artery.
16. *Video 16*
17. *Video 17:* Transgastric modified hepatic vein view showing anterior vena cava, hepatic veins and right atrium.
18. *Video 18:* Transgastric two chamber view showing left ventricle and atrium coronary sinus and mitral valve.
19. *Video 19:* Transgastric apical short-axis view showing left and right ventricle.
20. *Video 20:* Transgastric basal long-axis view showing mitral leaflets, mitral subvalvular apparatus, left ventricle (anteroseptal and inferolateral walls: basal and mid segments), LV outflow tract, aortic valve and proximal ascending aorta.
21. *Video 21:* Transgastric basal short-axis view showing mitral and tricuspid valve.
22. *Video 22:* Transgastric mid-papillary short-axis view showing left and right ventricles and papillary muscles.
23. *Video 23:* Transgastric right ventricle inflow-outflow view showing right atrium, PV and TV, RV.
24. *Video 24:* Transgastric right ventricle inflow view showing right ventricle and atrium, tricuspid valve: Chordae and papillary muscles.
25. *Video 25:* Transgastric basal right ventricle outflow view showing LV, RV, TV and PV.
26. *Video 26:* Deep transgastric long-axis view showing left ventricle and outflow tract, interventricular septum, aortic valve and ascending aorta, left atrium, mitral valve, right ventricle, pulmonic valve.
27. *Video 27:* Upper esophageal aortic arch long-axis view showing aortic arch, innominate vein and mediastinal tissue.
28. *Video 28:* Upper esophageal aortic arch short-axis view showing aortic arch, left brachiocephalic vein, pulmonary artery and pulmonic valve.

Chapter 4

TEE FOR ATRIAL SEPTAL DEFECT

S. No. Video Name

1. *Video 1:* 2D assessment of atrial septal defect. Midesophageal 4 chamber view (probe rotated to right) showing interatrial septal aneurysm and an ostium secundum atrial septal defect. The repair of the defect in such a scenario is done by excising the interatrial septum aneurysm and closing the atrial septal defect with a prosthetic or pericardial (in case of associated mitral regurgitation) patch. Also seen is the tricuspid value and superior vena cava.
2. *Video 2:* 2D assessement of mitral valve in atrial septal defect. Transgastric basal view showing the anterior mitral leaflet, postcleft repair in a patient with ostium primum atrial septal defect and moderate mitral regurgitation.
3. *Video 3:* Color Doppler assessment of atrial septal defect. Midesophageal bicaval view showing superior vena cava type sinus venosus atrial septal defect shunting from left to right.
4. *Video 4:* 2D echo showing percutaneous closure of an ostium secundum atrial septal defect. The catheter containing the amplatzer ductal occluder device is seen traversing the atrial septal defect.
5. *Video 5:* 2D and Color Doppler assessment of atrial septal defect. Midesophageal bicaval view showing superior vena cava type sinus venosus atrial septal defect shunting from left to right.
6. *Video 6:* Color Doppler echocardiography in a patient for percutaneous atrial septal defect closure. The catheter containing the amplatzer septal occluder is seen traversing the atrial septal defect. A small mosaic jet is seen along the catheter.
7. *Video 7:* Color Doppler in midesophageal right ventricle inflow-outflow view showing the deployed amplatzer septal occlude device without any residual shunt across the atrial septal defect. In this view it may appear that the left rim of the device is resting on the aortic valve but this finding is just because of the angle at which the device is being imaged. In the midesophageal 4 chamber view it was clear that the aortic valve is free from the device.
8. *Video 8:* Color Doppler in midesophageal 4 chamber view showing a fully deployed and well approximated amplatzer septal occluder with no residual shunt and free of mitral valve annulus.
9. *Video 9:* Color Doppler in midesophageal right ventricle inflow-outflow view showing a fully deployed and well approximated amplatzer septal occluder with no residual shunt and free of mitral valve annulus.
10. *Video 10:* Color Doppler in midesophageal descending thoracic aortic long axis view showing blood flow through abdominal aorta on cardiopulmonary bypass when perfused via a femoral artery cannula during Robotic cardiac surgery.
11. *Video 11:* 2D echo for percutaneous cannulation of superior vena cava. Midesophageal bicaval view showing superior vena cava cannula for robotic atrial septal defect closure. The cannula tip is in the right atrium which is the incorrect position of the cannula.
12. *Video 12:* 2D echo for percutaneous cannulation of superior vena cava. Midesophageal bicaval view showing superior vena cava cannula for robotic atrial septal defect closure. The cannula tip is at the junction of right atrium and superior vena cava which is the correct position of the cannula.
13. *Video 13:* 2D echocardiography showing midesophageal descending thoracic aorta short axis view progressing to long axis view. This is the ideal view to visualize the retrograde guidewire insertion during cannulation of femoral artery in Redo surgeries, Robotic cardiac surgeries and placement of intra-aortic counterpulsation balloon. The tip of intra-aortic counterpulsation balloon may also be located in this view.
14. *Video 14:* Color Doppler echocardiography showing blood flow in the midesophageal descending thoracic aorta long axis view. Note the nonpulsatile nature of blood flow because the patient is on cardiopulmonary bypass. The flow is from left side of image towards right side of image.
15. *Video 15:* Color Doppler echocardiography showing blood flow in the midesophageal descending thoracic aorta long axis view. Note the pulsatile nature of blood flow and the flow is from right of image towards left of image.
16. *Video 16:* 2D echo showing the placement of guidewire in descending thoracic aorta for cannulation of the femoral artery. The arterial cannula is not visible because it rarely traverses the abdominal aorta.
17. *Video 17:* Color Doppler in midesophgeal descending thoracic aortic long axis view showing blood flow through abdominal aorta on cardiopulmonary bypass when perfused via a femoral artery cannula.
18. *Video 18:* 2D echocardiography in midesophgeal bicaval view showing the placement of guidewire for percutaneous placement of superior vena cava cannula. The guidewire is hitting the interatrial septum causing arrhythmias.
19. *Video 19:* 2D echo for percutaneous inferior vena cava cannulation. Modified hepatic vein view showing guidewire placement for the placement of inferior vena cava cannula. The cannula should be 1 cm proximal to the inferior vena cava right atrial junction.
20. *Video 20:* Color Doppler in modified hepatic vein view showing the confluence of hepatic and portal vein to form the inferior vena cava.

21. *Video 21:* 2D echocardiography in modified hepatic vein view showing the placement of guidewire for percutaneous cannulation of inferior vena cava cannula.
22. *Video 22:* Color Doppler echocardiography showing the draining of inferior vena cava into right atrium in the modified deep transgastric view.
23. *Video 23:* 2D echocardiography in midesophageal view showing left atrial hematoma after minimally invasive cardiac surgery.
24. *Video 24:* 2D echo for percutaneous cannulation of superior vena cava. Midesophageal bicaval view showing superior vena cava cannula for robotic atrial septal defect closure. The cannula tip is at the junction of right atrium and superior vena cava which is the correct position of the cannula.
25. *Video 25:* 2D echo for percutaneous cannulation of superior vena cava. Midesophageal bicaval view showing superior vena cava cannula for robotic atrial septal defect closure. The cannula tip is in the right atrium which is the incorrect position of the cannula.

Chapter 5
TEE FOR VENTRICULAR SEPTAL DEFECT

S. No. Video Name

1. *Video 1:* Color Doppler midesophageal aortic valve short axis view showing left superior pulmonary vein stenosis in a patient with VSD.
2. *Video 2:* Color Doppler modified midesophageal aortic valve short axis view showing flow across left superior pulmonary vein after resection of membrane.
3. *Video 3:* 2D assessement of mitral valve in atrial septal defect. Transgastric basal view showing the anterior mitral leaflet postcleft repair in the same patient with ostium primum atrial septal defect and moderate mitral regurgitation.
4. *Video 4:* 2D echocardiography in midesophageal aortic valve short axis view showing prolapse of septal leaflet of TV into subaortic VSD causing closure of ventricular septal defect.
5. *Video 5:* 3D echocardiography in deep transgastric view showing a subaortic ventricular septal defect just adjoining the septal leaflet of tricuspid valve.
6. *Video 6:* 2D echocardiography in deep transgastric view showing a subaortic ventricular septal defect just adjoining the septal leaflet of tricuspid valve.
7. *Video 7:* 2D echocardiography in deep transgastric view showing a subaortic ventricular septal defect just adjoining the septal leaflet of tricuspid valve and beneath the aortic valve.
8. *Video 8:* 2D echocardiography in deep transgastric view showing subaortic membrane (complete) just below aortic valve.
9. *Video 9:* 2D echocardiography in deep transgastric view showing (closer look) subaortic membrane (complete) just below aortic valve.
10. *Video 10:* Color Doppler in midesophageal long axis view showing subaortic membrane (partial) just below aortic valve.
11. *Video 11:* 2D echocardiography in deep transgastric view showing a supramitral ring (complete).

Chapter 7
TEE FOR PULMONARY STENOSIS

S. No. Video Name

1. *Video 1:* Tetralogy of Fallot in pulmonary stenosis.
2. *Video 2:* Double chamber right ventricular in pulmonary stenosis.
3. *Video 3:* Pulmonary insufficiency.
4. *Video 4:* Transesophageal echocardiography of pulmonary stenosis.
5. *Video 5:* Atrial septal defects in pulmonary stenosis.

Chapter 8
TEE FOR DOUBLE-CHAMBERED RIGHT VENTRICLE

S. No. Video Name

1. *Video 1:* 2D echo in midesophageal right ventricle inflow-ouflow view showing a perimembranous ventricular septal defect and a muscle bundle obstructing the flow in right ventricular outflow tract in a patient with double chambered right ventricle.
2. *Video 2:* 2D echo in midesophageal right ventricle inflow-ouflow view showing the repair of ventricular septal defect with a Dacron patch and resection of the muscle bundle leading to a patent right ventricular outflow tract.

Chapter 9
TEE FOR PATENT DUCTUS ARTERIOSUS

S. No. Video Name

1. *Video 1:* Color flow Doppler in modified ME descending thoracic aorta short axis view (Probe rotated to right to visualize left pulmonary artery) showing patent ductus arteriosus.

Chapter 11
TEE FOR TETRALOGY OF FALLOT

S. No. Video Name

1. *Video 1:* 2D echo deep transgastric view showing a subaortic ventricular septal defect and aortic over-ride

in a patient with Tetralogy of Fallot. The aortic root is always enlarged because of the over-ride.

2. *Video 2:* 2D echocardiography in mid papillary transgastric view showing normal left ventricular function.
3. *Video 3:* 2D echocardiography in upper esophageal ascending aortic short axis view showing pulmonic valve stenosis.
4. *Video 4:* Color Doppler in midesophageal long axis view showing a subaortic ventricular septal defect shunting from left to right and infundibular pulmonary stenosis in a patient with Tetralogy of Fallot.
5. *Video 5:* 2D echo in midesophageal right ventricle inflow-outflow view showing subaortic ventricular septal defect and infundibular pulmonary stenosis in a patient with Tetralogy of Fallot.
6. *Video 6:* Color Doppler in midesophageal right ventricle inflow-outflow view showing subaortic ventricular septal defect and infundibular pulmonary stenosis in a patient with Tetralogy of Fallot.

Chapter 12
TEE FOR DOUBLE-OUTLET RIGHT VENTRICLE

S. No. Video Name

1. *Video 1:* 2D echocardiography in midesophageal long axis view showing a subaortic ventricular septal defect with over-riding of aorta (>50% in this case) in a patient with double-outlet right ventricle.
2. *Video 2:* 2D echocardiography in deep transgastric long axis view showing a subaortic ventricular septal defect with over-riding of aorta (>50% in this case) in a patient with double-outlet right ventricle. Because of so much of over-ride the right ventricle ejects directly into the aorta. Note the mitral valve in its cross-section.

Chapter 13
TEE FOR TRANSPOSITION OF GREAT ARTERIES

S. No. Video Name

1. *Video 1:* 2D echo for assessment of ventricular septal defect in transposition of great arteries. The echocardiogram shows an anterior muscular ventricular septal defect with a subpulmonic extension. In transposition of great arteries, the pulmonary artery is arising from left ventricle, hence the extension towards systemic outflow is no more subaortic but subpulmonic.
2. *Video 2:* 2D echo showing the atrial baffle post-double switch operation. Left atrium (constructed by pericardium posteriorly is now directed to the left ventricle and the left ventricle now ejects into the aorta (arterial switch done).
3. *Video 3:* 2D echo for evaluation of regressed left ventricle in transposition of great arteries. Transgastric midpapillary short axis view showing the comparative shape and size of both the right and left ventricles. Note the banana shaped left ventricle and well developed right ventricle.
4. *Video 4:* 2D echo for evaluation of regressed left ventricle in transposition of great arteries. Midesophageal 4 chamber view showing a restrictive upper muscular ventricular septal defect in a patient with transposition of great arteries.
5. *Video 5:* 2D echo for assessment of ventricular septal defect in transposition of great arteries. The midesophageal 4 chamber view shows a large inlet ventricular septal defect with both the ventricles lying side by side.
6. *Video 6:* 2D echo and color Doppler assessment of transposition of great arteries. The midesophageal long axis view shows accessory mitral tissue in the left ventricular tract causing obstruction and gradient across left ventricular outflow tract.
7. *Video 7:* 2D echo for assessment of transposition of great arteries. The midesophageal long axis view showing the connection from left atrium to left ventricle to pulmonary artery.
8. *Video 8*: 2D echo for assessment of transposition of great arteries. The midesophageal long axis view showing the connection from right atrium to right ventricle to aorta.

Chapter 14
TEE FOR CONGENITALLY CORRECTED TRANSPOSITION OF GREAT ARTERIES

S. No. Video Name

1. *Video 1:* 2D echo in midesophageal long axis view showing the relation between aorta and pulmonary artery. Right ventricle ejects into aorta which is anterior to pulmonary artery.
2. *Video 2:* 2D echo in midesophageal 4-chamber view showing perimembranous ventricular septal defect with right atrium opening into left ventricle and left ventricle ejecting into pulmonary artery.
3. *Video 3:* 2D echocardiography in midesophageal 4-chamber view, of a patient who has undergone "Double Switch Operation", showing an atrial baffle made from atrial wall. The neo left atrium made from pericardium is seen opening into the left ventricle and the left ventricle ejecting into the aorta.
4. *Video 4:* 2D echo in transgastric midpapillary short axis view showing left and right ventricles (crescent-shaped) after a Double Switch Operation. Note the underfilled morphologic right ventricle.
5. *Video 5:* 2D echocardiography in deep transgastric view showing the cross-section of tricuspid valve morphological right ventricle ejecting in the aorta in a patient with congenitally corrected transposition of great arteries.

6. *Video 6:* 2D echo post-Double Switch Operation (Senning + Rastelli procedure) showing pulmonary artery conduit arising from right ventricle on left side of screen.
7. *Video 7:* Color Doppler post-Double Switch Operation (Senning + Rastelli procedure) showing unobstructed blood flow through pulmonary artery conduit arising from right ventricle on left side of screen
8. *Video 8:* Color Doppler post-Double Switch Operation (Senning + Rastelli procedure) showing unobstructed blood flow from inferior vena cava to the right atrium.
9. *Video 9:* 2D echo post-Double Switch Operation (Senning + Rastelli procedure) showing a Dacron patch between the atria used to create the baffle.
10. *Video 10:* Color Doppler post-Double Switch Operation (Senning + Rastelli procedure) showing unobstructed blood flow in the left atrium.
11. *Video 11:* 2D echo in a patient with congenitally corrected transposition of great arteries showing the corrected anatomy after the Double Switch Operation (Senning + Rastelli procedure).

Chapter 15
TEE FOR EBSTEIN'S ANOMALY

S. No. Video Name

1. *Video 1:* TEE image of a patient with Ebstein's anomaly showing apical displacement of the TV leaflet and the thin, "atrialized" portion of the affected right ventricular wall.
2. *Video 2 to 6:* The septal leaflet of the TV was tethered to the ventricular septum. Showing the dilated RV and "dubble appearance".

Chapter 16
TEE FOR DOUBLE-INLET LEFT VENTRICLE

S. No. Video Name

1. *Video 1:* 2D echo in transgastric basal view showing both the atrioventricular valves opening into the single large morphological left ventricle (seen from the apex of heart).
2. *Video 2:* 2D echocardiography in midesophageal 4 chamber view showing a dextroposed aorta from morphological left ventricle in a patient with double-inlet left ventricle.
3. *Video 3:* TEE in bicaval view showing discard out LV instead of RV.

Chapter 17
TEE FOR UNIVENTRICULAR HEART

S. No. Video Name

1. *Video 1:* 2D echo in midesophageal bicaval view (probe turned to right) showing thrombus in the conduit of the Fontan circulation. Note the spontaneous echo contrast proximal to the thrombus.
2. *Video 2:* 2D echo in midesophageal bicaval view (probe turned to right) showing thrombus in the conduit of the Fontan circulation.
3. *Video 3:* Color Doppler echocardiography, in modified midesophageal bicaval view (probe turned to right), showing stenosis of the anastomosis between prosthetic conduit and inferior vena cava in a patient who has undergone Fontan operation.
4. *Video 4:* Color Doppler echocardiography, in modified midesophageal bicaval view (probe turned to right), showing stenosis of the anastomosis between prosthetic conduit and inferior vena cava in a patient who has undergone Fontan operation.

Chapter 18
TEE FOR TOTAL ANOMALOUS PULMONARY VENOUS CONNECTION

S. No. Video Name

1. *Video 1:* 2D echo in midesophageal 4 chamber view showing a dilated coronary sinus which is present in coronary sinus total anomalous pulmonary vein connection.
2. *Video 2:* Color Doppler in midesophageal 4 chamber view showing increased blood flow through the coronary sinus indicative of coronary sinus total anomalous pulmonary vein connection.

Chapter 20
TEE FOR LEFT SUPERIOR VENA CAVA

S. No. Video Name

1. *Video 1:* 2D echo in midesophageal modified aortic valve short axis view (probe rotated to left) showing left superior vena cava as a distinct entity near the left atrial appendage.
2. *Video 2:* 2D echo in midesophageal 4 chamber view showing a distinct vessel near the lateral annulus of mitral valve. Left superior vena cava is seen (arrow).
3. *Video 3:* Color Doppler in midesophageal modified aortic valve short axis view (probe rotated to left) showing blood flow in left superior vena cava near the left atrial appendage.

All above videos do not have voice over

Abbreviations

A	:	Anterior
Ao	:	Aorta
ASD	:	Atrial Septal Defect
ASO	:	Anti-Streptolysin O
ATL	:	Anterior Tricuspid Leaflet
AV	:	Atrioventricular
AVSD	:	Atrioventricular Septal Defect
CCTGA	:	Congenitally Corrected Transposition of the Great Arteries
CHF	:	Congestive Heart Failure
CVP	:	Central Venous Pressure
DORV	:	Double-Outlet Right Ventricle
ECG	:	Electrocardiogram
ESM	:	Ejection Systolic Murmur
ECHO	:	Echocardiogram
IAS	:	Interatrial Septum
IVC	:	Inferior Vena Cava
IVS	:	Interventricular Septum
LA	:	Left Atrium
LAA	:	Left Atrial Appendage
LAX view	:	Long-axis View
LPA	:	Left Pulmonary Artery
LSPV	:	Left Superior Pulmonary Vein
LSVC	:	Left Superior Vena Cava
LV	:	Left Ventricular
LVOT	:	Left Ventricular Outflow Tract
ME	:	Midesophageal
MPA	:	Main Pulmonary Artery
MPAP	:	Mean Pulmonary Artery Pressure
MV	:	Mitral Valve
P	:	Posterior Leaflet of the Tricuspid Valve
PA dilatation	:	Pulmonary Artery Dilatation
PAD	:	Peripheral Artery Disease
PAH	:	Pulmonary Arterial Hypertension

PAP	:	Pulmonary Artery Pressure
PAV	:	Partial Atrioventricular/Posteroanterior View
PBS	:	Pulmonary Branch Stenosis
PDA	:	Patent Ductus Arteriosus
PEDP	:	Pulmonary Artery End-diastolic Pressure
Pre-CPB	:	Pre-cardiopulmonary Bypass
PS	:	Progressive Supranuclear
PV	:	Pulmonary Valve
PVR	:	Pulmonary Vascular Resistance
PW Doppler	:	Pulsed Wave (PW) Doppler
RA	:	Right Atrium
RPA	:	Right Pulmonary Artery
RUPV	:	Right Upper Pulmonary Vein
RV	:	Right Ventricle
RVH	:	Right Ventricular Hypertrophy
RVOT	:	Right Ventricular Outflow Tract
RVSP	:	Right Ventricular Systolic Pressure
S	:	Septal Leaflet of the Tricuspid Valve
SAX view	:	Short-axis View
SPAP	:	Systolic Pulmonary Artery Pressure
STL	:	Septal Tricuspid Leaflet
SVA	:	Systemic Venous Atrium
SVC	:	Superior Vena Cava
SVR	:	Systemic Vascular Resistance
TAPSE	:	Tricuspid Annular Plane Systolic Excursion
TGA	:	Transposition of the Great Arteries
TOF	:	Tetralogy of Fallot
TEE	:	Transesophageal Echocardiography
TTE	:	Transthoracic Echocardiography
TRV	:	Tricuspid Regurgitation Jet Velocity
TV	:	Tricuspid Valve
VSD	:	Ventricular Septal Defect
XC	:	Cor Triatriatum Chamber

Chapter 1

Introduction to TEE for Congenital Heart Disease

Usha Kiran, Poonam Malhotra Kapoor, Sarvesh Pal Singh, Ajay Jha

Chapter Outline

INTRODUCTION

The guidelines for performing transesophageal echocardiography in patients with congenital heart disease state that "the intraoperative transesophageal echocardiography (TEE) should not stand alone as the sole diagnostic study since there are inherent limitations in imaging certain important structures that are otherwise identified best by transthoracic echocardiography (i.e. transverse aortic arch, aortic isthmus, distal left pulmonary artery, and collateral pulmonary vessels). Additional constraints specific to intraoperative TEE include limited potential for optimal Doppler alignment, limited time to perform a complete study, and suboptimal ambient lighting".

It is also a recommendation that any echocardiographer doing TEE for congenital heart disease should be well versed with the TTE and must have performed at least 50 echocardiographic examinations independently.

It is the author's opinion and experience that rather than concentrating of any particular finding or diagnosis it is better to perform a systematic TEE examination and understand the various structural defects along with the relationship of different intracardiac structures with one another.

INDICATIONS FOR TEE IN PATIENTS WITH CONGENITAL HEART DISEASE

Diagnostic Indications

- Patient with suspected congenital heart disease (CHD) and nondiagnostic TTE

- Presence of patent foramen ovale (PFO) and direction of shunting as possible etiology for stroke
- Patent foramen ovale (PFO) evaluation with agitated saline contrast to determine possible right-to-left shunt, prior to transvenous pacemaker insertion
- Evaluation of intra- or extracardiac baffles following Fontan, Senning or Mustard procedure.

Aortic Dissection

- Intracardiac evaluation for vegetation or suspected abscess
- Pericardial effusion or cardiac function evaluation and monitoring postoperative patient with an open sternum or poor acoustic windows
- Evaluation for intracardiac thrombus prior to cardioversion for atrial flutter/fibrillation
- Evaluating status of prosthetic valve.

Perioperative Indications

Immediate preoperative definition of cardiac anatomy and function.

TEE GUIDED INTERVENTIONS

- Guidance for placement of atrial septal defect (ASD) or ventricular septal defect (VSD) occlusion device
- Guidance for blade or balloon atrial septostomy
- Catheter tip placement for valve perforation and dilation in catheterization laboratory
- Guidance during radiofrequency ablation procedure
- Results of minimally invasive surgical incision or video-assisted cardiac procedure.

CONTRAINDICATIONS FOR THE USE OF TEE (TABLE 1)

Absolute

- Unrepaired tracheoesophageal fistula
- Esophageal obstruction or stricture
- Perforated hollow viscus
- Poor airway control
- Severe respiratory depression
- Uncooperative, unsedated patient.

Relative

- History of prior esophageal surgery
- Esophageal varices or diverticulum
- Gastric or esophageal bleeding
- Vascular ring, aortic arch anomaly with or without airway compromise
- Oropharyngeal pathology
- Severe coagulopathy
- Cervical spine injury or anomaly.

DEFINITIONS

- *Situs:* Site or position.
- *Solitus:* Usual or normal.
- *Situs solitus:* Normal position.
- *Inversus:* Reverse or opposite.
- *Situs inversus:* Opposite or reverse of normal.
- *Ambiguus:* Uncertain, indeterminant.
- *Situs ambiguus:* Uncertain, indeterminant or ambiguous position.

TABLE 1 List of absolute and relative contraindications to transesophageal echocardiography

Absolute contraindications	*Relative contraindications*
• Perforated viscus • Esophageal stricture • Esophageal tumor • Esophageal perforation, laceration • Esophageal diverticulum • Active upper GI bleed	• History of radiation to neck and mediastinum • History of GI surgery • Recent upper GI bleed • Barrett's esophagus • History of dysphagia • Restriction of neck mobility (severe cervical arthritis, atlantoaxial joint disease) • Symptomatic hiatal hernia • Esophageal varices • Coagulopathy, thrombocytopenia • Active esophagitis • Active peptic ulcer disease

- *Cardiac position:* Refers to the intrathoracic location of the heart as left-sided (levocardia), right-sided (dextrocardia), or midline (mesocardia).
- *Cardiac malposition:* An abnormal intrathoracic location of the heart, or a location that is abnormal (inappropriate) relative to the position (situs) of the abdominal viscera.
- *Chamber designations:* Right and left refer to morphology rather than position, as right or left atrium, right or left ventricle.
- *Isomerism: (Gr) isos = equal; meros = part.* Refers to the morphologic similarity of bilateral structures that are normally dissimilar such as right and left atrial appendages, right and left bronchi, right and left lungs.
- *Ventricular loop:* The right or left bend (loop) that forms in the straight heart tube of the embryo.
- *d-Loop:* The normal *rightward (dextro = d) bend in the* embryonic heart tube. The d-loop designation as applied to the developed heart indicates that the sinus or inflow portion of the morphologic right ventricle lies to the right of the morphologic left ventricle **(Fig. 1)**.
- *l-Loop:* A *leftward (levo = l) bend in the embryonic heart* tube. The l-loop designation as applied to the developed heart indicates that the sinus or inflow portion of the morphologic right ventricle lies to the left of the morphologic left ventricle.
- *Concordant: (L) concordare = to agree*, i.e. agreeing or appropriate.
- *Malposition of the great arteries:* Refers to abnormal spatial relationships of the aorta and the pulmonary trunk to each other. Malpositions can be in either the lateral or the anteroposterior plane. The great arteries are *malposed* but not *transposed because ventricular—great arterial* concordance is maintained.

SIGNIFICANCE

- Situs inversus with dextrocardia (complete situs inversus, mirror image dextrocardia) usually occurs without coexisting congenital heart disease **(Fig. 2)**.
- Situs inversus with levocardia is consistently associated with coexisting congenital heart disease.
- Situs solitus with dextrocardia is only occasionally associated with a structurally normal heart.

IMAGING PLANES AND ORIENTATION

Understanding the orientation of the imaging plane is crucial for both acquisition of the desire images and correct interpretation of the displayed cardiac anatomy. Although TEE is limited to the confines of the esophagus and stomach, the ability to alter the position and orientation of the ultrasound beam allows a broad view of the cardiac anatomy.

GOALS OF THE EXAMINATION

TEE examinations, whether comprehensive or abbreviated, should display all pertinent structures in the heart. Each cardiac chamber and valve should be visualized in at least two orthogonal planes. All segments of the myocardium should be visualized. This approach helps ensure the diagnosis of any significant abnormalities and minimizes the incorrect identification of artifacts.

Echocardiographers differ in their approach to a diagnostic TEE examination. Many prefer to start with

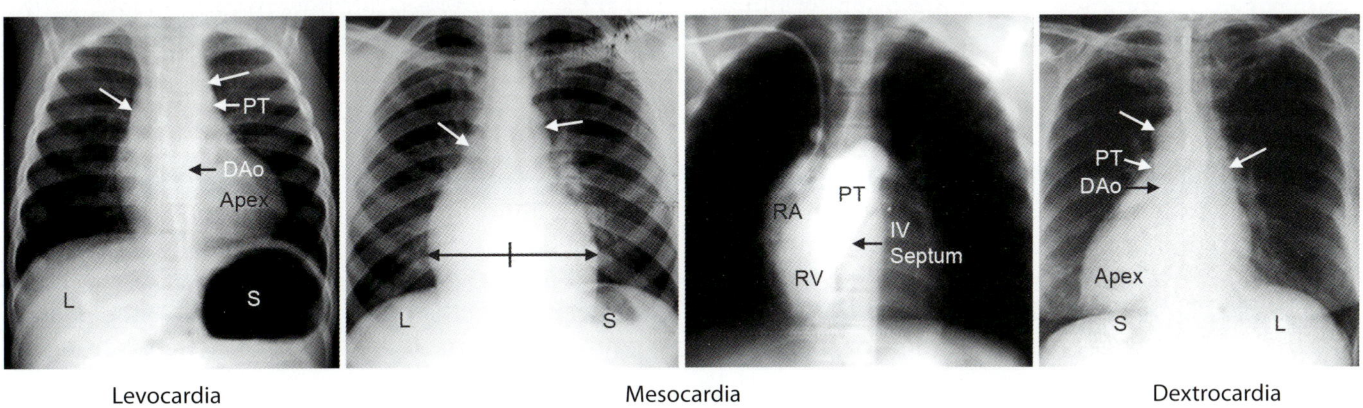

Figure 1 X-ray chest PAV typically seen in levocardia, mesocardia and dextrocardia

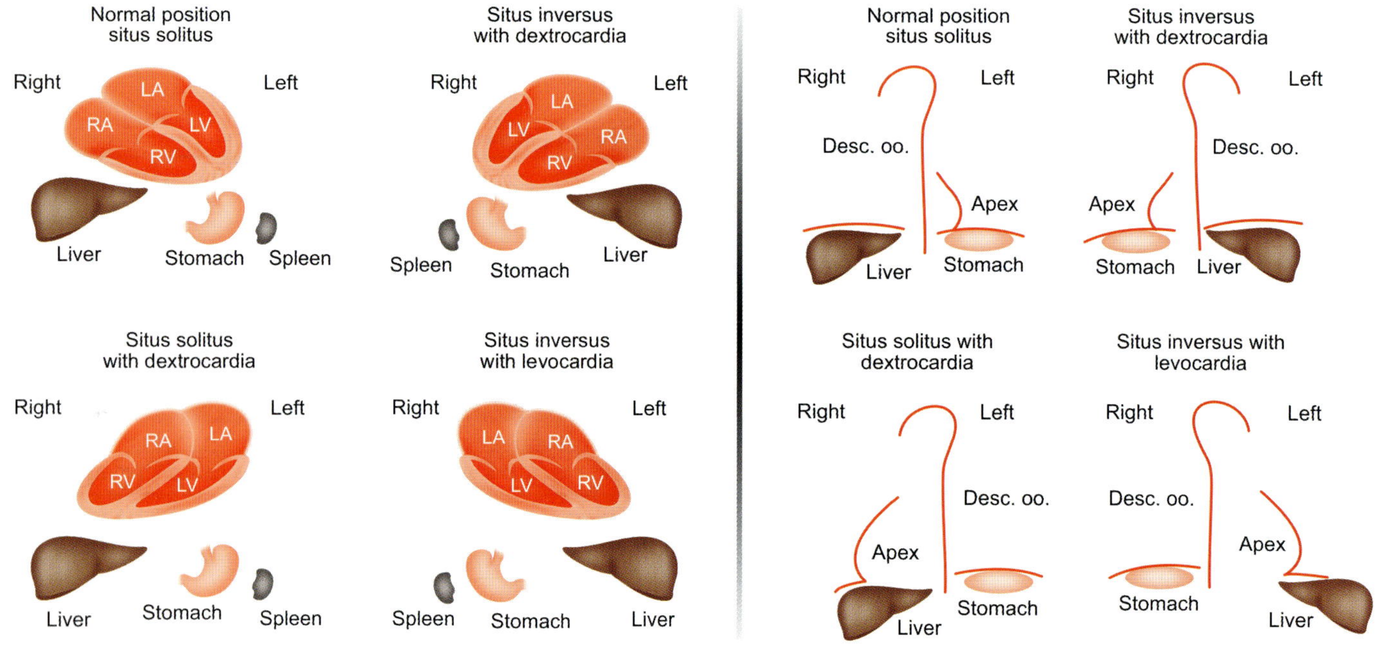

Figure 2 Diagrammatic representation in situs solitus and situs inversus

those views that examine known pathology. Other believe the examination should first systematically examine for unknown pathology before the area of concern is evaluated. A common approach starts with TG views of the left ventricle because of the frequent abnormalities detected with these views. Each of these approaches has of any approach must be a complete examination of all structures of the heart. A joint task force including members of the American Society of Echocardiography and the Society of Cardiovascular Anesthesiologists has published guidelines for performing a comprehensive intraoperative multiplane TEE examination. However, additional views are often required to assess a particular abnormality and no consensus has been reached regarding whether all 20 cross-sections described in the guidelines should be acquired in every surgical patient.

The examination is based on progressive esophageal advancement of the probe to evaluate cardiac anatomy and function followed by progressive withdrawal for the evaluation of the aorta. This approach minimizes manipulation of the TEE probe, thereby shortening the examination time. This author has not found the depth of probe insertion to be reliable tool for identifying intracardiac anatomy. The preferred approach is to report the location of cardiac anatomy/pathology relative to known intracardiac structures and standard cross-sectional views. The progressive advancement/removal of the probe provides a systematic anatomic orientation (avoiding disorientation as to the displayed imaging plane) and allows for easy description of anatomy relative to other cardiac structures. Pathology in the aorta can be referred to the depth of probe insertion but this has more value in the long-term outpatient evaluation of lesions and, we believe, little value in the intraoperative examination.

PROBE INSERTION

The TEE probe is passed into the esophagus in the same manner in which an orogastric tube is placed. The easiest way to insert the probe is to perform a jaw lift by grabbing the mandible with the left hand inserting the probe with the right. The probe is inserted with constant gentle pressure in addition to a slight turning back and forth and from left to right to find the esophageal opening. If resistance is encountered, the cause most often is excessive extension of the head and neck. Advancement of the probe is stopped after the head of the probe has passed the larynx and cricopharyngeus muscle, where a distinct loss of resistance of felt. The imaging head will lie in the upper esophagus.

PROBE MANIPULATION

Once in the esophagus, the transducer should be gently guided and the operator should never apply undue force.

There are 4 probe manipulations for optimal image acquisition **(Fig. 3)**. The probe manipulation described here is made with reference to the operator standing at the patient's head and looking towards the patient's feet.

- *Advance, withdraw:* Pushing or pulling the tip of the TEE probe.
- *Turn to right; turn to left (also referred to as clockwise and anticlockwise):* Rotating the anterior aspect of the TEE probe to the right or left of the patient.
- *Anteflex, retroflex:* Anteflex is flexing the tip of the TEE probe anteriorly by turning the large control wheel clockwise. Retroflex is flexing the tip of the TEE probe posteriorly by turning the large wheel anticlockwise.
- *Flex to right, flex to left:* Flexing the tip of the TEE probe with the small control wheel to the patient's right or left. The probe flexion to the right and left may not be necessary and should be avoided to minimize trauma to the esophagus.

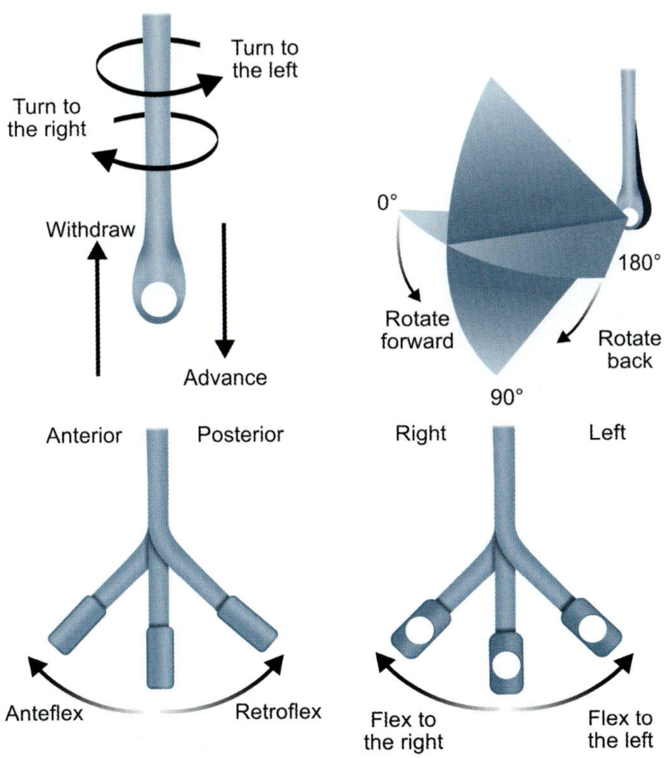

Figure 3 Different TEE probe movement while withdrawing and advancing the probe into the esophagus

Terminology of TEE Probe Manipulation

A large no. of complications are not seen with TEE, if the procedure for insertion are followed some complicate noted are as shown in **Table 2**.

ACHD: TRANSESOPHAGEAL ECHOCARDIOGRAPHIC IMAGING ALGORITHM

Equally important is the process of care of patients with ACHD undergoing TEE. Younger patients with ACHD and/or those with extensive cardiac interventions may have higher sedation requirements than those with acquired heart disease. If high sedation requirement is

TABLE 2 List of complications reported with TEE and the incidence of these complications during diagnostic TEE and intraoperative TEE[1-8]

Complication	*Diagnostic TEE (%)*	*Intraoperative TEE (%)*
Overall complication rate	0.18–2.8	0.2
Mortality	<0.01–0.02	0
Major morbidity	0.2	0–1.2
Major bleeding	<0.01	0.03–0.8
Esophageal perforation	<0.01	0–0.3
Heart failure	0.05	
Arrhythmia	0.06–0.3	
Tracheal intubation	0.02	
Endotracheal tube malposition		0.03
Laryngospasm	0.14	
Bronchospasm	0.06–0.07	
Dysphagia	1.8	
Minor pharyngeal bleeding	0.01–0.2	0.01
Severe odynophagia		0.1
Hoarseness	12	
Lip injury	13	
Dental injury	0.1	0.03

anticipated or there is a history of difficulty achieving adequate sedation during prior procedures, it would be prudent to ask for support from anesthesia and perform TEE in a setting with more intensive monitoring (such as a postanesthetic recovery room or critical care unit). The importance of achieving satisfactory sedation cannot be overstated in the ACHD population, as evaluation of primary and associated congenital abnormalities will often prolong the study.

REFERENCES

1. Daniel WG, Erbel R, Kasper W, et al. Safety of transesophageal echocardiography. A multicenter survey of 10,419 examinations. Circulation. 1991;83:817-21.
2. Khandheria BK, Seward JB, Tajik AJ. Transesophageal echocardiography. Mayo Clin Proc. 1994;69:856-63.
3. Hilberath JN, Oakes DA, Shernan SK, et al. Safety of transesophageal echocardiography. J Am Soc Echocardiogr. 2010;23(11):1115-27.
4. Seward JB, Khandheria BK, Oh JK, et al. Critical appraisal of transesophageal echocardiography: limitations, pitfalls, and complications. J Am Soc Echocardiogr. 1992;5:288-305.
5. Lennon MJ, Gibbs NM, Weightman WM, Leber J, EeHC, Yusoff IF. Transesophageal echocardiography-related gastrointestinal complications in cardiac surgical patients. J Cardiothorac Vasc Anesth. 2005;19:141-5.
6. Owall A, Stahl L, Settergren G. Incidence of sore throat and patient complaints after intraoperative transesophageal echocardiography during cardiac surgery. J Cardiothorac Vasc Anesth. 1992;6:15-6.
7. Chan KL, Cohen GI, Sochowski RA, et al. Complications of transesophageal echocardiography in ambulatory adult patients: analysis of 1500 consecutive examinations. J Am Soc Echocardiogr. 1991;4:577-82.
8. Practice guidelines for perioperative transesophageal echocardiography. A report by the American Society of Anesthesiologists and the Society of Cardiovascular Anesthesiologists Task Force on Transesophageal Echocardiography. Anesthesiology. 1996;84:986-1006.

Chapter 2

Chambers, Valves and Normal Dimensions

Sandeep Chauhan, Poonam Malhotra Kapoor, Jitin Narula, Rajshekhar

Chapter Outline

- Left Ventricular Measurements
- Right Ventricular Dimensions
- Nadas' Criteria
- Reference Values for Normal Adult Transesophageal Echocardiography Measurements

The major challenge in transesophageal echocardiography (TEE) for congenital heart disease is to identify the chambers and great arteries. Also a good echocardiographer should be able to predict with reasonable accuracy the development of all the structures he is examining. The dimensions of chambers and vessels in children undergoing surgery are compares with standard values studied in normal children based on the basis of body weight and body surface area.

The differences between various chambers are compared in **Table 1**.

Many researchers have studied and prepared tables for normal values of different cardiac structures, e.g. aortic valve annulus, left ventricular diameters for various age groups **(Tables 2 to 5)**. It is for the institution to decide which normograms to follow based on which the adequacy of development of various chambers and structures may be classified. Since much of the existing data has been derived from transthoracic echocardiogram (TTE) it may not apply exactly to TEE but minor differences are acceptable in paucity of data from TEE examinations.

TABLE 1 Right atrium (RA) vs left atrium (LA)

RA morphology	*LA morphology*
Wide-necked appendage	Narrow-necked hook like appendage
Extensive pectinate muscles	Smooth-walled except appendage
Valves of IVC and coronary sinus	

TABLE 2 Right ventricle vs left ventricle

	Right ventricle	*Left ventricle*
Atrioventricular valve	Trileaflet	Bileaflet (unless AML cleft)
Leaflet attachment	Septum	No septal
Annulus location	More apical	More basal
Apex	Prominent	Less prominent trabeculations
Moderator band	Present	Absent
Infundibulum	Present	Absent

TABLE 3 Different dimensions of right and left ventricles for different weight and body surface area

Wt	*BSA*	*LVIDd (–2 Z)*	*LVIDd (+2 Z)*	*LVESD (–2 Z)*	*LVESD (+2 Z)*	*IVSd (–2 Z)*	*IVSd (+2 Z)*	*LVPWd (–2 Z)*	*LVPWd (+2 Z)*	*RVDD (–2 Z)*	*RVDD (+2 Z)*	*LAd (–2 Z)*	*LAd (–2 Z)*
3.0	0.21	15	21	9	14	2.3	4.9	2.4	4.6	4.1	12.9	9.4	15.1
3.6	0.23	15.4	22.2	9.5	14.3	2.3	5.1	2.5	4.7	4.1	13.1	10.2	16.2
4.0	0.245	16.4	23.6	10.2	16.2	2.4	5.2	2.6	4.6	4.2	13.2	10.5	17.5
4.6	0.27	17	25.4	10.4	16.8	2.4	5.2	2.7	4.9	4.2	13.2	11.5	18.7
5.5	0.30	18	25.8	10.8	18.8	2.5	5.3	2.8	5.4	4.2	13.2	11.5	19.1
7.0	0.36	19	27.2	10.8	18.8	2.5	5.3	2.8	5.4	4.3	13.3	12	20.6
8.5	0.42	21	31	12	20.1	2.6	5.6	2.9	5.5	4.4	13.4	13	20.6
10	0.47	22	32.1	13	21	2.6	5.8	3.1	6.1	4.5	13.5	13.8	21.8
12	0.54	23.4	34.6	14	22	2.7	5.9	3.1	6.1	4.8	13.8	14.5	22.9
13	0.57	25.6	36.4	15	23.6	3.1	6.1	3.3	6.3	5	14	15.3	24.1
15	0.64	26	37.2	15.4	24.4	3.3	6.3	3.3	6.3	5.2	14	16.1	24.1
17	0.70	27.2	39.2	15.7	25.1	3.3	6.3	3.4	6.4	5.5	14.3	16.1	25.5
19	0.76	27.4	40.4	16.1	26.5	3.5	6.5	3.5	6.9	5.7	14.5	16.2	26.2
23	0.88	29.6	42	17.7	27.7	3.6	6.8	3.6	7.8	5.8	15.2	16.5	28.5
28	1.0	31	43.2	18	29.2	3.8	7.4	3.7	8.1	6.4	15.6	17	29.4
32	1.1	31.7	45.3	18.6	30.2	4	7.6	3.7	8.1	6.4	16	19.2	30.8

Abbreviations: Wt–weight; BSA–body surface area; LVIDd–left ventricle internal dimension diastole; LVESD–left ventricle end systolic diameter, IVSd–interventricular septum diastole; LVPWd–left ventricle posterior wall diastole; RVDD–right ventricle diastolic diameter; LAd–left atrium diastole.

TABLE 4 Mitral and tricuspid valve diameters by 2D echocardiography: Mean (95% confidence intervals)

BSA	0.2	0.25	0.3	0.4	0.5	0.6	0.7	0.8	0.9	1.0	1.2	1.4
Wt	2	3	4	7	10	13	16	19	23	28	37	46
MV (PL)	10 (7–13)	12 (9–15)	13 (10–16)	16 (13–19)	18 (15–21)	19 (16–23)	21 (18–24)	22 (18–26)	23 (19–26)	24 (20–27)	25 (22–28)	26 (23–30)
MV (A4C, S4C)	12 (7–17)	15 (10–20)	17 (12–22)	20 (16–25)	23 (18–28)	25 (20–31)	27 (22–32)	29 (23–35)	31 (25–36)	32 (26–37)	35 (28–40)	36 (31–42)
TV (A4C, S4C)	12 (8–17)	15 (10–19)	17 (12–22)	21 (16–26)	23 (18–29)	26 (20–31)	27 (22–33)	29 (33–36)	31 (24–37)	32 (25–38)	34 (25–42)	36 (28–44)

Abbreviations: BSA–body surface area; Wt–weight; MV–mitral valve; PL–parasternal long axis view; A4C–apical 4 chamber view; S4C–subcostal 4 chamber view; TV–tricuspid valve.

TABLE 5 Two-dimensional echocardiographic measurements of valve annuli in neonates (mm)

Body weight (kg)	0.5	1.0	1.5	2.0	2.5	3.0	3.5	4.0	4.5	5.0
Aortic valve (PL)	4–5.5	4.5–6	4.5–6.5	5–7	5.5–7.5	6–8	6.5–8.5	7–9	7.5–9	8–9.5
Pulmonary valve (PL)	4–7.5	4.5–8	5.5–9	6–9.5	6.5–10	7.5–11	8–11.5	8.5–12	9.5–13	10–13.5
Mitral valve (PL)	5.5–9.5	6–10	6.5–11	7–11.5	8–12	8.5–13	9–13.5	9.5–14	10–14.5	11–15.5
Mitral valve (apical view)	6–9.5	6.5–10	7.5–11	8–11.5	8.5–12	9–12.5	9.5–13	10.5–14	11–14.5	11.5–15
Tricuspid valve (apical view)	6.5–9.5	7–10.5	8–11	8.5–12	9.5–12.5	10–13.5	11–14	11.5–15	12–15.5	13–16

Abbreviation: PL–parasternal long axis view.

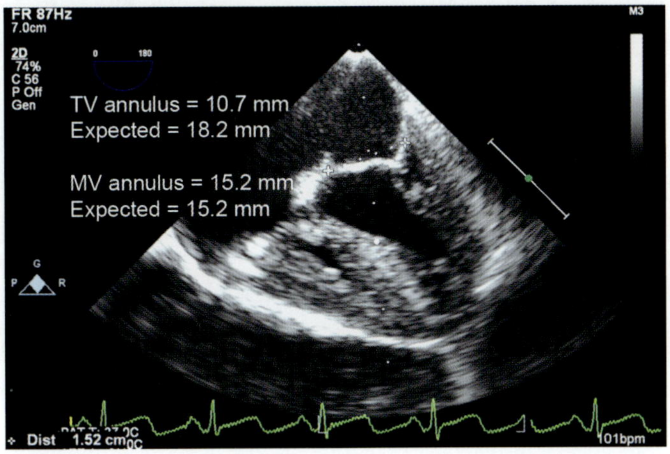

Figure 1 2D echo in midesophageal 4 chamber view showing a hypoplastic tricuspid valve and right ventricle

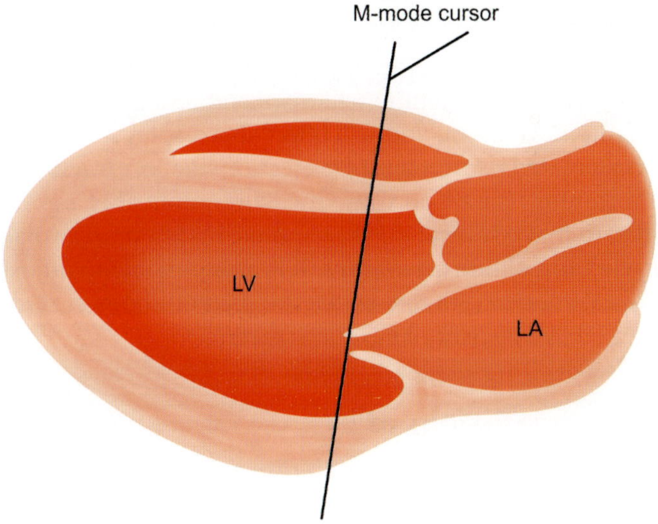

Figure 2 Positioning of M-mode cursor for measurement of LV dimension

LEFT VENTRICULAR MEASUREMENTS (TABLE 2)

Some measurements of the left ventricular (LV) wall and cavity dimensions in both systolic and diastolic. Linear LV measurements can be taken directly from a 2D echo image **(Fig. 1)** or using M-mode echo **(Fig. 2)** if you prefer, in either ME-4 chamber or ME-2 chamber view at the level of the mitral valve leaflet tips. Although M-mode has the advantage of high temporal resolution, making it easier to visualize motion of the endocardium, it is nonetheless easier to ensure correct alignment of your measurements (i.e. at 90° to the long axis of the LV cavity) if you take them directly from the 2D image. Whatever technique you prefer, be sure to identify end-diastole and end-systole and the endocardial/epicardial borders correctly.

Starting at the right ventricular (RV) border of the interventricular septum, use the callipers to measure the diastolic LV dimension **(Fig. 3)**:

- IVSd (interventricular septal wall dimension—diastole)
- LVIDd (LV internal dimension—diastole)
- LVPWd (LV posterior wall dimension—diastole)

Then repeat the process for the systolic LV dimensions:

- IVSs (interventricular septal wall dimension—systole)
- LVIDs (LV internal dimension—systole)
- LVPWs (LV posterior wall dimension—systole).

In the past, it has been recommended that such M-mode measurements be taken from leading edge to leading edge, but the improved resolution of

TABLE 6 RV, RVOT and PA diameters—references ranges

	Normal	*Mild*	*Moderate*	*Severe*
Modified apical 4-chamber view				
Basal RV diameter (cm)	2.0–2.8	2.9–3.3	3.4–3.8	≥3.9
Mid RV diameter (cm)	2.7–3.3	3.4–3.7	3.8–4.1	≥4.2
Base to apex length (cm)	7.1–7.9	8.0–8.5	8.6–9.1	≥9.2
Parasternal short axis view				
RVOT at AV level (cm)	2.5–2.9	3.0–3.2	3.3–3.5	≥3.6
RVOT at PV annulus (cm)	1.7–2.3	2.4–2.7	2.8–3.1	≥3.2
Main PA (cm)	1.5–2.1	2.2–2.5	2.6–2.9	≥3.0

contemporary echo machines means that measurements can instead be taken directly from the tissue-blood interface. The echo machine will display the measurements as you make them, and will often also display a number of calculated parameters (e.g. ejection fraction, fractional shortening) based on these measurements. It is a good idea to make several measurements on different cardiac cycles and obtain an average. It is also possible to adjust the LV internal dimensions for the patient's body surface area (BSA), measured in square meters.

Common Pitfalls of LV

Pitfalls in the assessment of LV dimensions include:

Failure to take measurements at the correct time points (end-diastole).

Failure to identify the endocardium correctly—be particularly carefully to avoid mistaking chordate tendinease for the endocardium of the LV posterior wall.

RIGHT VENTRICULAR DIMENSIONS (TABLE 6)

Assessment of RV dimensions is commonly made qualitatively by 'eyeball' particularly in the modified apical 4 chamber view. In this view, the RV is normally around two-thirds the size of the left ventricle; if two ventricles appears to be the same size, the RV is dilated.

RV size can also be assessed quantitatively, and because of its complex morphology it is possible to obtain RV diameters from several different points. Use 2D imaging to take measurements at end-diastole as follows:

- Modified apical 4 chamber view
  - Basal RV diameter (RVD1)
  - Mid RV diameter (RVD2)
  - RV base-to-apex (long axis) length (RVD3)

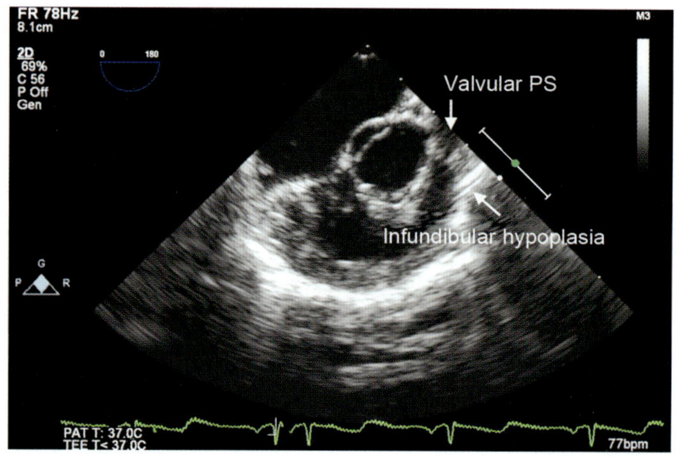

Figure 3 2D echo in midesophageal right ventricle inflow-outflow view showing a hypoplastic right ventricle infundibulum and pulmonic valvular stenosis

- Parasternal short axis view—aortic valve levels
  - RV outflow tract diameter at aortic valve level
  - RVOT diameter at pulmonary valve annulus level
  - Main pulmonary artery diameter.

Right Ventricular Function (Fig. 3)

Assessment of RV function is often made qualitatively, using 'eyeball' assessment of RV contractility from several different views. Inspect the RV carefully for evidence of regional wall motion abnormalities (normokinesia, hypokinesia, akinesia, dyskinesia) and describe the regions(s) affected (RV free wall, RV apex, interventricular septum (IVS), RVOT anterior wall). A more quantitative approach to RV function can also be taken, using one more of the following parameters:

- Fractional area change
- Tricuspid annular plane systolic excursion
- Tei index.

NADAS' CRITERIA

Assessment for Presence of Heart Disease in Children

Major Criteria

- Systolic murmur > grade III
- Diastolic murmur
- Cyanosis
- CCF.

Minor Criteria

- Systolic murmur, < grade III
- Abnormal S2
- Abnormal ECG
- Abnormal CXR
- Abnormal BP.

Presence of 1 major or 2 minor criteria → significant

REFERENCE VALUES FOR NORMAL ADULT TRANSESOPHAGEAL ECHOCARDIOGRAPHY MEASUREMENTS

Parameter		*Mean ± SO (mm)*	*Range (mm)*
Left atrial appendage	Right pulmonary artery diameter	17 ± 3	12–22
	Left upper pulmonary vein diameter	11 ± 2	7–16
	Length	28 ± 5	15–43
	Diameter	16 ± 5	10–28
	Superior vena cava diameter	15 ± 3	8–20
	Right ventricular outflow tract diameter	27 ± 4	16–36
Left atrium	Anteroposterior diameter	38 ± 6	20–52
	Medial-lateral diameter	39 ± 7	24–52
Right atrium	Anteroposterior diameter	38 ± 5	28–52
	Medial-lateral diameter	38 ±6	29–53
	Tricuspid annular diameter	28 ± 5	20–40
	Mitral annular diameter	29 ± 4	20–38
	Coronary sinus diameter	6.6 ± 1.5	4–10
Left ventricle	Anteroposterior diameter (diastole)	43 ± 7	33–55
	Medial-lateral diameter (diastole)	42 ± 7	23–54
	Anteroposterior diameter (systole)	28 ± 6	18–40
	Medial-lateral diameter (systole)	27 ± 6	18–42
	Aortic root diameter	28 ± 3	21–34
Descending thoracic aorta diameter	Proximal	21 ± 4	14–30
	Distal	20 ± 4	13–28

Chapter 3

TEE Views in Congenital Heart Disease

Sarvesh Pal Singh, Poonam Malhotra Kapoor

Chapter Outline

- Midesophageal Four Chamber View
- Midesophageal Two Chamber View
- Midesophageal Bicommissural View
- Midesophageal Long-axis View
- Midesophageal Aortic Valve Long-axis View
- Midesophageal Aortic Valve Short-axis View
- Midesophageal Bicaval View
- Midesophageal Descending Thoracic Aorta Long-axis View
- Midesophageal Descending Thoracic Aorta Short-axis View
- Midesophageal Ascending Aorta Long-axis View
- Midesophageal Ascending Aorta Short-axis View
- Midesophageal Left Atrial Appendage View
- Midesophageal Modified Bicaval View
- Midesophageal Right Pulmonary Vein View
- Midesophageal Right Ventricle Inflow-Outflow View
- Lower Esophageal Coronary Sinus View
- Transgastric Views
- Probe Manipulation to Achieve Transgastric Views
- Transgastric Modified Hepatic Vein View
- Transgastric Two Chamber View
- Transgastric Apical Short-axis View
- Transgastric Basal Long-axis View
- Transgastric Basal Short-axis View
- Transgastric Mid-papillary Short-axis View
- Transgastric Right Ventricle Inflow-Outflow View
- Transgastric Right Ventricle Inflow View
- Transgastric Basal Right Ventricle Outflow View
- Deep Transgastric Long-axis View
- Upper Esophageal Aortic Arch Long-axis View
- Upper Esophageal Aortic Arch Short-axis View

INTRODUCTION

Transesophageal echocardiography (TEE) has the unique advantage of portability and the ability to obtain high-resolution images of the abnormal cardiovascular anatomy, function and is relatively easy to perform with a low risk of complications.

Transesophageal echocardiography use has become an integral part in the care of cardiac surgical patients.

This is evolving to be used in other subspecialties. The purpose of this article is to introduce the novice echocardiographer to a stepwise approach in image orientation and acquisition in TEE for CHD. This chapter is based on the ASE Guidelines (J Am Soc Echocardiogr. 2013;26:921-64) which give 28 essential TEE views for a comprehensive TEE examination in a child/infant/neonate, which is a step up from the previous 20 essential TEE views **(Tables 1 to 3)**.

TABLE 1 Recommended transesophageal echocardiography

Window (depth from incisors)	*Cross section*	*Multiplane angle range*	*Structure imaged*
UE (20–25 cm)	Aortic arch LAX Aortic arch SAX	0° 90°	Aortic arch, left brachiocephalic vein Aortic arch, PA, PV, left brachiophalic vein
Midesophageal (30–40 cm)	Four chamber Mitral commissural Two chamber LAX RV inflow-outflow AV SAX AV LAX Bicaval Ascending aortic SAX Ascending aortic LAX Descending aorta SAX Descending aorta LAX	0°–20° 60°–70° 80°–100° 120°–160° 60°–90° 30°–60° 120°–160° 80°–110° 0°–60° 100°–150° 0° 90°–110°	LV, LA, RA, MV, TV, IAS MV, LV, LA, LAA LV, LA, LAA, MV LV, LA, AV, LVOT, MV, ascending aorta RV, RA, TV, RVOT, PV, PA AV, IAS, coronary ostia, LVOT, PV AV, LVOT, proximal ascending aorta, right PA RA, SVC, IVC, IAS, LA, CS Ascending aorta, SVC, PA, right PA Ascending aorta, right PA Descending thoracic aorta, left pleural space Descending thoracic aorta, left pleural space
TG (40–50 cm)	Basal SAX Mid – SAX Two chamber LAX RV inflow	0°–20° 0°–20° 80°–100° 0°–120° 100°–120°	LV, MV, RV, TV LV, RV, papillary muscles LV, MV, chordae, papillary muscle, CS, LA LVOT, AV, MV RV, TV, RA, TV chordae, papillary muscle
Deep TG (45–50 cm)	LAX	0°–20°	LVOT, AV, ascending aorta, arch

TABLE 2 Minimal perioperative transesophageal echocardiography study (II)

YOE view		*Structure seen*	*Information provided*
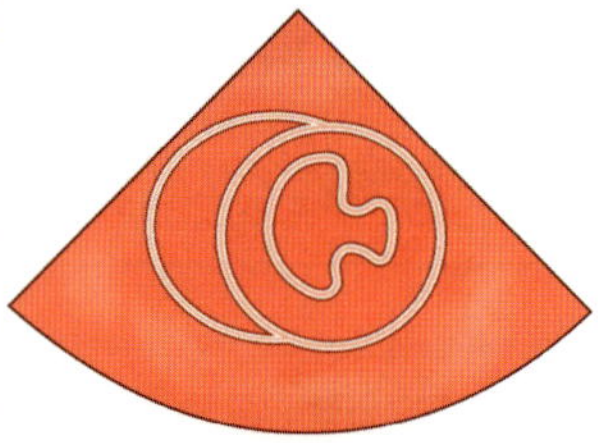	TG mid SAX	RV free wall; ventricular septum; LV anterior, lateral, inferior, posterior wall	Global and regional LV and RV function, wall thickness. Hypertrophy? Preload?
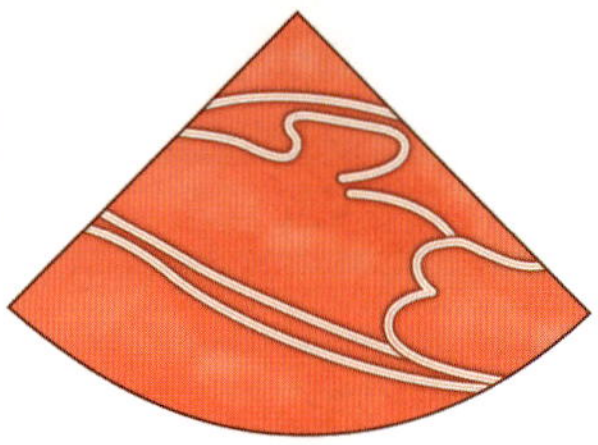	TG LAX	LV posterior wall, anterior septum, papillary muscles, mitral valve, LVOT, aortic valve	Global and regional LV function, aortic flow (Doppler). LVOT obstruction? Aortic stenosis? Aortic regurgitation?
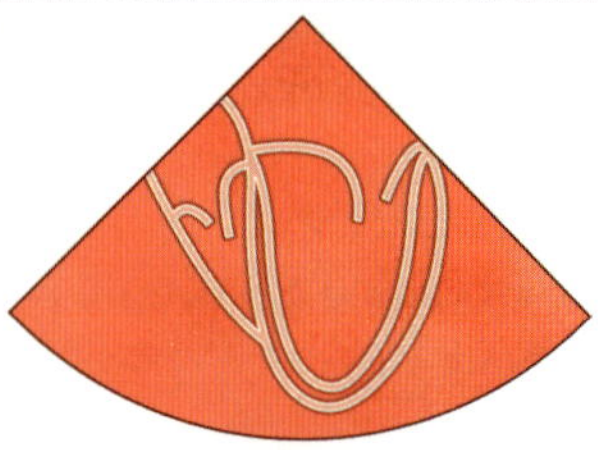	MOE four chamber	RA, tricuspid valve, RY, atrial and ventricular septum, LA, mitral valve, LV lateral wall	Global and regional RV and LV function, LA, RA size, function, masses, septal shape, transmitral flow (Doppler). Tricuspid. mitral regurgitation? Mitral stenosis? SAM?
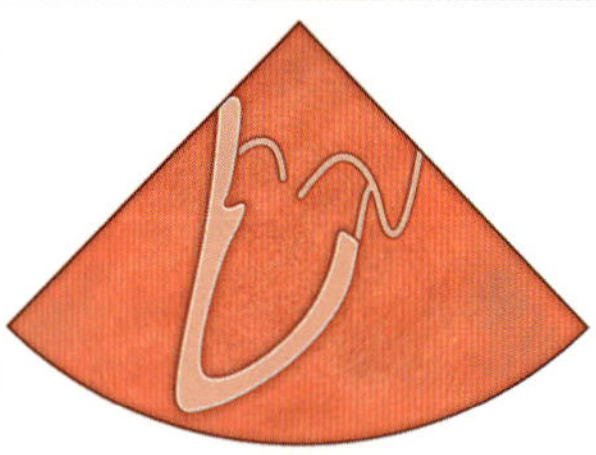	MOE two chamber	LA, LA appendage, mitral valve, LV inferior and anterior wall	Global and regional LV function, transmitral flow (Doppler). Mitral regurgitation, stenosis?
	MOE LAX	LA, mitral valve. LVOT, aortic valve, LV anteroseptal and posterior wall	Global and regional LV function, SAM? Aortic stenosis, regurgitation?

TABLE 3 Minimal perioperative transesophageal echocardiography study (II)

YOE view		*Structure seen*	*Information provided*
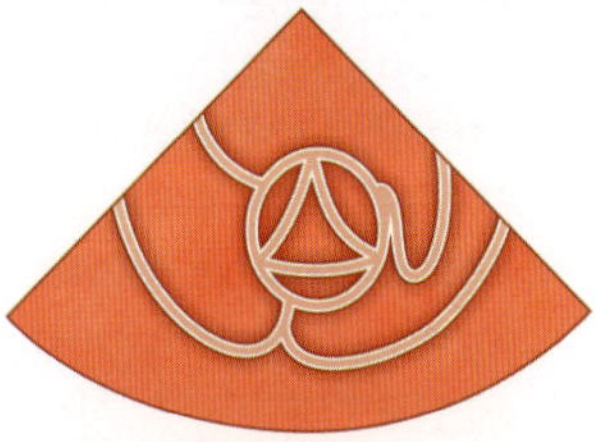	MOE AV SAX	AV, cusps, sinuses of Valsalva, coronary ostia	Tricuspid or bicuspid valve? Cusp mobility, valve opening area. Aortic stenosis? Vegetations?
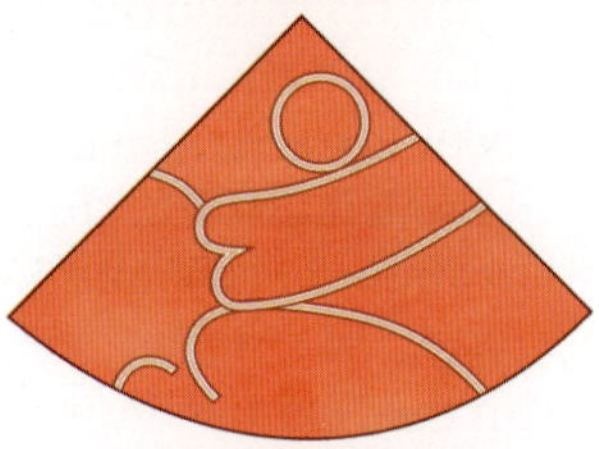	MOE AV LAX	AY, cusps, aortic root, sinotubular junction, ascending aorta, right pulmonary artery SAX	Aortic dimensions, wall composition, cusp mobility. Aortic stenosis, regurgitation? Dissection? Aneurysm? Atheroma?
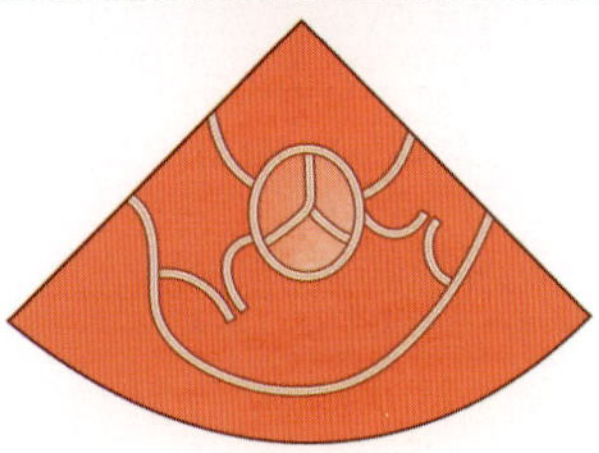	MOE RV inflow-outflow	RA, tricuspid valve, RV inflow and outflow tract, pulmonary valve, main pulmonary artery LAX	RV global and regional function. Tricuspid, pulmonary regurgitation? RV systolic pressure (Doppler), thrombi? Foreign bodies
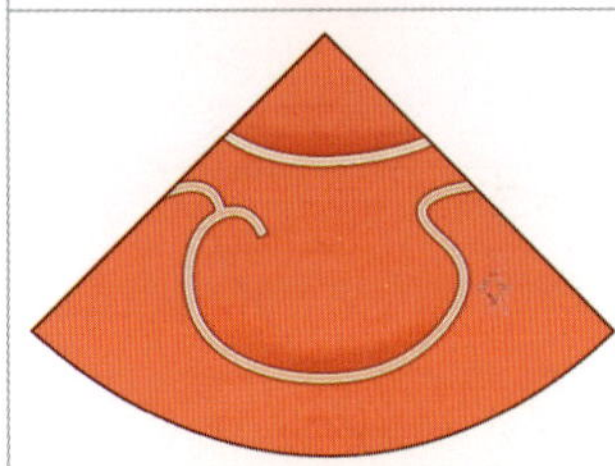	MOE bicaval	LA, atrial septum, inferior and superior caval veins, RA	Septum shape and motion. Open foramen ovale? Atrial septum defect? Thrombi?
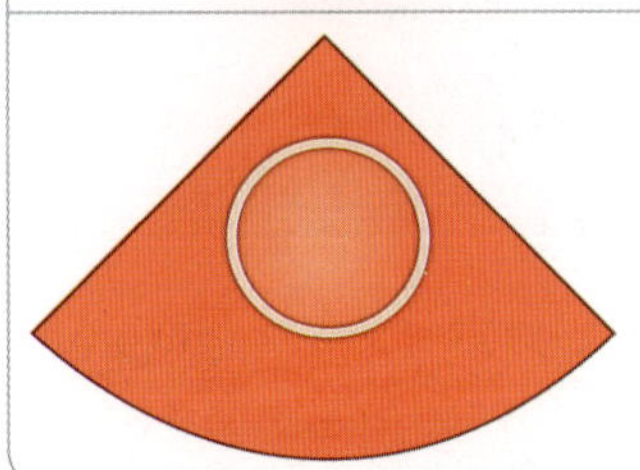	Descending aortic SAX	Aortic wall and lumen, posterior mediastinum	Aneurysm? Dissection? Rupture? Atheroma? Interamural/periaortic hematoma? Effusion?

MIDESOPHAGEAL FOUR CHAMBER VIEW

- **Multiplane angle range:**
  - 0–20 degrees
  - *Sector depth:* ~ 12–14 cm
- **Anatomy imaged:**
  - Left ventricle and atrium
  - Right ventricle and atrium
  - Mitral and tricuspid valves
  - Interatrial and interventricle septum
- **Clinical utility (Figs 1A to C):**
  - *Ventricle function:* Global and regional
  - *Intracardiac chamber masses:* Thrombus, tumor, air, foreign bodies
  - *Mitral and tricuspid valve evaluation:* Pathology, pathophysiology
  - Congenital or acquired interatrial and ventral septal defects
  - Hypertrophic obstructive cardiomyopathy evaluation.

Probe Manipulation

- The ME four-chamber view is obtained by turning the probe to the left (counterclockwise rotation of the probe) or to the right (clockwise rotation of the probe) is performed to center the mitral valve (MV) and left ventricle in the sector display.
- The image depth is then adjusted to ensure viewing of the left ventricular (LV) apex. The multiplane angle should be rotated to approximately 10 to 20 until the aortic valve (AV) or LV outflow tract (LVOT) is no longer in the display and the tricuspid annular dimension is maximized. Because the apex is at a slightly inferior plane to the left atrium, slight retroflexion may be required to align the MV and LV apex.

A color flow Doppler sector with the Nyquist limit set at 50 to 60 cm/sec should be placed over both the MV and TV to aid in the identification of valvular pathology (regurgitation and/or stenosis), as well as to the IAS to identify shunt flow.

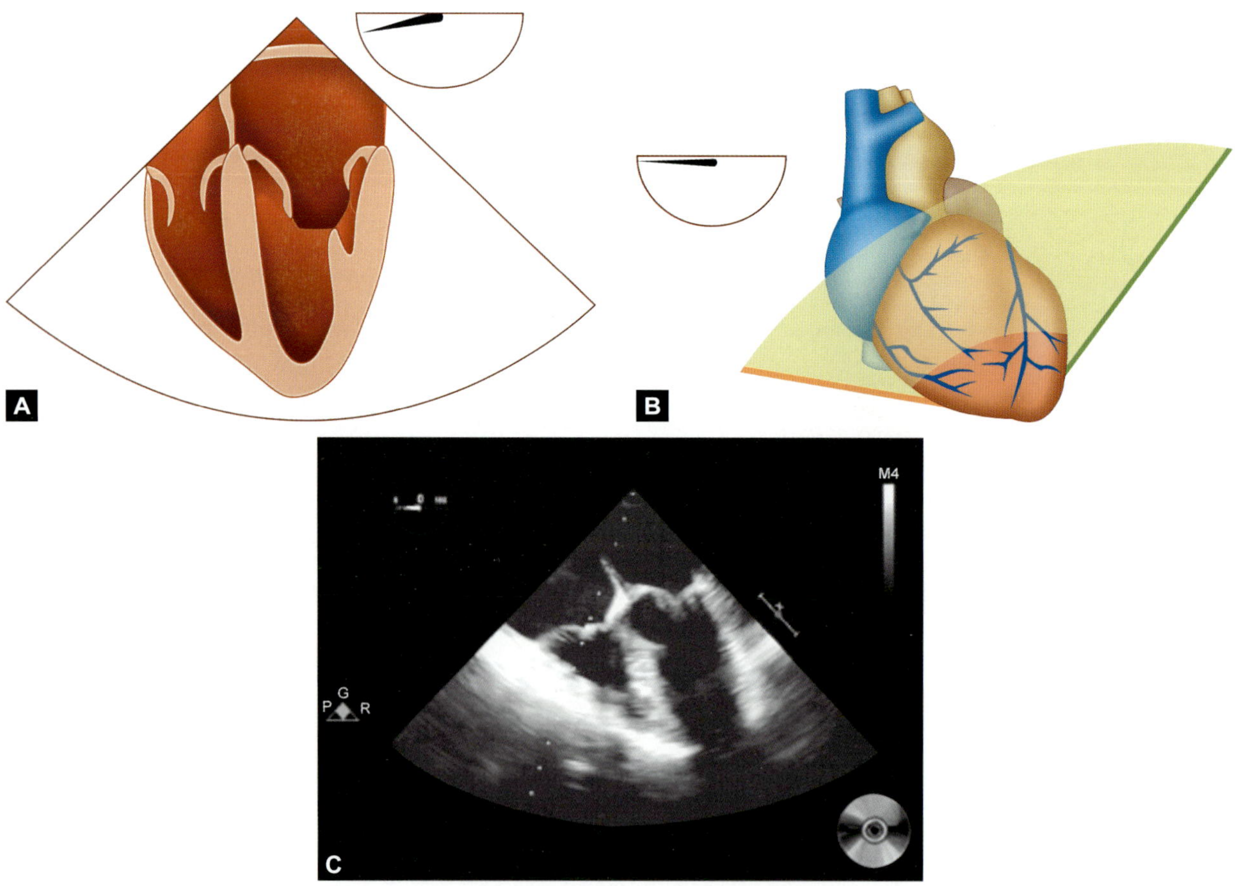

Figures 1A to C (A) Midesophageal four chamber view; (B) Animation of midesophageal four chamber view; (C) **(Video 1)** Midesophageal four chamber view for identification of four chambers, IAS, IVS, MV and TV

MIDESOPHAGEAL TWO CHAMBER VIEW

- **Multiplane angle range:**
  - 80–100 degrees
  - *Sector depth:* ~ 12–14 cm
- **Anatomy imaged left ventricle, atrium, and atrial appendage:**
  - Mitral valve
  - *Left pulmonary veins:* Turning probe to left
  - Coronary sinus (short-axis or long-axis by turning probe tip to left)
  - Left atrium
  - Left ventricle
  - Left atrial appendage
- **Clinical utility (Figs 2A and B):**
  - *Left ventricle function:* Global and regional
  - *Left ventricle and atrial masses:* Thrombus, tumor, air, foreign bodies
  - *Mitral valve evaluation:* Pathology, pathophysiology
  - Ventricular diastolic evaluation via transmitral and pulmonary vein Doppler flow profile analysis
  - *Coronary sinus evaluation:* Coronary sinus catheter placement; dilation secondary to persistent left superior vena cava.

Probe Manipulation

- From the ME four-chamber view, rotating the multiplane angle forward to between 80 and 100 degrees until the right ventricle disappears from the image the ME two-chamber view will develop.
- Diagnostic information obtained from this view includes global and regional LV function, MV function, and regional assessment of the LV anterior and inferior walls.
- The basal inferior and mid inferior wall segments are perfused by the RCA, whereas the apical inferior, apical cap, apical anterior, mid anterior, and basal anterior wall segments are perfused by the LAD coronary artery.

A color flow Doppler sector with the Nyquist limit at 50 to 60 cm/sec should be applied over the MV to aid in the identification of valvular pathology (regurgitation and/or stenosis). The coronary sinus is seen in short-axis (SAX), as a round structure immediately superior to the basal inferior LV segment.

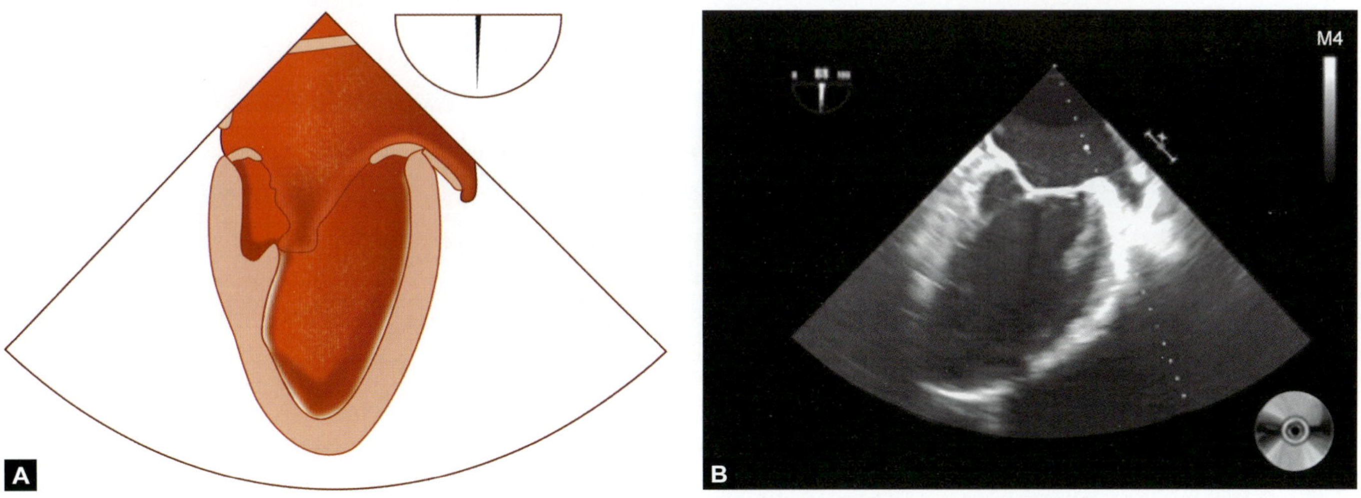

Figures 2A and B (A) Outline of midesophageal two chamber view; (B) **(Video 2)** Midesophageal two chamber view to show the LV and LA and also provide detailed evaluation of the mitral valve and regional assessment of the LV anterior and inferior walls

MIDESOPHAGEAL BICOMMISSURAL VIEW

- **Multiplane angle range:**
  - 60–70 degrees
  - *Sector depth:* ~ 12 cm
- **Anatomy imaged:**
  - Left ventricle and atrium
  - Mitral valve
- **Clinical utility (Figs 3A to D):**
  - *Left ventricle function:* Global and regional
  - *Left ventricle and atrial masses:* Thrombus, tumor, air, foreign bodies
  - *Mitral valve evaluation:* Pathology, pathophysiology
  - Ventricular diastolic evaluation via transmitral Doppler flow profile analysis.

Probe Manipulation

- From the ME four-chamber view, rotating the transducer angle to between 60 and 70 will generate the ME mitral commissural view.
- Extreme turning of the probe to the right and left enables visualization of parts of the MV annulus (or sewing ring of prosthetic valves).
- In addition, the anterolateral and posteromedial papillary muscles with their corresponding chordae are prominent structures in the ME commissural view.
- Diagnostic information obtained from this view includes regional LV function, anterior/anterolateral and inferior/inferolateral walls and MV function and left atrial appendage.

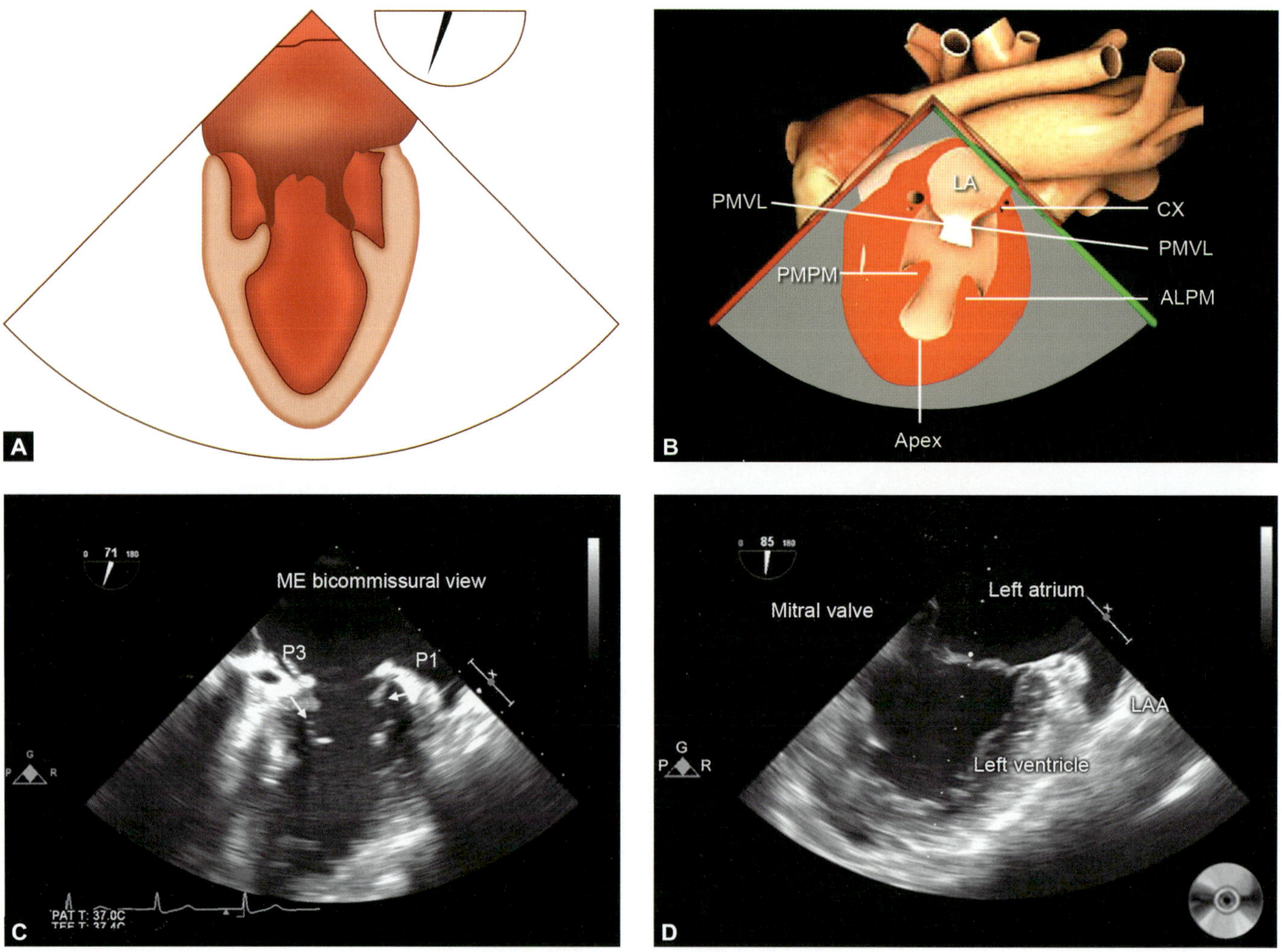

Figures 3A to D (A) Outline of midesophageal bicommissural view; (B) Simulator of midesophageal bicommissural view; (C) Midesophageal bicommissural view; (D) **(Video 3)** Midesophageal bicommissural view for a detailed view of LA, LV and MV leaflets and their scallops

MIDESOPHAGEAL LONG-AXIS VIEW

- **Transducer angle:**
  - 120 degrees
- **Level:**
  - Midesophageal
- **Maneuver (from prior image):**
  - Anteflex
- **Clinical utility (Figs 4A to C):**
  - LV function
  - MV disease
  - AV and aortic root disease
  - Interventricular septum pathology.

Probe Manipulation

Increasing the omni, while slightly rotating the probe counterclockwise brings in the long-axis view, with similar structures seen as that in the parasternal long-axis and apical long-axis of transthoracic echo. This is the best view to look at the LVOT and anteroseptum as well as A2 and P2 of the mitral valve.

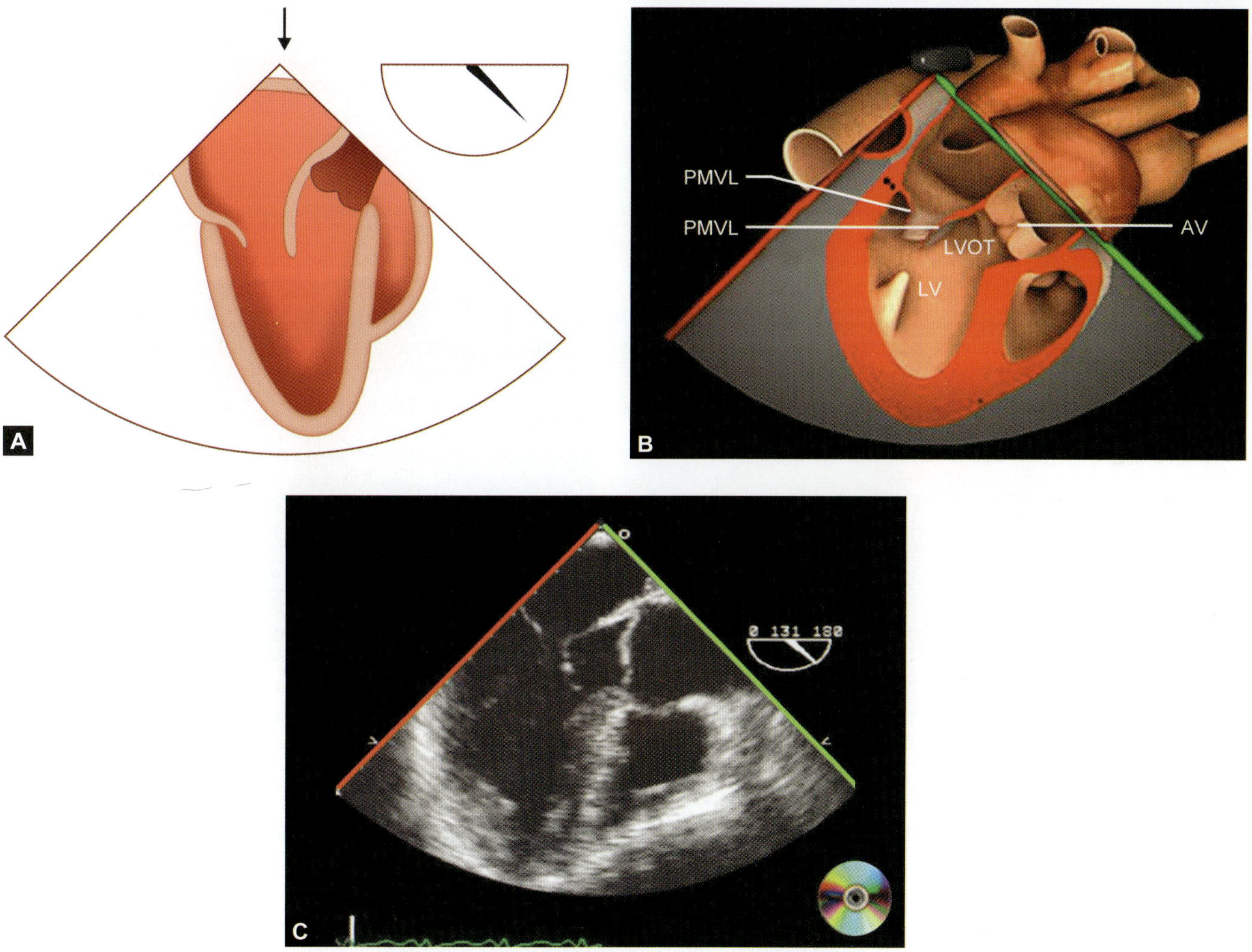

Figures 4A to C (A) Outline of midesophageal long-axis view; (B) Simulator of midesophageal long-axis view; (C) **(Video 4)** Midesophageal long-axis view for LV function, MV disease, AV and aortic root disease to view the aortic over-ride and IVS in detail

MIDESOPHAGEAL AORTIC VALVE LONG-AXIS VIEW

- **Multiplane angle range:**
  - 120–160 degrees
  - *Sector depth:* ~ 8–10 cm
- **Anatomy imaged:**
  - Aortic valve
  - Proximal ascending aorta
  - Left ventricular outflow tract
  - Mitral valve
  - Right pulmonary artery
- **Clinical utility (Figs 5A to C):**
  - *Aortic valve:* Pathology, pathophysiology
  - *Ascending aorta pathology:* Atherosclerosis, aneurysms and dissections
  - *Mitral valve evaluation:* Pathology, pathophysiology.

The AV LAX view is suitable for assessing the grade of AR with color Doppler. Application of color Doppler in the normal AV demonstrates no transvalvular flow during diastole but laminar flow during systole.

Probe Manipulation

- From the ME two-chamber view, rotating the multiplane angle forward to between 120 and 160 until the LVOT and AV come into the display develops the ME LAX view.
- Visualized structures include the left atrium, MV, left ventricle, LVOT, AV, and proximal ascending aorta.
- This view offers diagnostic information regarding chamber volume and function, MV and AV function, LVOT pathology, and regional assessment of the left ventricle.

Color flow Doppler can be applied to the MV, LVOT, and AV to aid in the identification of valvular pathology (regurgitation and/or stenosis).

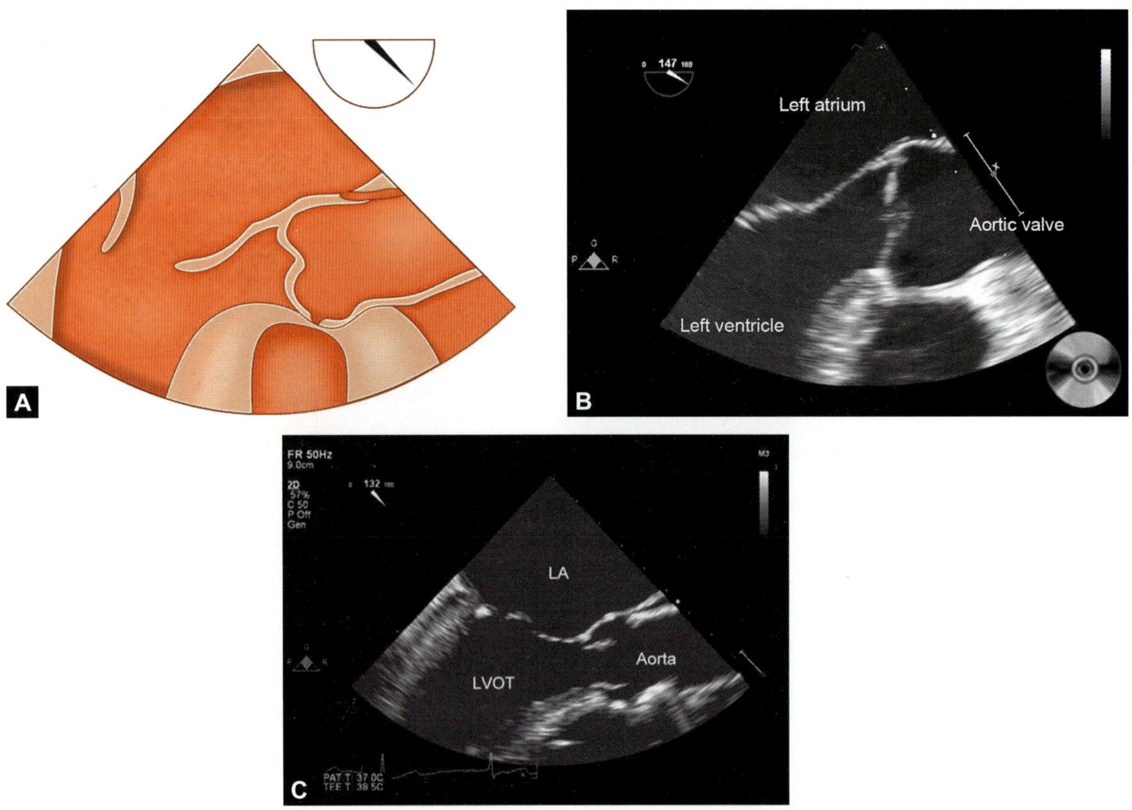

Figures 5A to C (A) Outline of midesophageal aortic valve long-axis view; (B) **(Video 5)** Midesophageal aortic valve long-axis view showing the aortic and mitral valves and regional assessment of LV, also excellent for aortic annulus and AML length; (C) Midesophageal aortic valve long-axis view in systole

MIDESOPHAGEAL AORTIC VALVE SHORT-AXIS VIEW

- **Multiplane angle range:**
  - 30–60 degrees
  - *Sector depth:* ~ 10–12 cm
- **Anatomy imaged aortic valve:**
  - Interatrial septum
  - Coronary ostia and arteries
  - Right ventricular outflow tract
  - Pulmonary valve
- **Clinical utility (Figs 6A to C):**
  - *Aortic valve:* Pathology, pathophysiology
  - *Ascending aorta pathology:* Atherosclerosis, aneurysms and dissections
  - *Left and right atrial masses:* Thrombus, embolus, air, tumor, foreign bodies
  - Congenital or acquired interatrial septal defects evaluation.

Probe Manipulation

- At 40–60° the characteristic short-axis view of the aortic valve (MOE AV SAX) is obtained. The right coronary cusp and sinus are located at the bottom, contiguous with the RV wall; the non-coronary sinus lies on the left and the left coronary sinus on the right.
- The AV cusps should be clearly identified. For a trileaflet valve, the left coronary cusp should be posterior and on the right side of the image. The noncoronary cusp is adjacent to the IAS.
- The right coronary cusp is anterior and adjacent to the RVOT.

Color flow Doppler can be applied over the AV to aid in identifying aortic regurgitation and seeing the VC width and the aortic annulus.

The systolic orifice area can be measured by planimetry (or calculated via the continuity equation using other views). "Normal" individuals may have a tiny jet of trace aortic regurgitation (AR), often located in the center of the AV. In the presence of AR, the SAX view is particularly useful in defining the locus of the regurgitant orifice. Slight withdrawal of the TEE probe demonstrates the proximal ascending aorta. Advancement of the probe depicts the LVOT.

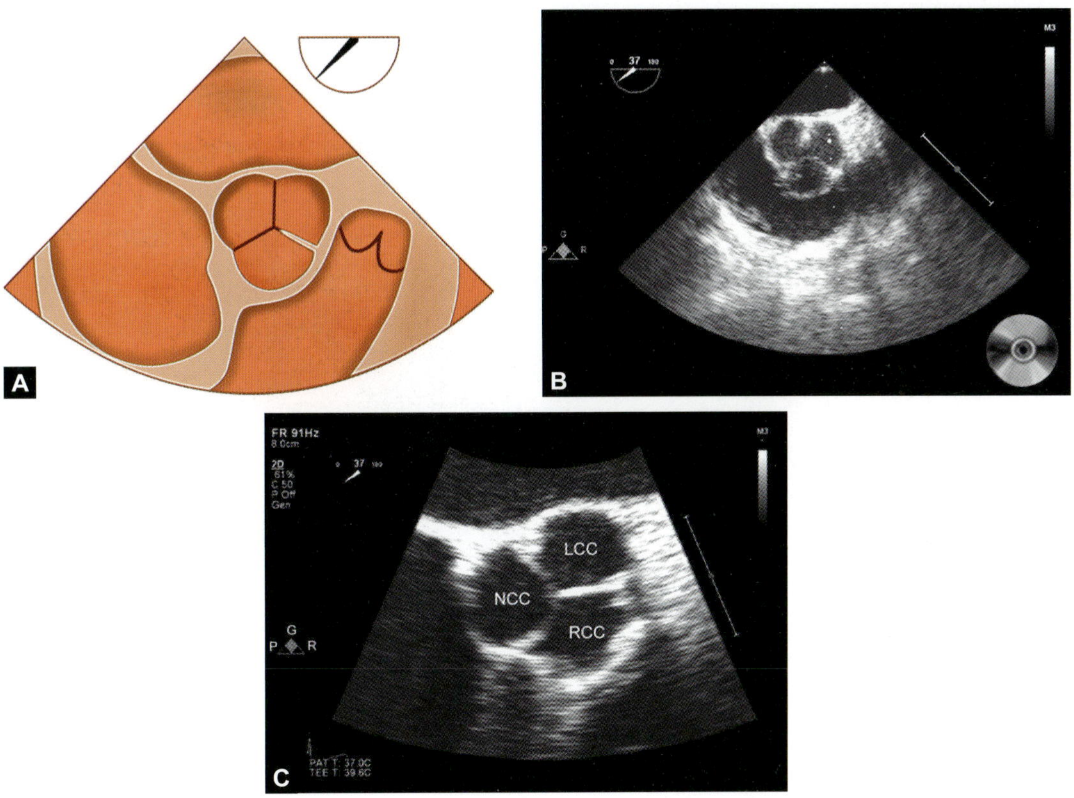

Figures 6A to C (A) Midesophageal aortic valve short-axis view with AV in center; (B) **(Video 6)** Midesophageal aortic valve short-axis view the 3 cusps of AV, calcification in the 3 cusps, presence and quantification of AS and AR; (C) Midesophageal aortic valve short-axis view in diastole

MIDESOPHAGEAL BICAVAL VIEW

- **Multiplane angle range:**
  - 80–110 degrees
  - *Sector depth:* ~ 8–10 cm
- **Anatomy imaged:**
  - Right and left atrium
  - Superior vena cava (long-axis)
  - *Inferior vena cava orifice:* Advance probe and turn to right to visualize inferior vena cava in the long-axis, liver, hepatic and portal veins
  - Interatrial septum
  - *Right pulmonary veins:* Turn probe to right
- **Clinical utility (Figs 7A and B):**
  - *Right and left atrial masses:* Thrombus, embolus, air, tumor, foreign bodies
  - *Superior vena cava pathology:* Thrombus, sinus venosus atrial septal defect
  - Inferior vena cava pathology (thrombus, tumor)
  - Femoral venous line placement
  - Coronary sinus catheter line placement
  - *Right pulmonary vein evaluation:* Anomalous return, Doppler evaluation for left ventricular diastolic function.

Probe Manipulation

- From the ME RV inflow-outflow view, the multiplane angle is rotated forward to 80 to 110 and the probe is turned clockwise to the ME bicaval view.
- From this view, catheters or pacing wires entering the right atrium from the superior vena cava are well imaged.

Color Doppler of the IAS, including the use of a lower Nyquist limit setting, may be used to assess the presence of a low-velocity interatrial shunt. Agitated saline may also be injected after the administration of a Valsalva maneuver for further documentation of a right-to-left component.

The inferior and superior vena cava are seen entering the right atrium. This bicaval view can also be obtained at the mid-esophageal level as the ME bicaval view. By rotating the imaging plane to 100–110°, the junction of the inferior vena cava, with the right atrium on the left and the right atrial appendage on the right, can be seen. The fine linear and usually quite mobile structure arising from the junction is Eustach's valve.

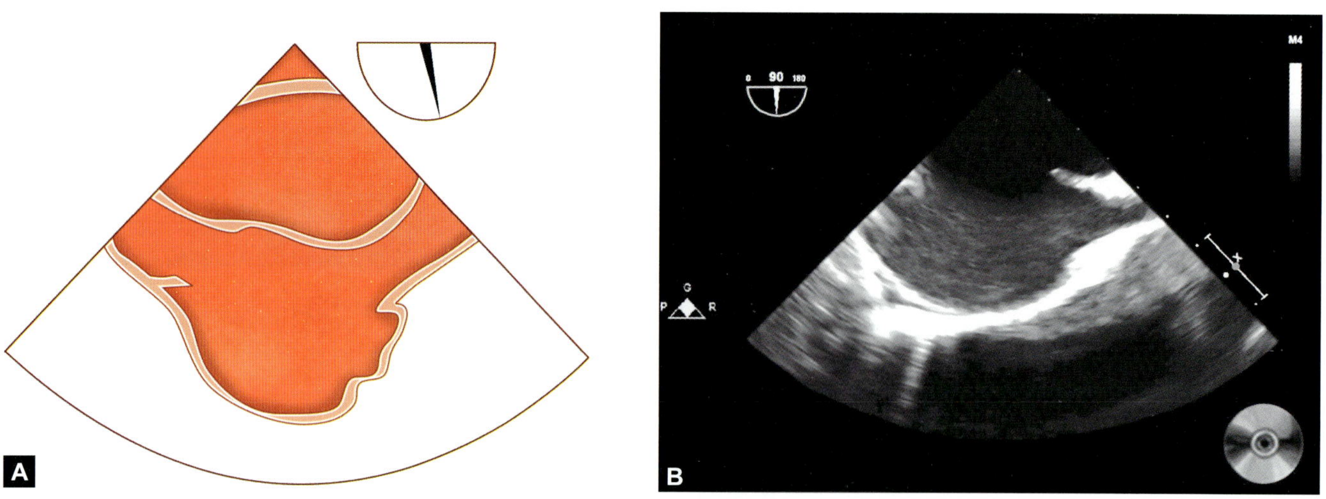

Figures 7A and B (A) Outline of midesophageal bicaval view; (B) **(Video 7)** Midesophageal bicaval view outline and video to see the IAS

MIDESOPHAGEAL DESCENDING THORACIC AORTA LONG-AXIS VIEW

- **Multiplane angle range:**
  - 90 degrees
  - *Sector depth:* ~6
- **Probe adjustments**
  - Neutral
- **Anatomy imaged:**
  - Descending aorta in long-axis in longitudinal plane
- **Clinical utility (Figs 8A to C):**
  - Aortic atherosclerosis
  - Aortic dissection
  - Intra-aortic balloon pump (IABP) placement.

Probe Manipulation

- The LAX view is obtained at a transducer angle of approximately 90 to 100 degrees. Image depth should be decreased to enlarge the size of the aorta and the focus set to be in the near field. Finally, gain should be adjusted in the near field to optimize imaging.
- While keeping the aorta in the center of the image, the probe can be advanced or withdrawn to image the entire descending aorta **(Figs 8A to C)**. Because there are no internal anatomic landmarks in the descending aorta, describing the location of pathology is difficult.
- One approach to this problem is to identify the location in terms of distance from the incisors. The descending thoracic aorta is located posterior and to the left of the esophagus and when imaging this structure the transesophageal echocardiographic probe faces the left thoracic cavity. Thus, intercostal arteries are typically seen arising from the aorta toward the right side of the screen.
- When imaging the descending thoracic aorta, the hemiazygous vein (which drains the left posterior thorax) may be seen in the far field of imaging. In the mid to upper thorax, this vein joins the azygous vein (which drains the right posterior thorax). This venous structure is typically parallel to the aorta and aortic arch, eventually draining into the superior vena cava.

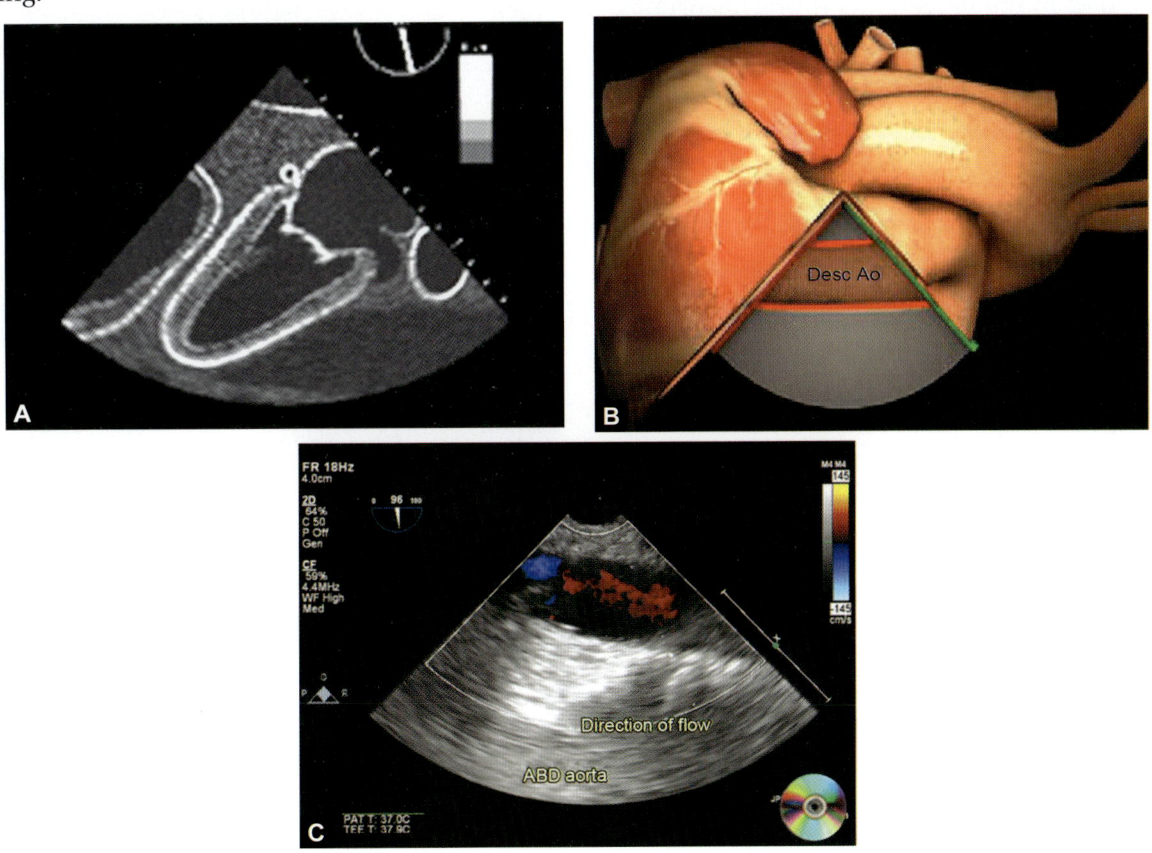

Figures 8A to C (A) The diagrammatic view of midesophageal descending thoracic aorta long-axis view; (B) Simulator view of midesophageal descending thoracic aorta long-axis view; (C) **(Video 8)** Midesophageal descending thoracic aorta long-axis view showing the descending thoracic aorta in the center

MIDESOPHAGEAL DESCENDING THORACIC AORTA SHORT-AXIS VIEW

- **Multiplane angle range:**
  - 0 degree
  - *Sector depth:* ~ 6 cm
- **Anatomy imaged:**
  - Descending thoracic aorta
  - Left pleural space
- **Clinical utility (Figs 9A and B):**
  - *Descending aorta pathology:* Atherosclerosis, aneurysms, and dissections
  - Intra-aortic balloon placement evaluation
  - Left pleural effusion.

The entire thoracic descending aorta is not well visualized by TTE. A short-axis view of the descending aorta can be imaged posteriorly to the left atrium in the parasternal long-axis view. From the apical window, a short-axis cross-section of the descending aorta is seen lateral to the left atrium in the four-chamber view and a long-axis stretch in the two-chamber view. By 908 transducer, a rotation long-axis view is obtained and a mid part of the descending thoracic aorta may be visualized. Although a partial assessment of the size of the descending aorta and detection of large abnormal structures such as dissection membranes are possible in these views, the descending aorta lies far from the transducer and the assessment is incomplete, suboptimal and not accurate. However, in acute aortic syndrome with left pleural effusion, scanning from the back may provide good or optimal views of the descending aorta.

Probe Manipulation

- From the TG LAX view, the transducer angle is returned to 0 to 10 and the probe turned to the left (counterclockwise).
- Although one can begin imaging the descending aorta below the diaphragm (typically beginning at the celiac artery), abdominal gas and variable aortic position may prevent adequate imaging, and withdrawing the probe to just above the diaphragm allows imaging of the descending thoracic aorta. This is at a sector depth of 6 cm.

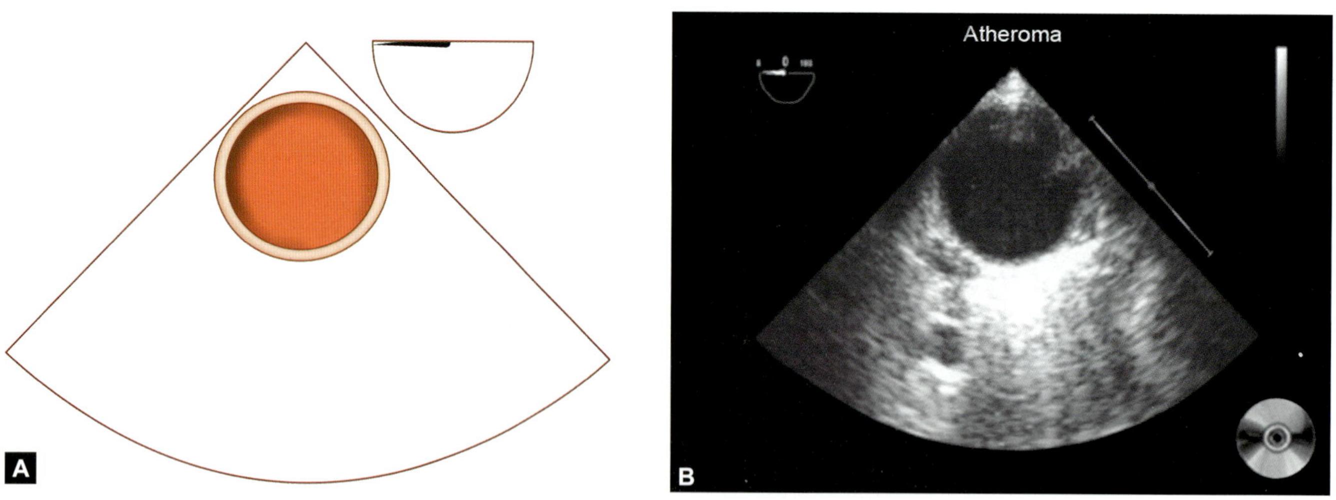

Figures 9A and B (A) Outline of midesophageal descending aorta short-axis view; (B) **(Video 9)** Midesophageal descending thoracic aorta short-axis view showing the descending thoracic aorta. Ideal for IABP placement evaluation and see left pleural effusion

MIDESOPHAGEAL ASCENDING AORTA LONG-AXIS VIEW

- **Multiplane angle range:**
  - 100–150 degrees
  - *Sector depth:* ~ 12 cm
- **Anatomy imaged:**
  - Ascending aorta
  - Right pulmonary artery
- **Clinical utility (Figs 10A to C):**
  - *Ascending aorta pathology:* Atherosclerosis, aneurysms, and dissections
  - Anterograde cardioplegia delivery evaluation
  - Pulmonary embolus/thrombus.

Probe Manipulation

- Probe tip depth (from lips) upper esophageal (20–25 cm)
- Withdrawing the probe from the ME LAX view allows imaging of the LAX of the ascending aorta.
- The right pulmonary artery (PA) is adjacent to the esophagus and posterior to the ascending aorta.
- When the image is centered on this structure, counterclockwise rotation results in LAX imaging of the main PA and the pulmonic valve (PV).
- Because the LAX of the PA is parallel to the insonation beam, this is an optimal view for pulsed-wave or continuous-wave Doppler of the RV outflow tract (RVOT) or PV.
- Proximal pulmonary emboli can sometimes be seen from this view.

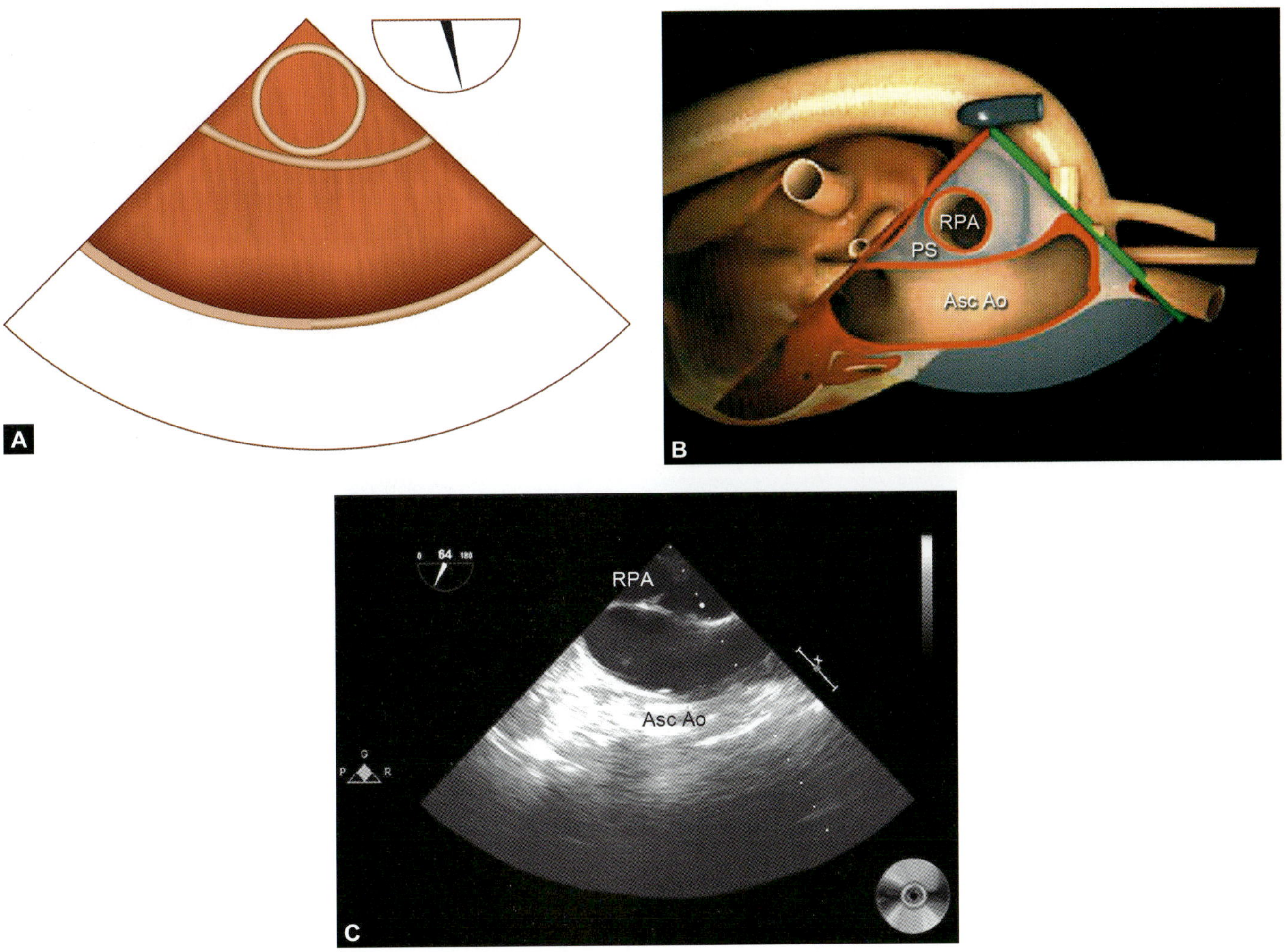

Figures 10A to C (A) Outline of midesophageal ascending aorta long-axis view; (B) Simulator view of midesophageal ascending aorta long-axis view; (C) **(Video 10)** Midesophageal ascending aorta long-axis view showing the relation of the RPA and aorta

MIDESOPHAGEAL ASCENDING AORTA SHORT-AXIS VIEW

- **Multiplane angle range:**
  - 0–60 degrees
  - *Sector depth:* ~ 12 cm
- **Anatomy imaged:**
  - Ascending aorta
  - Superior vena cava (short-axis)
  - Main pulmonary artery
  - Right pulmonary artery
  - Left pulmonary artery (turn probe tip to left)
  - Pulmonic valve.
- **Clinical utility (Figs 11A to C):**
  - *Ascending aorta pathology:* Atherosclerosis, aneurysms, and dissections
  - *Pulmonic valve:* Pathology, pathophysiology
  - Pulmonary embolus/thrombus evaluation
  - *Superior vena cava pathology:* Thrombus, sinus venosus atrial septal defect
  - Pulmonary artery catheter placement.

Probe Manipulation

- From the image of the main PA, rotating the multiplane angle back to 20 to 40 degrees images the bifurcation of the PA, the SAX view of the ascending aorta, and the SAX view of the superior vena cava, ME ascending aortic SAX.

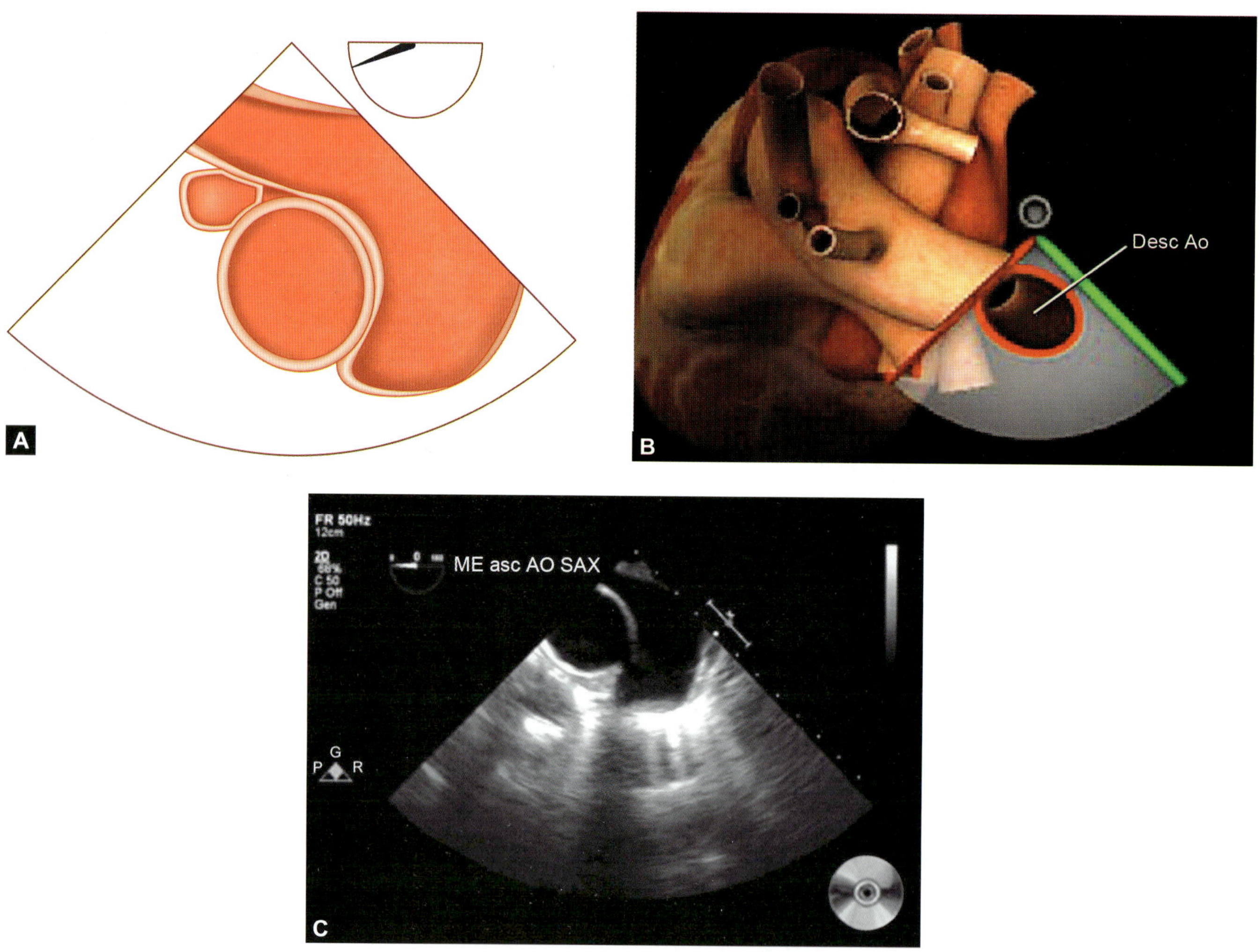

Figures 11A to C (A) Outline of midesophageal ascending aorta short-axis view; (B) Simulator view of midesophageal ascending aorta short-axis view; (C) **(Video 11)** Midesophageal ascending aorta short-axis view showing the ascending aorta, superior vena cava (short-axis), main pulmonary artery, right pulmonary artery, left pulmonary artery (turn probe tip to left), pulmonic valve

MIDESOPHAGEAL LEFT ATRIAL APPENDAGE VIEW

- **Transducer angle:**
  - 90–110 degrees
- **Level:**
  - Midesophageal
- **Maneuver (from prior image):**
  - Advanced
- **Clinical utility (Figs 12A to C):**
  - Left atrial appendage
  - Left upper pulmonary vein.

Probe Manipulation

- From the ME left pulmonary vein view (at a transducer angle of 90 to 110), turning the probe to right (clockwise) with possible advancement and/or anteflexion of the probe will open the LA appendage for the ME LA appendage view.
- The left superior pulmonary vein is also imaged. Given the complex and highly variable anatomy of the LA appendage, a complete assessment of morphology typically requires imaging the LA appendage in multiple views.
- Backward rotating from 90 to 0 while imaging the LA appendage and/or simultaneous multiplane imaging should be performed.

Color flow Doppler and pulsed-wave Doppler may be useful, particularly for assessment of emptying velocities.

- In a normal LAA spectral Doppler trace, four waves are seen during sinus rhythm (Figure 12C):
  1. During atrial systole, LAA contraction and emptying is seen above the baseline. Velocity is 60 ±14 cm/sec.
  2. During early systole, LAA filling is seen below the baseline. Velocity is 52 ± 13 cm/sec.
  3. Passive flow during the remainder of systole is seen as alternating small waves on both sides of the baseline.
  4. Early diastolic LAA emptying during LV early filling seen above the baseline. Velocity is 20 ± 11 cm/sec.
- An additional low velocity mid-diastolic wave from pulmonary venous filling may be seen below the baseline.

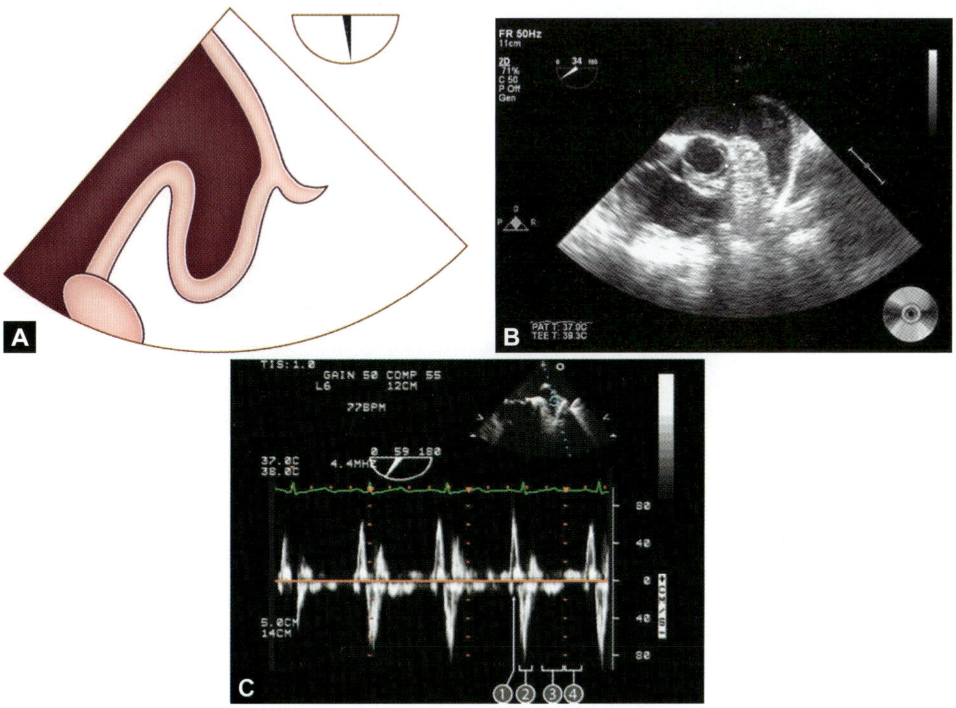

Figures 12A to C (A) Outline of midesophageal left atrial appendage view; (B) **(Video 12)** Midesophageal left atrial appendage view showing left atrial appendage and left upper pulmonary valve; (C) Spectral Doppler data acquired for blood flow in the left atrial appendage (LAA). In the upper right, a two dimensional TEE image of the midesophageal left atrial appendage view; the blue circle indicates the location of the sample volume within the LAA. In the lower half of the image, a spectral Doppler trace shows the relationship between red blood cell velocity and time. The baseline is orange. Four waves are seen during sinus rhythm

MIDESOPHAGEAL MODIFIED BICAVAL VIEW

- **Transducer angle:**
  - 50–70 degrees
- **Structures imaged:**
  - Right atrium
  - Left atrium
  - Interatrial septum
  - Inferior vena cava
  - Tricuspid valve
- **Probe adjustments:**
  - Probe rotated toward right as in bicaval view
- **Clinical utility (Figs 13A to C):**
  - For cannula placement in the superior vena cava (SVC)/(Inferior vena cava) IVC in all minimally invasive procedures, e.g. Robotic group.

Probe Manipulation

- From the ME RV inflow-outflow view, maintaining a transducer angle of 50 to 70, the probe is turned to the right (clockwise) until primarily the TV is centered in the view, resulting in the ME modified bicaval TV view.
- The left atrium, right atrium, interatrial septum, inferior vena cava, and TV are well imaged.
- The right atrial appendage as well as the superior vena cava will be seen. Because of the radially short septal TV leaflet, many tricuspid regurgitant jets are eccentric and directed toward the interatrial septum; from this view, the septal TV leaflet is imaged en face, and jets directed toward the interatrial septum may be parallel to the insonation beam.
- The orthogonal view (at 120–140) results in a LAX view of the TV which similarly may image an eccentric medial regurgitant jet parallel to the insonation beam.

Color flow Doppler and spectral Doppler (particularly continuous-wave Doppler) should be performed in these views.

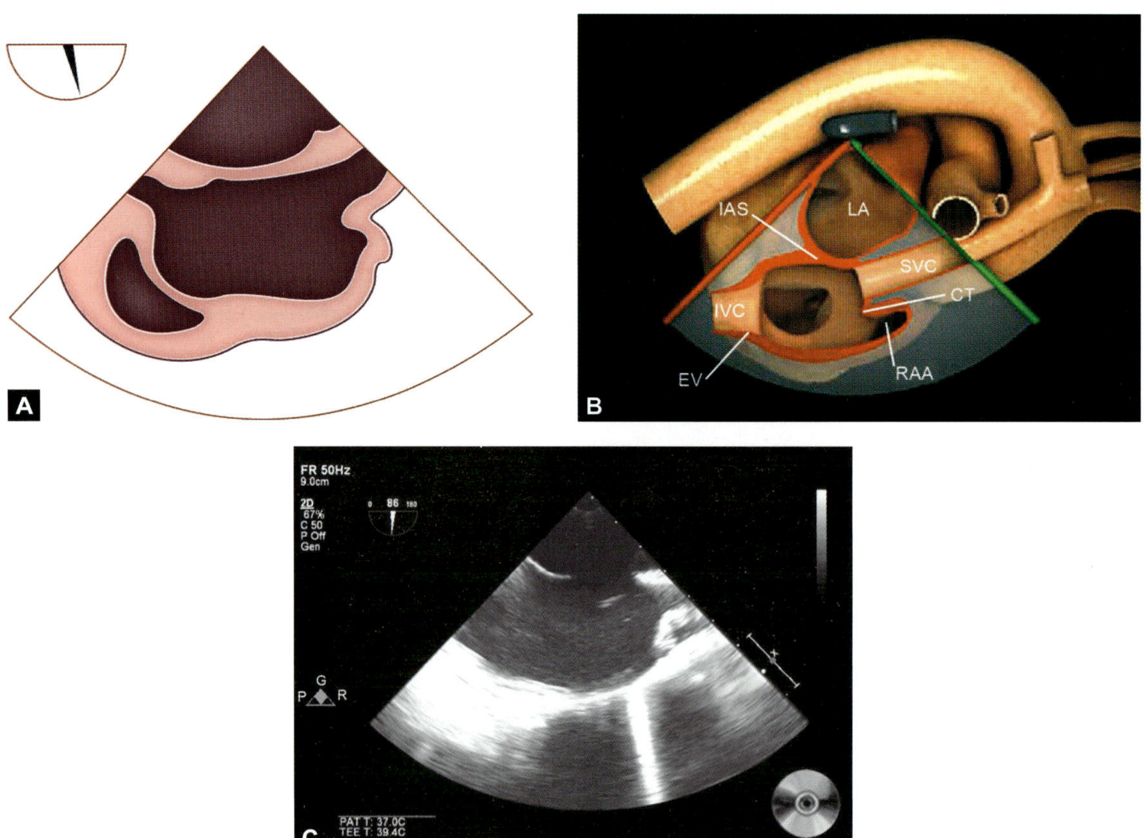

Figures 13A to C (A) Outline of Midesophageal modified bicaval view; (B) Simulator of midesophageal modified bicaval view; (C) **(Video 13)** midesophageal modified bicaval view showing right atrial appendage and superior vena cava

MIDESOPHAGEAL RIGHT PULMONARY VEIN VIEW

- **Transducer angle:**
  - 0–30 degrees
- **Level:**
  - Upper-esophageal
- **Maneuver (from prior image):**
  - Continuous wave (CW), advance
- **Clinical utility (Figs 14A and B):**
  - Mid-ascending aorta
  - Superior vena cava
  - Right pulmonary veins.

Probe Manipulation

- From the upper esophagus the pulmonary veins can be imaged as they enter the left atrium from their respected sides.
- The upper and lower pulmonary veins enter the atria at slightly different angles, the lower pulmonary veins run more in the posteromedial direction and the upper veins more in the anteromedial direction.
- The lower veins exhibit a more horizontal course and the upper veins a slightly vertical course. The left upper pulmonary vein is found easily at 0–30° between the left atrial appendage.

Localization of the pulmonary veins is facilitated by color Doppler imaging. If two left pulmonary veins are imaged simultaneously, then the vein adjacent to the left atrial appendage is the left upper pulmonary vein.

From the ME ascending aorta SAX view, advancing the probe and turning to the right (clockwise) will result in the ME right pulmonary vein view. The inflow of the inferior pulmonary vein is typically perpendicular to the insonation beam, but superior pulmonary vein inflow is typically parallel to the beam, and Doppler from this view can be performed. In addition to the right pulmonary veins, the superior vena cava (SAX view) and ascending aorta (SAX view) are also imaged.

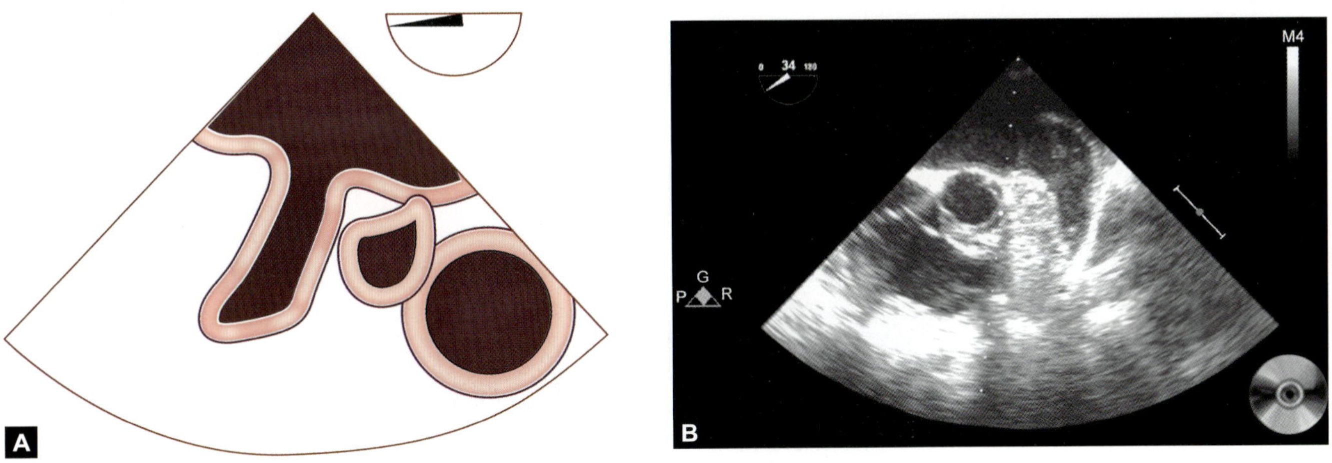

Figures 14A and B (A) Outline of midesophageal right pulmonary vein view; (B) **(Video 14)** Midesophageal right pulmonary vein view to show the position between aorta, superior vena cava and the right pulmonary artery, seen to the right side in figure B

MIDESOPHAGEAL RIGHT VENTRICLE INFLOW-OUTFLOW VIEW

- **Multiplane angle range:**
  - 60–90 degrees
  - *Sector depth:* ~ 10–12 cm
- **Anatomy imaged:**
  - Right ventricle and atrium
  - Left atrium
  - Right atrium
  - Tricuspid valve
  - Aortic valve
  - Right ventricular outflow tract
  - Pulmonic valve and main pulmonary artery
- **Clinical utility (Figs 15A to C):**
  - *Right ventricle and atrial masses and left atrial:* Thrombus, embolus, tumor, foreign bodies
  - *Pulmonic valve and subpulmonic valve:* Pathology, pathophysiology
  - Pulmonary artery catheter placement
  - *Tricuspid valve:* Pathology, pathophysiology.

Probe Manipulation

- At 60–100° the cross-sectional view of the aorta still remains in the middle of the image whereas, from left to right, the right atrium, tricuspid valve, RV, pulmonary valve, and main pulmonary artery become visible as they wind around the aorta. This view is called mid-esophageal RV inflow-outflow view (**Midesophageal Right Ventricle inflow-outflow**)
- It is indispensable for evaluating the right heart and congenital lesions involving the RV and pulmonary artery.

Color flow Doppler can be applied to the TV and PV to aid in the identification of valvular pathology insufficiency or stenosis. If a parallel Doppler beam alignment with the tricuspid regurgitation color jet is possible, the RV systolic pressure can be estimated using the modified Bernoulli equation.

RV systolic pressure = 4 × (tricuspid regurgitation peak velocity jet)2 + central venous pressure

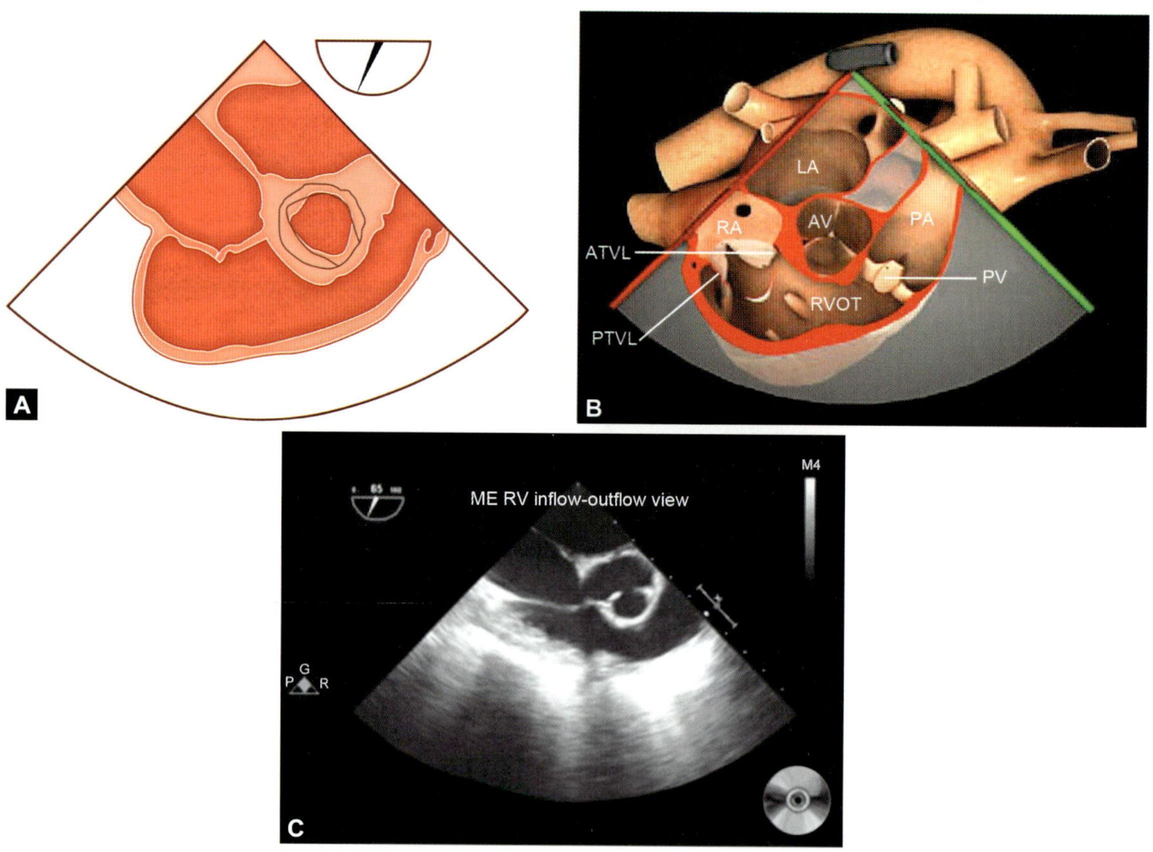

Figures 15A to C (A) Outline of midesophageal right ventricle inflow-outflow view; (B) Simulator of midesophageal right ventricle inflow-outflow view; (C) **(Video 15)** Midesophageal right ventricle inflow-outflow view showing the right ventricle and atrium, left atrium, right atrium tricuspid valve, aortic valve, right ventricle outflow tract, pulmonic valve and main pulmonary artery

LOWER ESOPHAGEAL CORONARY SINUS VIEW

- **Multiplane angle range:**
  - 0–10 degrees
  - *Sector depth:* ~ 12–14 cm
- **Primary diagnostic uses:**
  - Placement of retrograde cardioplegia cannula
- **Clinical utility (Figs 16A to C):**
  - Coronary sinus in LAX
  - TV (septal and posterior leaflets).

Probe Manipulation

These views are obtained during withdrawal of the probe from the proximal gastric level to the low esophageal level and by rotating the imaging plane from 0° to 10°. These views are useful in the evaluation of right heart anatomy, function, and pathology. The function of the right ventricular free wall, as well as the morphology of coronary sinus, atrial septum, tricuspid valve, and right atrial appendage, can be assessed. At 90° the velocity of tricuspid regurgitation can be measured as required for the estimation of right ventricular systolic pressure. The views are also useful for detection of masses (thrombi, vegetations) and for localisation of catheters, cannulas, and electrodes in the right heart.

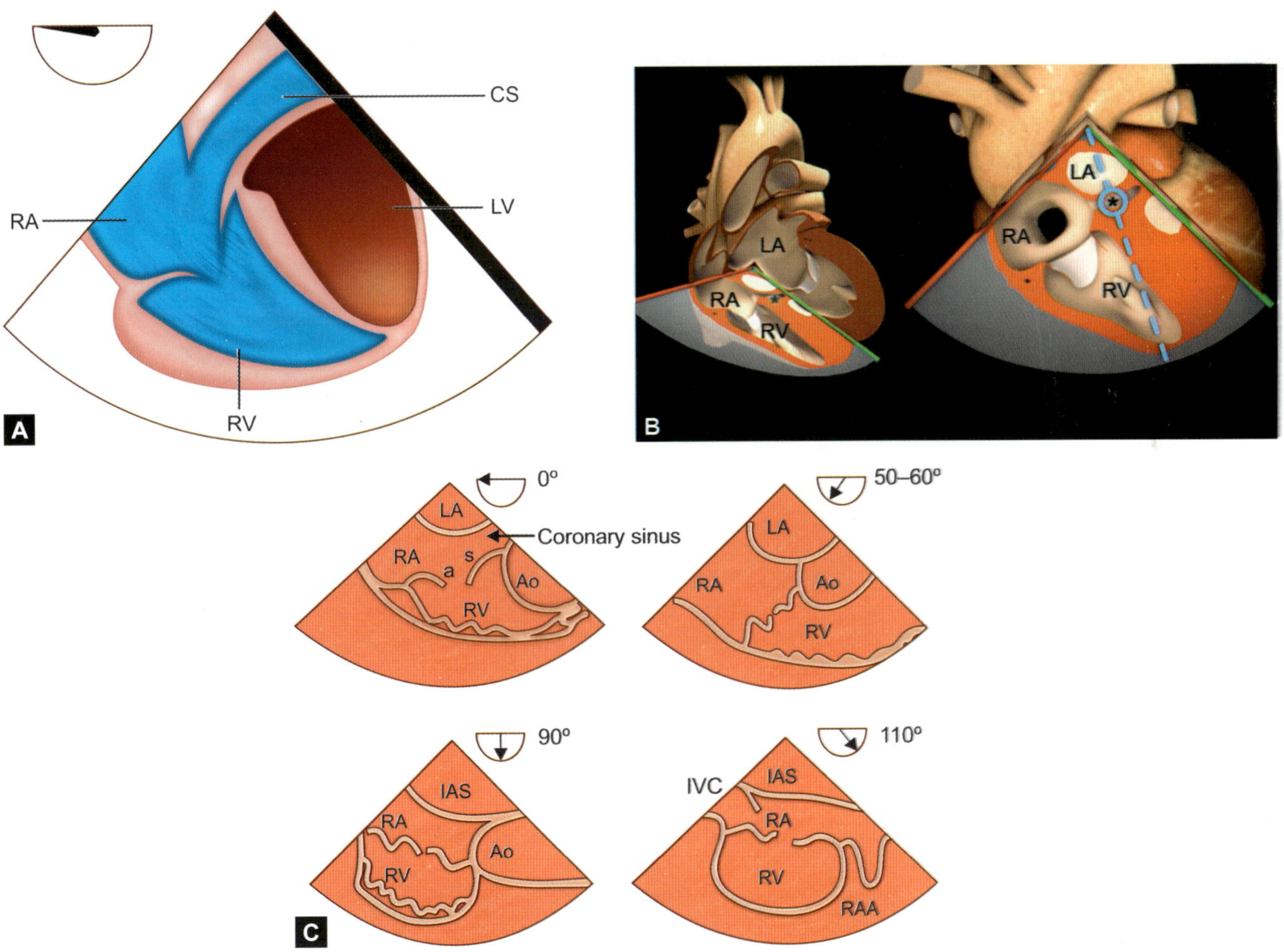

Figures 16A to C (Video 16) (A) Outline of lower esophageal coronary sinus view; (B) Simulator of lower esophageal coronary sinus view; (C) Lower esophageal coronary sinus view

Abbreviations: a = anterior leaflet of the tricuspid valve, Ao = aorta, IAS = atrial septum, IVC = inferior vena cava, LA = left atrium, RA = right atrium, RAA = right atrial appendage, RV = right ventricle, s = septal leaflet of the tricuspid valve

TRANSGASTRIC VIEWS

The deep transgastric left ventricular long-axis **(deep TG LAX)** view resembles the transthoracic apical view and requires maximal anteflexion of the transesophageal echocardiography probe tip. The transgastric two chamber **(TG two chamber)** view allows for evaluation of the basal and middle anterior and inferior wall motion and the mitral valve apparatus, including both papillary muscles in their long axes. The transgastric long-axis **(TG LAX)** view offers good alignment of ultrasound beam and blood flow across the aortic valve, which is a prerequisite for reliable Doppler measurements of aortic flow velocity. Alternatively, aortic blood flow velocity can also be measured in the deep transgastric planes, particularly in the **deep TG right ventricular (RV) view**. Flows in the RV outflow tract, across the pulmonary valve, and in the pulmonary artery can also be measured here using Doppler. The tricuspid valve can be interrogated in the transgastric RV inflow **(TG RV inflow)** view in its long-axis and at approximately 30° in its short-axis **(TG TV SAX) (Fig. 17)**.

PROBE MANIPULATION TO ACHIEVE TRANSGASTRIC VIEWS

By advancing the probe deeper into the gastric fundus and maximizing the anteflexion of its tip with the beam at 0°, a modified transgastric 'apical' or five-chamber view of the heart can be obtained. At the top of the screen both ventricles (usually foreshortened) and at the bottom both atria can be seen. The RV is on the left and the LV is on the right of the screen. With minor adjustment, the view can be modified into a three-chamber view or deep transgastric long-axis view **(deep TG LAX)** with the para-apical region of the LV at the top, the left atrium at the bottom, and the LV outflow tract, aortic valve, and a proximal portion of the ascending aorta in the center (on the left of the left atrium). This view allows excellent alignment of the ultrasound beam with the blood flow out of the LV, which is a prerequisite to any quantitative Doppler measurements in the outflow tract and across the aortic valve. By clockwise rotation of the imaging plane, the right heart structures can be evaluated. The aorta remains in the center of the sector, and on its right the RV~ outflow tract with the pulmonary valve and the proximal main pulmonary artery will appear. The right atrium and tricuspid valve are localized on the left of the aortic cross-section. This view is useful for Doppler measurements of blood flow velocity across the RV outflow tract and the pulmonary valve.

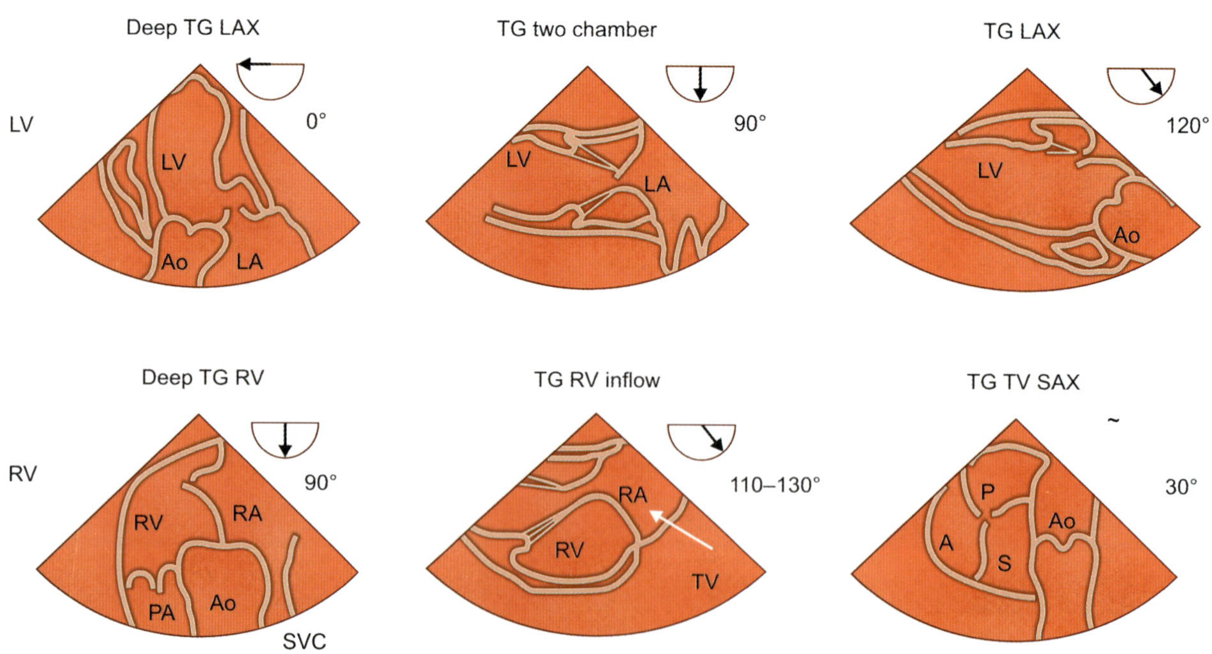

Figure 17 Probe manipulation to achieve transgastric views

TRANSGASTRIC MODIFIED HEPATIC VEIN VIEW

- **Transducer angle:**
  - 0–20 degrees
- **Level:**
  - Lower-esophageal
- **Maneuver (from prior image):**
  - Continuous wave (CW), advance
- **Clinical utility (Figs 18A to D):**
  - Interior vena cava (IVC)
  - Hepatic veins
  - Inferior vena cava (IVC) diameter for right atrium (RA) size.

Probe Manipulation

Three-dimensional heart model shown in cross-section to highlight the position of the TEE plane in the modified transgastric hepatic vein view. Posterior view of the heart and liver. The blue dotted line represents the orientation of the pulsed wave cursor, and the blue circle indicates the position of the sample box in the hepatic vein.

- A normal hepatic vein spectral Doppler trace has four peaks **(Figure 18D)**:
  1. **A wave**—a result of retrograde atrial systolic flow. It is seen below the baseline as blood flow is away from the transducer.
  2. **S wave**—a result of antegrade ventricular systolic flow. It is seen above the baseline as blood flow is towards the transducer.
  3. **V wave**—a result of retrograde end-ventricular systolic flow. It is seen below the baseline as blood flow is away from the transducer.
  4. **D wave**—a result of antegrade ventricular diastolic flow. It is seen above the baseline as blood flow is towards the transducer.

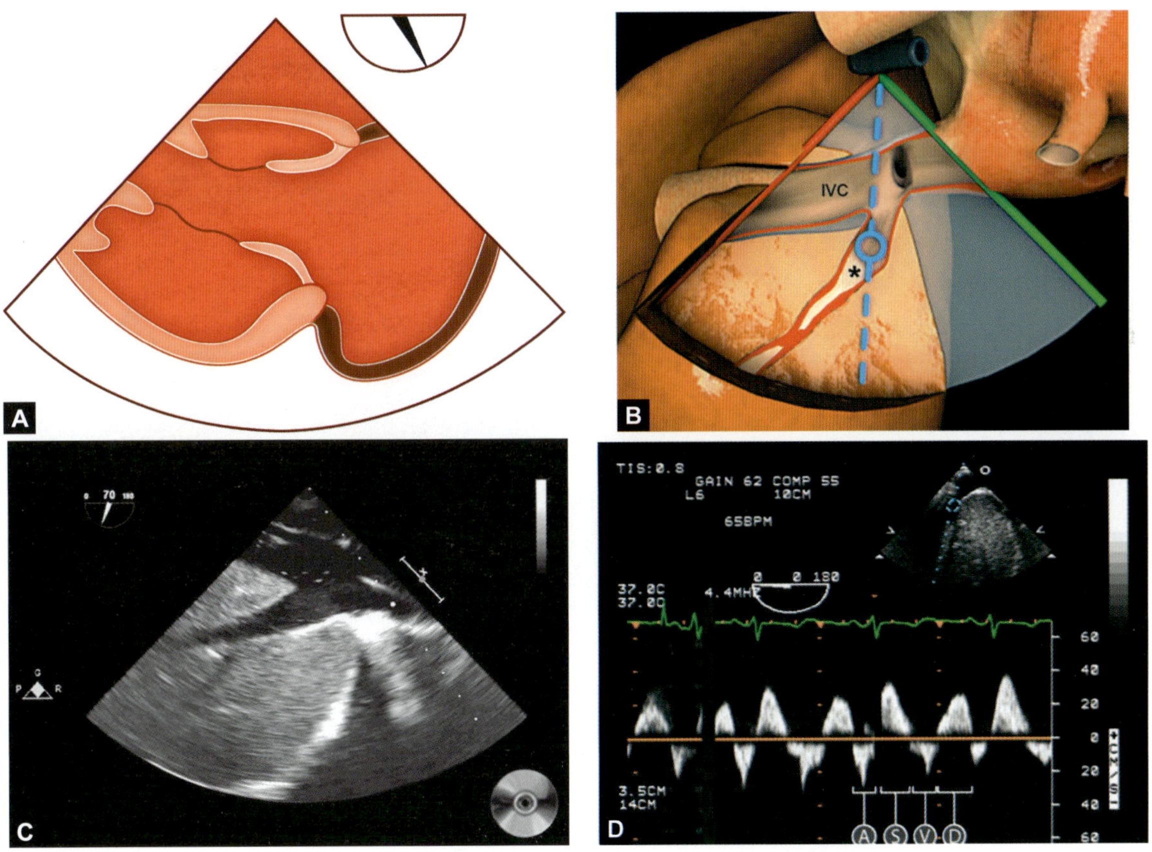

Figures 18A to D (A) Outline of transgastric modified hepatic vein view; (B) Simulator of transgastric modified hepatic vein view; (C) **(Video 17)** Transgastric modified hepatic vein view showing anterior vena cava, hepatic veins and right atrium; (D) Spectral Doppler data acquired for blood flow through the hepatic vein. In the upper right, a two dimensional TEE image of the modified-transgastric hepatic vein view: the blue circle indicates the location of the sample volume within the hepatic vein. In the lower half of the image, a spectral Doppler trace shows the relationship between red blood cell velocity and time. The baseline is orange.

Abbreviations: A = Atrial systolic flow wave, D = Ventricular diastolic flow wave, S = Ventricular systolic flow wave, V = End ventricular systolic flow wave, * = Hepatic vein, IVC = Inferior vena cava

TRANSGASTRIC TWO CHAMBER VIEW

- **Multiplane angle range:**
  - 80–100 degrees
  - *Sector depth:* ~ 12 cm
- **Anatomy imaged:**
  - Left ventricle and atrium
  - *Mitral valve:* Chordae and papillary muscles
  - Coronary sinus
- **Clinical utility (Figs 19A to C):**
  - Left ventricular regional and global function (including apex)
  - *Left ventricular and atrial masses:* Thrombus, embolus, air, tumor, foreign bodies
  - *Mitral valve:* Pathology and pathophysiology.

Starting out from the mid-papillary level and rotating the imaging plane to 90°, the LV transgastric two-chamber view is obtained. This longitudinal cross section shows the inferior wall at the top and the anterior wall at the bottom of the sector, whereas on the right we see the left atrium and the mitral valve and on the left the distal parts of the LV. The true apex can only rarely be imaged because the longitudinal imaging plane tends to run either in front of or behind the apex through the adjacent wall.

Probe Manipulation

- The probe is returned to the TG midpapillary SAX view, and the transducer angle is rotated to approximately 90 to 110 to obtain the TG two-chamber view.
- The anterior and inferior walls of the left ventricle are imaged in addition to the papillary muscles, chordae, and MV.
- Although the left atrium and LA appendage are often seen, far-field imaging may not allow accurate assessment of LA appendage pathology.

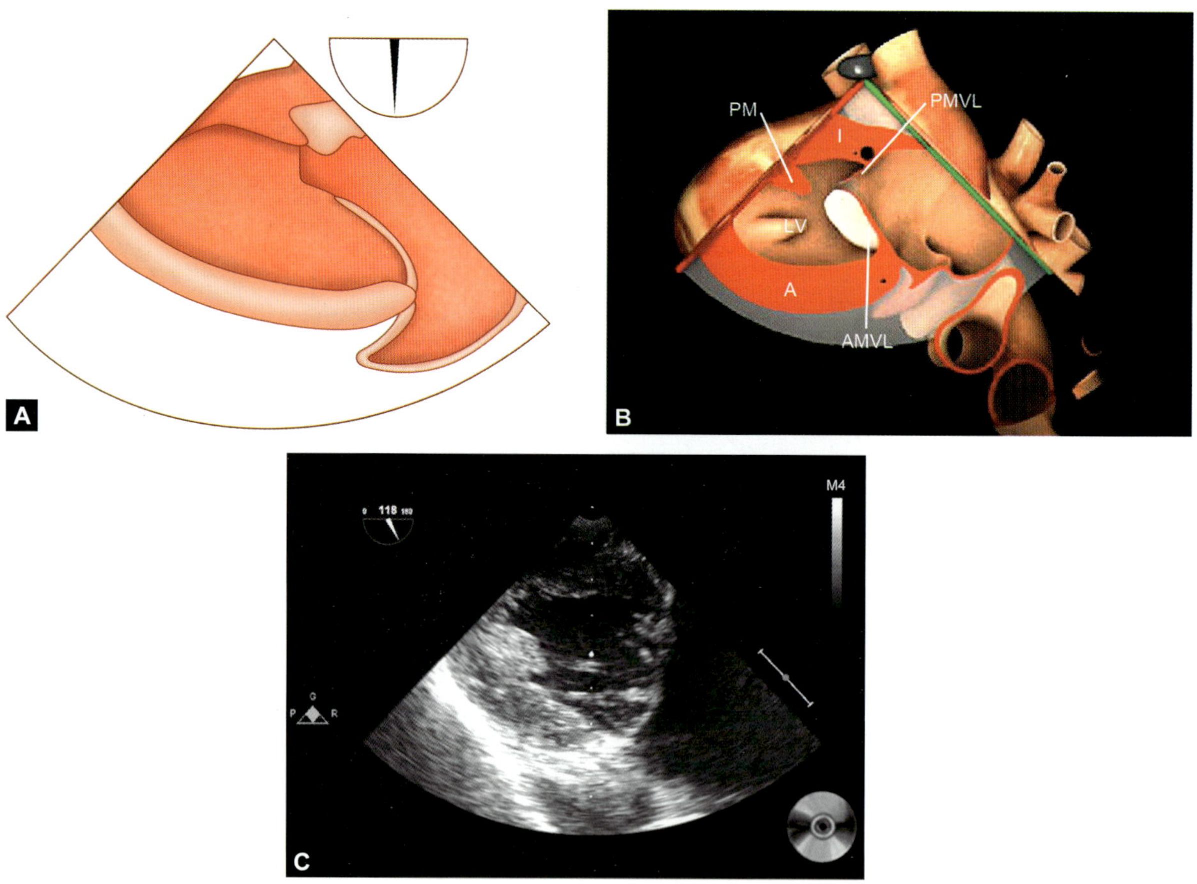

Figures 19A to C (A) Outline of transgastric two chamber view; (B) Simulator of transgastric two chamber view; (C) **(Video 18)** Transgastric two chamber view showing left ventricle and atrium coronary sinus and mitral valve

TRANSGASTRIC APICAL SHORT-AXIS VIEW[1]

- **Transducer angle:**
  - 0–20 degrees
  - Transgastric
- **Anatomy imaged:**
  - Left ventricle (apex)
  - Right ventricle (apex)
- **Clinical utility (Figs 20A to C):**
  - From the TG midpapillary short-axis (SAX) view (0–20), the probe is advanced while maintaining contact with the gastric wall, to obtain the TG apical short-axis (SAX) view
  - The right ventricle (RV) apex is imaged from this view by turning to the right (clockwise). This view allows evaluation of the apical segments of the left and right ventricles.

Probe Manipulation

The 17-segment model for regional LV assessment and coronary arterial distribution.

From base to the apex, the LV is divided into basal, mid and apical thirds corresponding to the proximal, middle and apical segments of the coronary arteries. The scheme divides the ventricle into 17 segments, six segments both in the basal and mid portions (anteroseptal, inferoseptal, anterior, anterolateral, inferolateral and inferior walls) and five at the apex (septal, anterior, lateral, inferior and apical). As these segments can be recorded from three SAX and several longitudinal views, it is possible (and useful) to evaluate a segment from more than one view **(Fig. 20C)**.

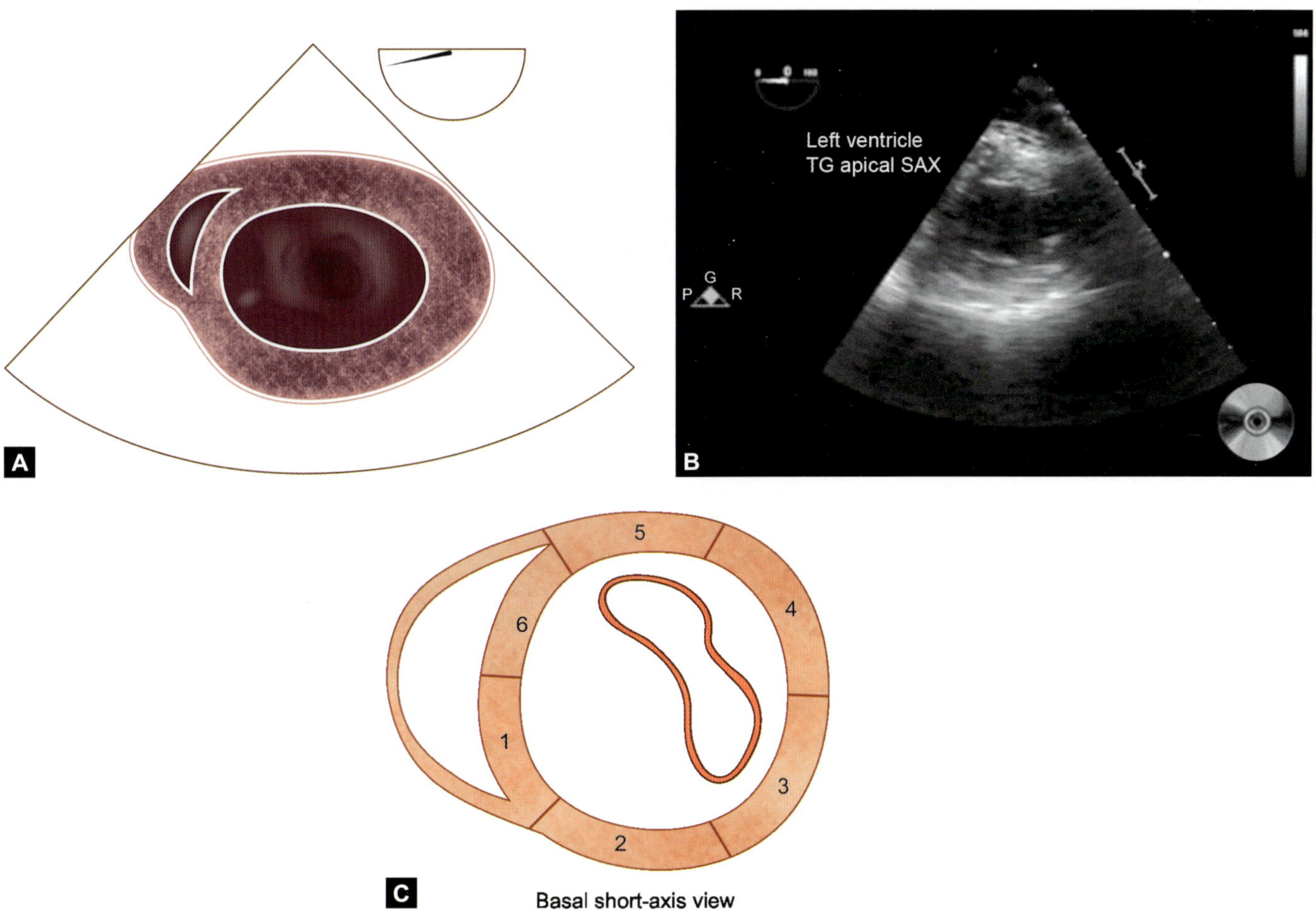

Figures 20A to C (A) Outline of transgastric apical SAX view; (B) **(Video 19)** Transgastric apical short-axis view showing left and right ventricle; (C) For viewing the apical 17th segment on TEE

TRANSGASTRIC BASAL LONG-AXIS VIEW[2]

- **Multiplane angle range:**
  - 110–130 degrees
  - *Sector depth:* ~12 cm
- **Probe adjustments:**
  - Neutral leftward
- **Anatomy imaged:**
  - Mitral leaflets
  - Mitral subvalvular apparatus
  - Left ventricle (anteroseptal and inferolateral walls: basal and mid segments)
  - LV outflow tract
  - Aortic valve and proximal ascending aorta
- **Clinical utility (Figs 21A and B):**
  - Left ventricular (LV) systolic dysfunction (anteroseptal and inferolateral walls)
  - Doppler interrogation of aortic valve.

Probe Manipulation

From the TG RV inflow view, turning to the left (counterclockwise) to return to the TG two-chamber view, then rotating the transducer angle to 110 to 130 degrees will result in the TG Basal LAX view. Sometimes, turning the probe slightly to the right is necessary to bring the LV outflow tract and AV into view.

Like the deep TG view, it allows for parallel alignment of the ultrasound beam with trans aortic flow, making it an excellent choice for spectral Doppler interrogation of the AV. In addition, ME views of the AV may be obscured by echo shadowing in patients with significant mitral annular calcification or in patients with prosthetic mitral valves and mitral annuloplasty rings. In these scenarios, both deep TG and TG LAX views often allow imaging of the AV without overlying shadowing.

Portions of the inferolateral wall and anterior septum are imaged, as well as the LV outflow tract, AV, and proximal aorta. With parallel Doppler beam alignment of the LV outflow tract, AV, and proximal aortic root, spectral and color Doppler interrogation of the LV outflow tract and AV is possible.

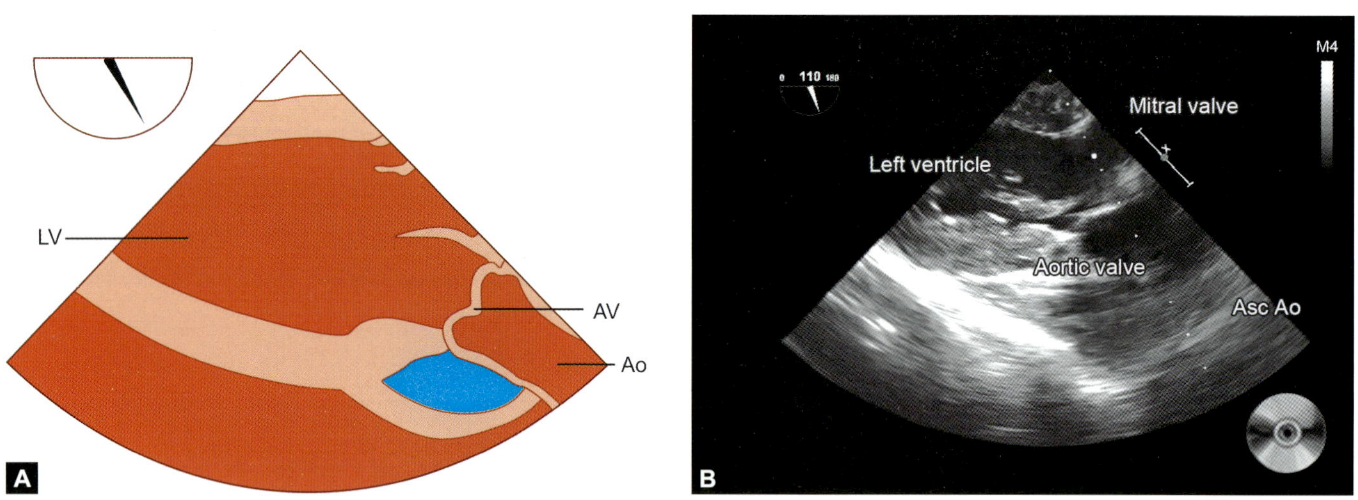

Figures 21A and B (A) Outline of TG LAX; (B) **(Video 20)** Transgastric basal long-axis view showing mitral leaflets, mitral subvalvular apparatus, left ventricle (anteroseptal and inferolateral walls: basal and mid segments), LV outflow tract, aortic valve and proximal ascending aorta

TRANSGASTRIC BASAL SHORT-AXIS VIEW

- **Multiplane angle range:**
  - 0–20 degrees
  - *Sector depth:* ~ 12 cm
- **Anatomy imaged left and right ventricle:**
  - Mitral valve
  - Tricuspid valve
- **Clinical utility (Figs 22A to C):**
  - *Mitral valve evaluation ("fish-mouth view"):* Pathology, pathophysiology
  - *Tricuspid valve evaluation:* Pathology, pathophysiology
  - Basal left ventricular regional function
  - Basal right ventricular regional function.

Probe Manipulation

- Toward the base of the ventricle the high papillary muscle view, with papillary muscles separated from the wall and circular in cross-section, can be obtained.
- A little more cranially, the chordae tendineae appear instead of the papillary muscles in the ventricular cavity (chordal view), only to be replaced shortly after by the mitral valve leaflets in this basal or mitral valve short-axis view **(TG basal SAX)**.
- The posterior leaflet is seen at the top right and the anterior leaflet at the bottom left of the sector. The anterolateral commissure is situated at about the 5 o'clock position, and the posteromedial commissure at about the 10 o'clock position of the sector.

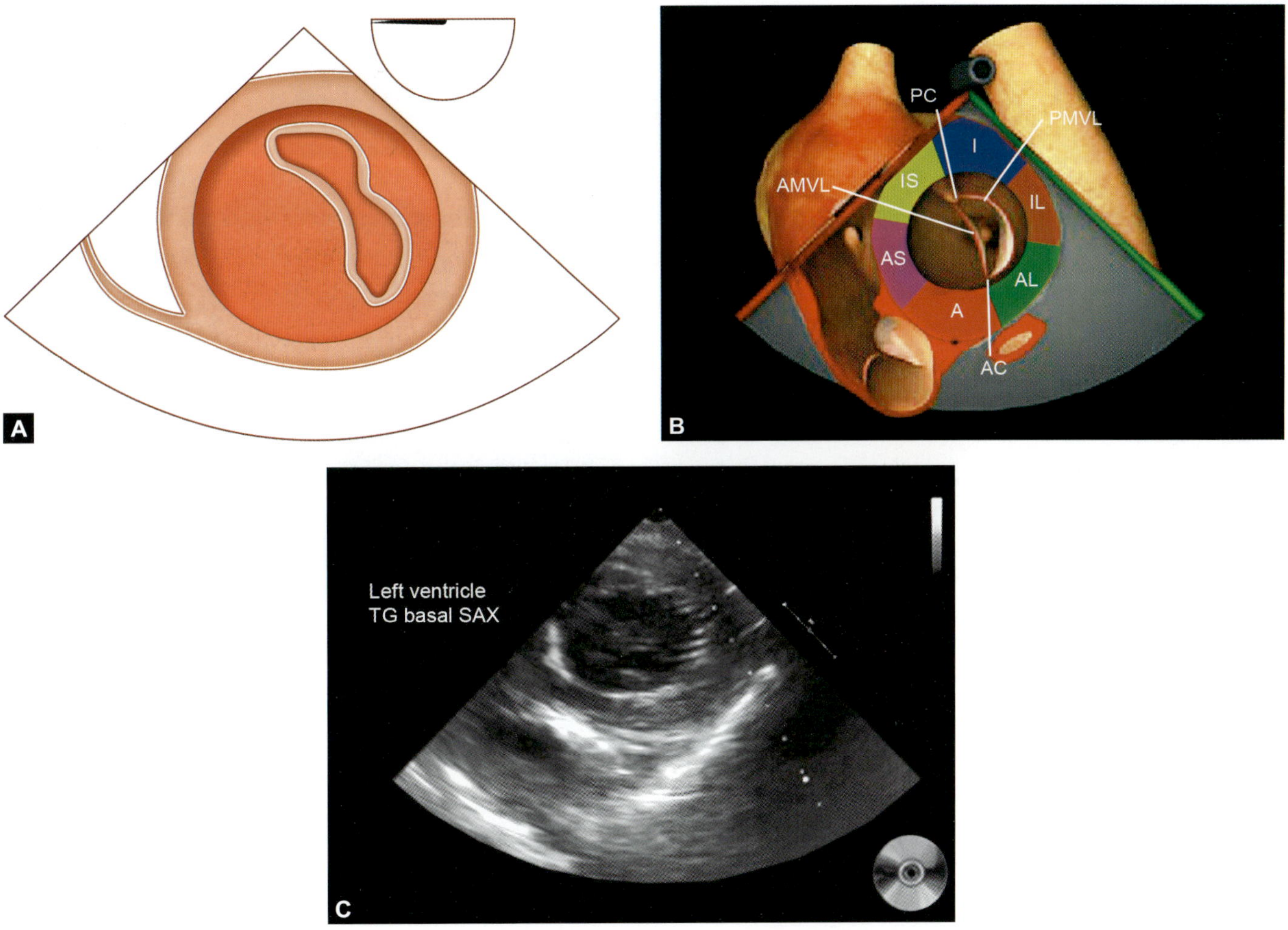

Figures 22A to C (A) Outline of TG basal SAX; (B) Simulator of TG basal SAX; (C) **(Video 21)** Transgastric basal short-axis view showing mitral and tricuspid valve

TRANSGASTRIC MID-PAPILLARY SHORT-AXIS VIEW

- **Multiplane angle range:**
  - 0–20 degrees
  - *Sector depth:* ~ 12 cm
- **Anatomy imaged:**
  - Left and right ventricles
  - Papillary muscles
- **Clinical utility (Figs 23A to C):**
  - Mid-left and right ventricular regional and global function
  - Intracardiac volume status.

Probe Manipulation

- While maintaining contact with the gastric wall, the anteflexed probe for the TG basal SAX view can be relaxed to a more neutral position, or the probe may be advanced further into the stomach to obtain the TG midpapillary SAX view.
- Proper positioning may require multiple probe manipulations using varying probe depths and degrees of anteflexion.
- The transducer angle should typically remain at 0 to 20. The TG mid papillary SAX view provides significant diagnostic information and can be extremely helpful in assessing LV size and volume status and global and regional function.
- This is the primary TG view for intraoperative monitoring of LV size and function because myocardium supplied by the left anterior descending, circumflex, and right coronary arteries can be seen simultaneously. Turning the probe to the right from this view will typically image the mid-RV in SAX.

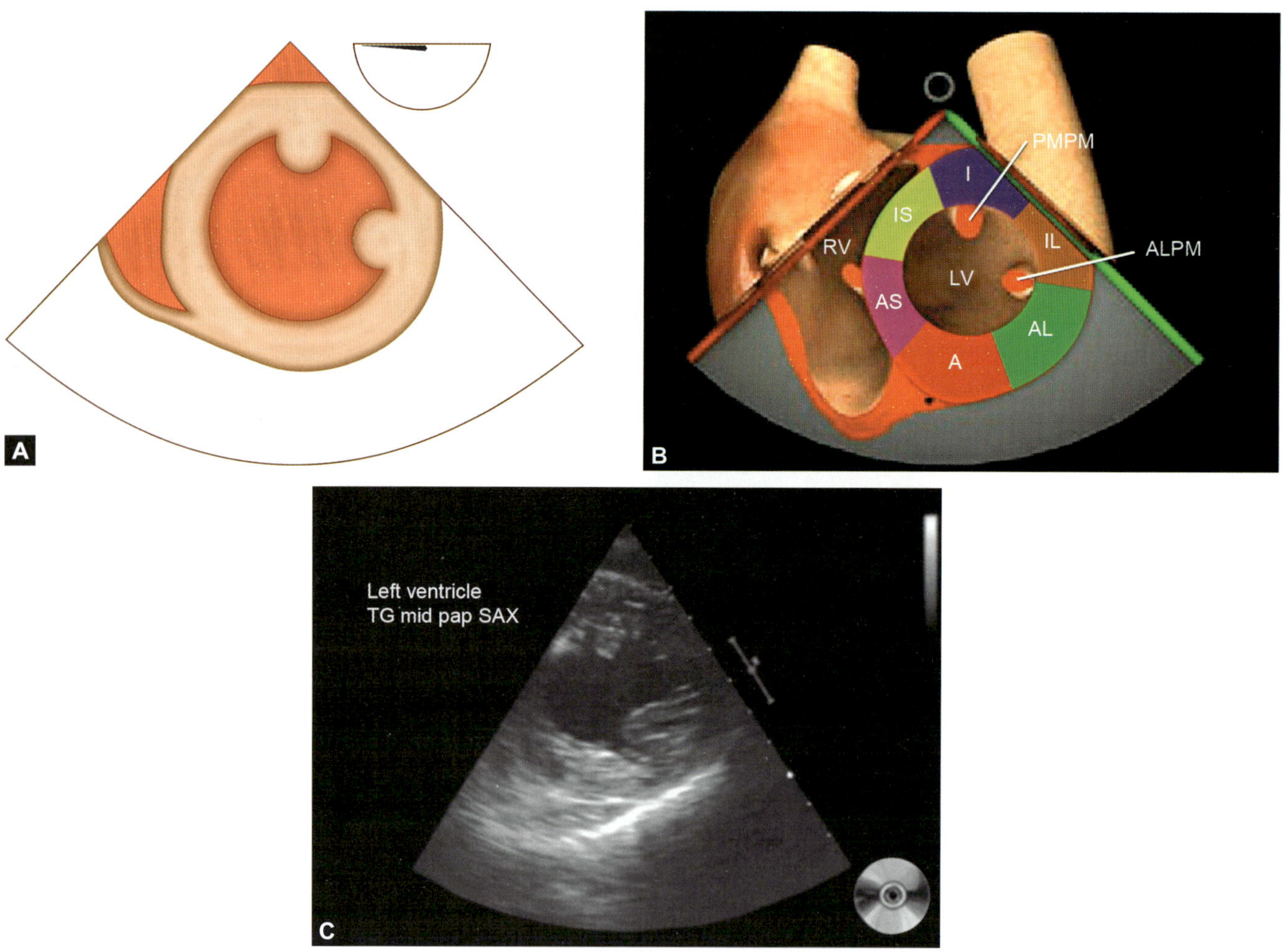

Figures 23A to C (A) Outline of TG mid SAX; (B) Simulator of TG mid SAX; (C) **(Video 22)** Transgastric mid-papillary short-axis view showing left and right ventricles and papillary muscles

TRANSGASTRIC RIGHT VENTRICLE INFLOW-OUTFLOW VIEW

- **Transducer angle:**
  - 0–20 degrees
- **Level:**
  - Transgastric
- **Maneuver (from prior image):**
  - Right-flex
- **Clinical utility (Figs 24A to C):**
  - Right atrium
  - Right ventricle
  - Right ventricular outflow tract
  - Pulmonary valve
  - Tricuspid valve.

Probe Manipulation

- From the ME AV SAX view, slight advancement of the probe and rotating the transducer angle to 50 to 70 until the RVOT and PV appear in the display results in the ME RV inflow-outflow view.
- From this view, one can evaluate RV size and function (with RVOT diameter), TV morphology and function, and PV morphology and function. Color flow Doppler as well as spectral Doppler of both valves should be performed.

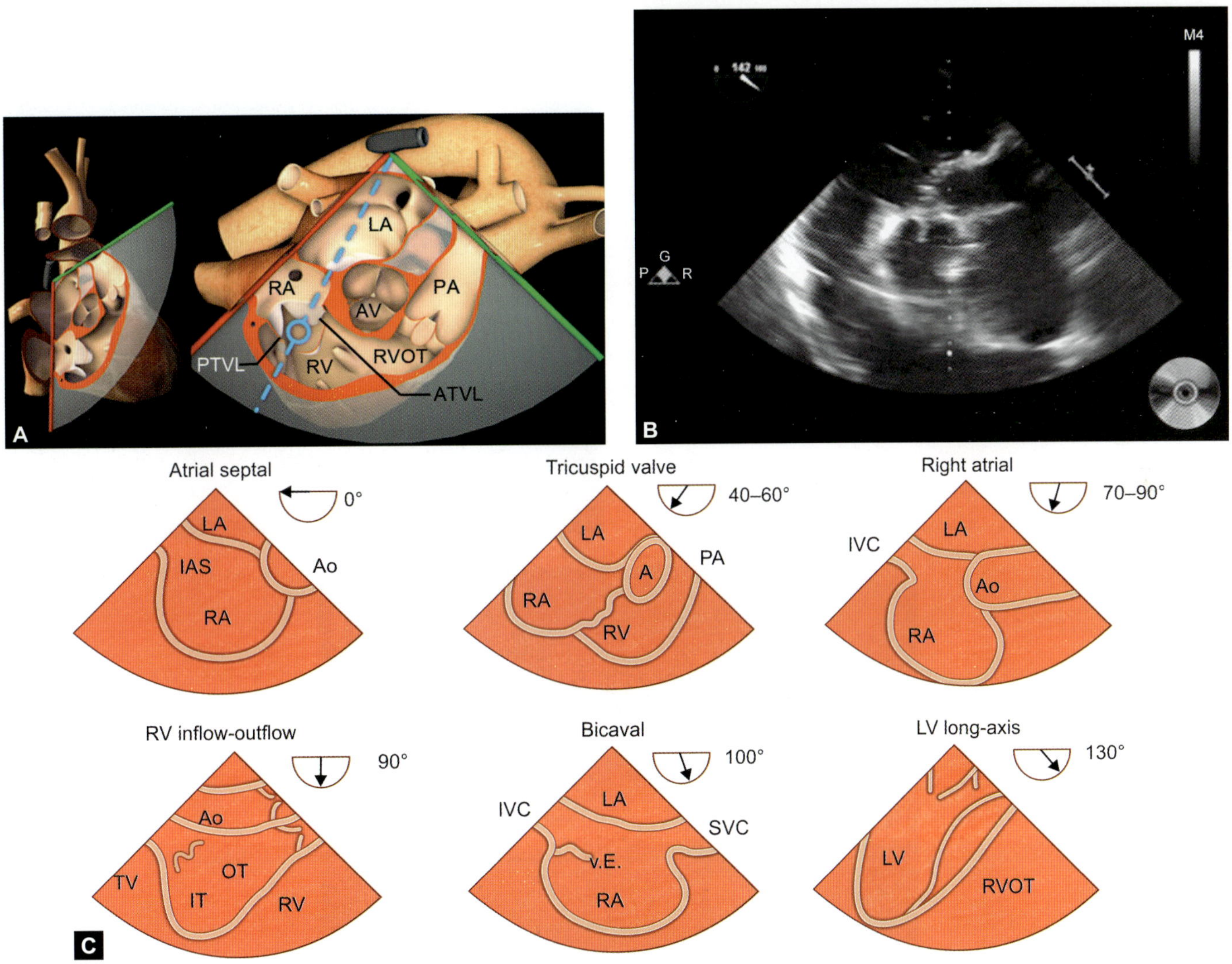

Figures 24A to C (A) Simulator of atrial septal; (B) **(Video 23)** Transgastric right ventricle inflow-outflow view showing right atrium, PV and TV, RV; (C) Lower and midesophageal views: In addition to the gastro-esophageal junction views, important right heart structures can also be interrogated at this level.

Abbreviation: Ao = aorta, IAS = atrial septum, IT = inflow tract, IVC = inferior vena cava, LA = left atrium, LV = left ventricle, OT = outflow tract, PA = pulmonary artery, RA = right atrium, RV = right ventricle, RVOT = right ventricular outflow tract, SVC = superior vena cava, TV = tricuspid valve, vE = valvula eustachi

TRANSGASTRIC RIGHT VENTRICLE INFLOW VIEW

- **Multiplane angle range:**
  - 100–120 degrees
  - *Sector depth:* ~ 12 cm
- **Anatomy imaged:**
  - Right ventricle and atrium
  - *Tricuspid valve:* Chordae and papillary muscles
- **Clinical utility (Figs 25A to C):**
  - Right ventricular regional and global function
  - *Right ventricular and atrium masses:* Thrombus, embolus, tumor, foreign bodies
  - *Tricuspid valve:* Pathology and pathophysiology.

Probe Manipulation

- Probe tip depth deep transgastric (45–50 cm)
  - From the TG two-chamber view (transducer angle of 90–110 degrees), turning to the right (clockwise) will result in the TG RV inflow (or RV two-chamber) view.
  - The anterior and inferior walls of the right ventricle are imaged in addition to the papillary muscles, chordae, and TV. The proximal RVOT is also frequently seen and slight advancement of the probe may allow imaging and Doppler interrogation of the PV.

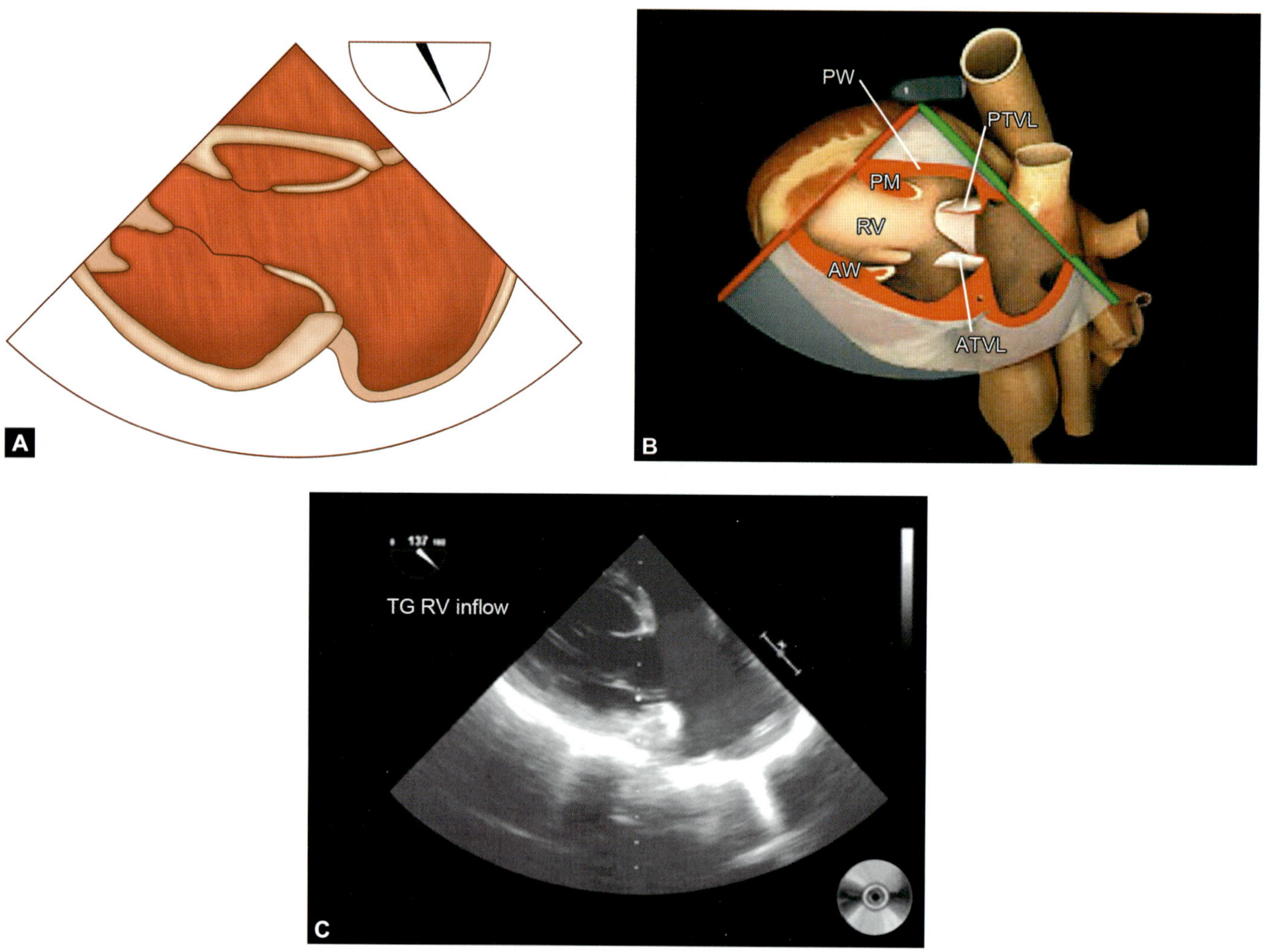

Figures 25A to C (A) Outline of TG RV inflow; (B) Simulator of TG RV inflow; (C) **(Video 24)** Transgastric right ventricle inflow view showing right ventricle and atrium, tricuspid valve: Chordae and papillary muscles

TRANSGASTRIC BASAL RIGHT VENTRICLE OUTFLOW VIEW[1]

- **Transducer angle:**
  - 0–20 degrees
- **Level:**
  - Transgastric
- **Maneuver (from prior image):**
  - Anteflex
- **Clinical utility (Figs 26A to C):**
  - Left ventricle (mid)
  - Right ventricle (mid)
  - Right ventricular outflow tract
  - Tricuspid valve (SAX)
  - Pulmonary valve.

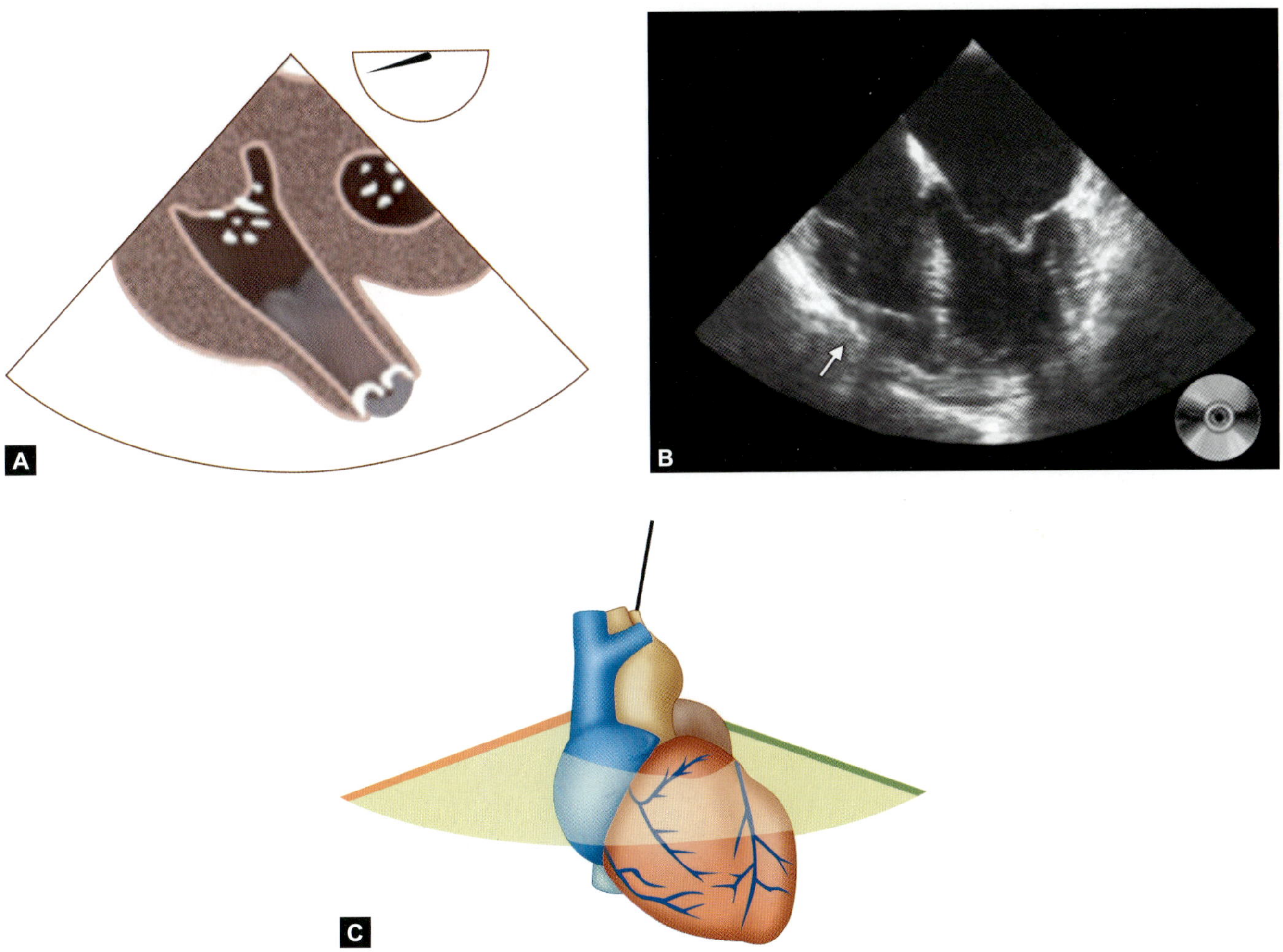

Figures 26A to C (A) Outline of transgastric basal right ventricle outflow view; (B) **(Video 25)** Transgastric basal right ventricle outflow view showing LV, RV, TV and PV; (C) Simulator view of transgastric basal right ventricle outflow view

DEEP TRANSGASTRIC LONG-AXIS VIEW

- **Multiplane angle range:**
  - 0–20 degrees (anteflexion)
  - *Sector depth:* ~16 cm
- **Anatomy imaged:**
  - Left ventricle and outflow tract
  - Interventricular septum
  - Aortic valve and ascending aorta
  - Left atrium
  - Mitral valve
  - Right ventricle
  - Pulmonic valve
- **Clinical utility (Figs 27A to D):**
  - Aortic valve and subaortic pathology and pathophysiology
  - Mitral valve pathology and pathophysiology
  - Left and right ventricle global function
  - *Left and right ventricle masses:* Thrombus, embolus, tumor
  - Foreign bodies
  - Congenital or acquired interventricular septal defect evaluation.

Probe Manipulation

The deep transgastric (TG) LAX view of the AV is obtained by insertion and anteflexion of the probe from the TG SAX imaging plane and can be difficult to attain without significant flexion of the probe in the stomach. However, the TG view can often align the transvalvular flow parallel to the ultrasound beam, rendering TEE reliable in detecting and quantifying transvalvular blood flow velocities. It is the preferred view for spectral Doppler measurements of flow velocities to generate estimates of AV gradients and spectral displays of regurgitant jets.

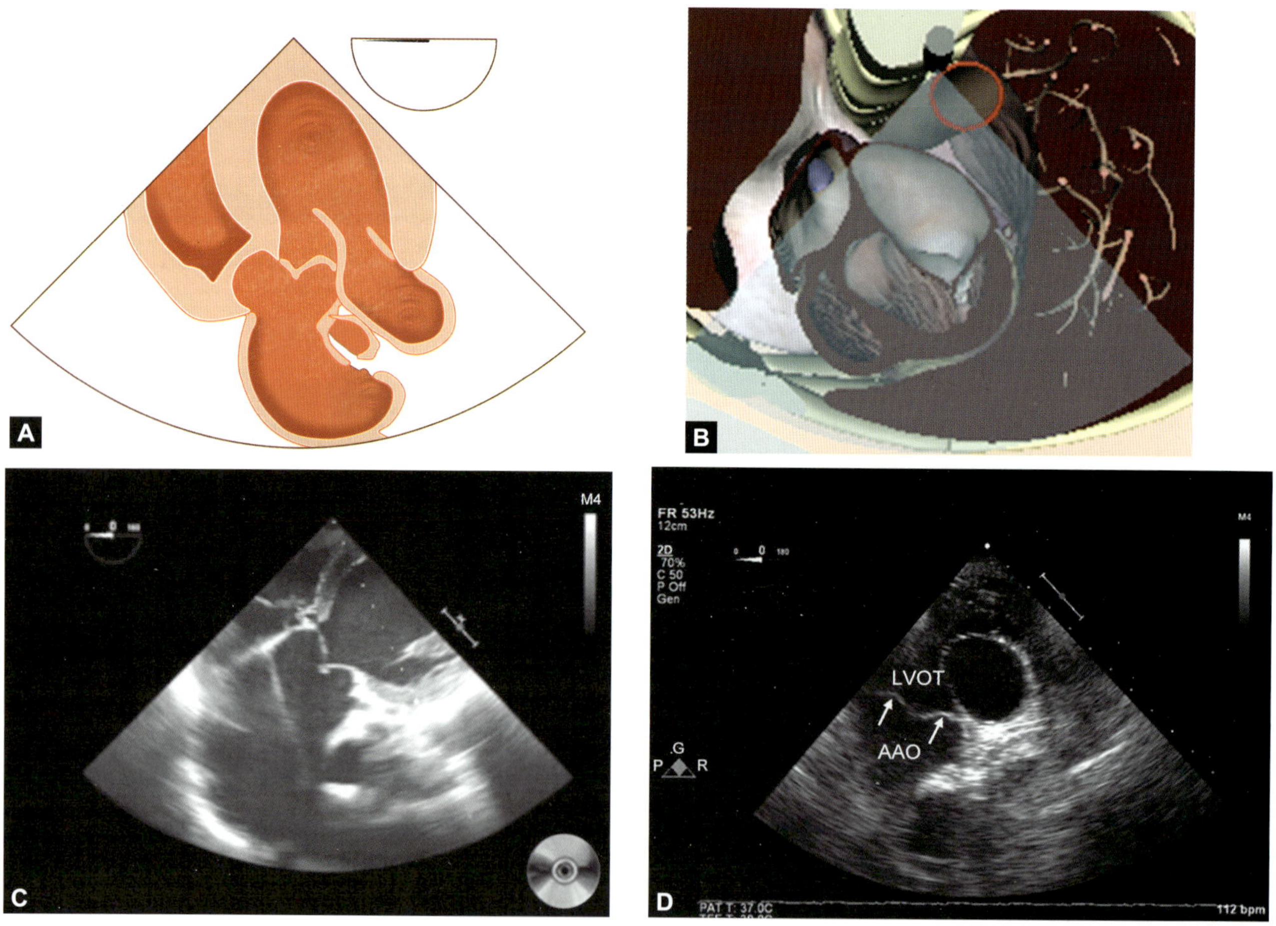

Figures 27A to D (A) Outline of deep TG LAX; (B) Simulator of deep TG LAX; (C) **(Video 26)** Deep transgastric long-axis view showing left ventricle and outflow tract, interventricular septum, aortic valve and ascending aorta, left atrium, mitral valve, right ventricle, pulmonic valve; (D) Deep transgastric long-axis view in diastole showing the LVOT and aortic valve. Excellent to measure the gradients across the aortic valve

UPPER ESOPHAGEAL AORTIC ARCH LONG-AXIS VIEW

- **Transducer angle:**
  - 0–10 degrees
- **Level:**
  - Upper esophageal
- **Maneuver (from prior image):**
  - Withdrawal
- **Clinical utility (Figs 28A to C):**
  - Aortic arch
  - Innominate vein
  - Mediastinal tissue.

Probe Manipulation

- While evaluating the descending aorta SAX view (transducer angle 0–10) and withdrawing the probe, the aorta will eventually become elongated, and the left subclavian artery may be imaged, indicating the beginning of the distal aortic arch.
- At this location, the aorta is positioned anterior to the esophagus, and thus the UE aortic arch LAX view is best imaged by then turning to the right (clockwise) so the probe faces anterior.
- This allows imaging of the mid aortic arch.
- In addition to the aorta, the left innominate vein is frequently imaged with venous flow by color flow Doppler. Because the left main stem bronchus typically crosses between the esophagus and the aorta, a portion of the proximal aortic arch and distal ascending aorta may not be visualized.

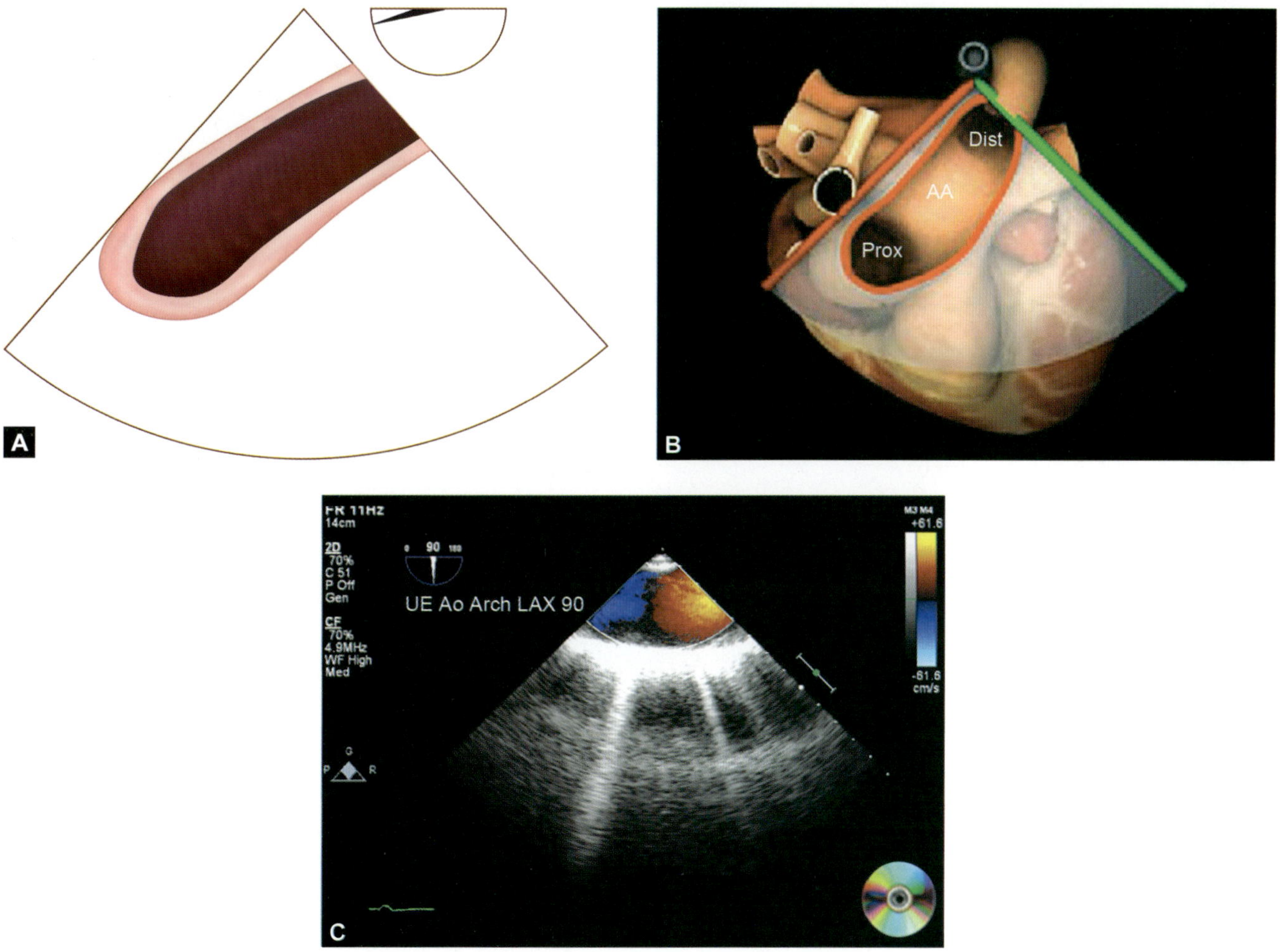

Figures 28A to C (A) Outline of upper esophageal aortic arch long-axis view; (B) Simulator view of upper esophageal aortic arch long-axis view; (C) **(Video 27)** Upper esophageal aortic arch long-axis view showing aortic arch, innominate vein and mediastinal tissue

UPPER ESOPHAGEAL AORTIC ARCH SHORT-AXIS VIEW

- **Multiplane angle range:**
  - 90 degrees
  - *Sector depth:* ~ 10 cm
- **Structures imaged:**
  - Aortic arch, left brachiocephalic vein; left subclavian and carotid arteries; right brachiocephalic artery, main pulmonary artery and pulmonic valve
- **Clinical utility (Figs 29 A to C):**
  - *Ascending aorta and arch pathology:* Atherosclerosis, aneurysms and dissections, pulmonary embolus, pulmonary valve evaluation (insufficiency, stenosis, Ross procedure); pulmonary artery catheter placement.

Probe Manipulation

- From the UE aortic arch LAX view, the transducer angle is rotated toward 70 to 90 to obtain the UE aortic arch SAX view.
- The main PA and PV can frequently be seen in LAX in the far field but may require adjustment of imaging depth, probe frequency and focal zone.
- Because of parallel Doppler beam alignment of the PV and main PA, spectral and color Doppler interrogation of the PV may be performed.
- Because of the curvature of the aorta, between the LAX and SAX view of the aortic arch, the right brachiocephalic and left common carotid arteries may be seen arising from the aorta, typically in the near field and to the right of the screen.

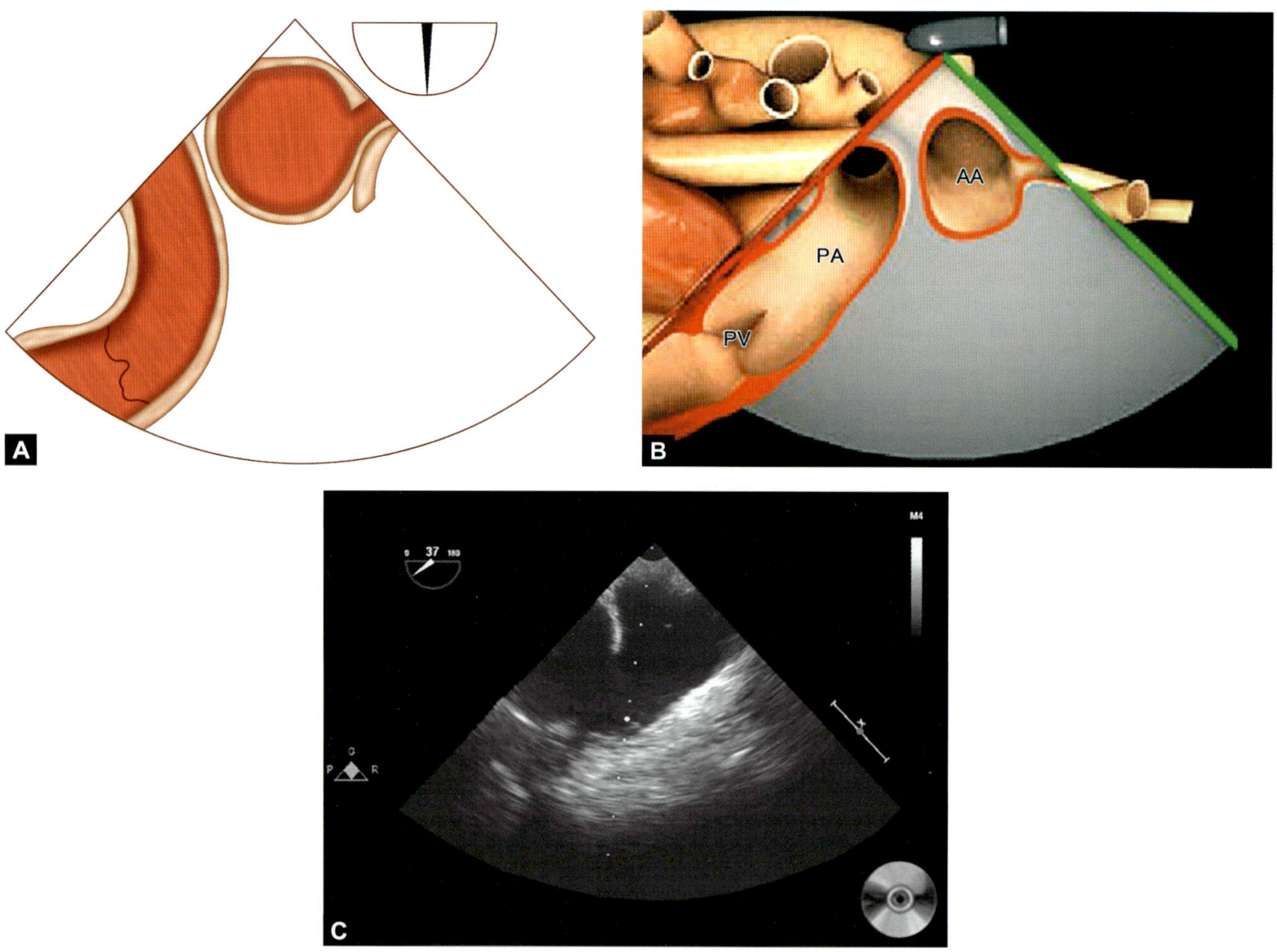

Figures 29A to C (A) Outline of upper esophageal aortic arch short-axis view; (B) Simulator view of upper esophageal aortic arch short-axis view; (C) **(Video 28)** Upper esophageal aortic arch short-axis view showing aortic arch, left brachiocephalic vein, pulmonary artery and pulmonic valve

CONCLUSION

Echocardiographic examination with congenital heart disease is a difficult task; the anatomy is grossly abnormal and the long lasting hemodynamic constraints have resulted in significant remodeling of the cardiac chambers. All possible planes and angles must be used in order to visualize properly the different structures. TEE provides important information on different views to visualize different valves, aorta and structures.

REFERENCES

1. Hahn RJ, Abraham T, Adams MS, et al. Guidelines for Performing a Comprehensive Transesophageal Echocardiographic Examination: Recommendations from the American Society of Echocardiography and the Society of Cardiovascular Anaesthesiologist. J Am Soc Echocardiogr. 2013;26:921-64.
2. Muralidhar K, Tempe D, Chakravarthy M, Shastry N, Kapoor PM, Tewari P, et al. Practical guidelines for perioperative transesophageal echocardiography. Recommendations of the Indian Association of Cardiovascular Thoracic Anaesthesiologists. Card Anaes. 2013;16(4):268-8.

Chapter 4

TEE for Atrial Septal Defect

Poonam Malhotra Kapoor, Vishwas Malik, Milind Hote, V Devagourou, Arun Subramaniam

Chapter Outline

DEFINITION

Atrial septal defect (ASD) is a communication between the left and right atrium due to a deficient interatrial septum. An ASD occurs when part of the atrial septum does not form properly **(Figs 1A and B).**

PATHOPHYSIOLOGY (FIG. 2A)

This allows blood to flow across the opening from the left atrium to the right atrium causing an increased volume of blood to be delivered to the right side of the heart, and subsequently to the lungs. Because it is receiving so much extra blood, the right side of the heart does more than its normal share of work. Over time, this extra blood volume can lead to enlargement of the right atrium and the right ventricle, decreased function of the right ventricle (due to volume overload), high pressures in the lungs (due to excess blood flow), and abnormalities of heart rhythm (due to the stretching and enlargement of the right atrium).

- *Pulmonary valve closes late:* P_2 delayed
- *RV fully loaded, so no increase in volume during inspiration:* Wide-fixed split.
- P_2 accentuated
- Lung fields plethoric due to increase in blood.

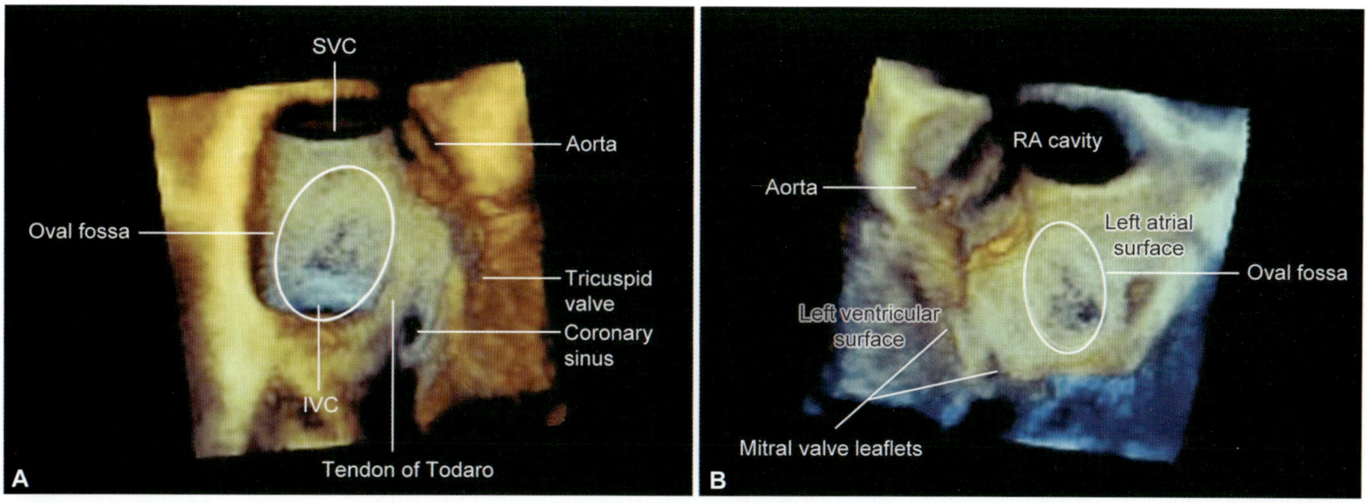

Figures 1A and B Normal atrial septum—3D transesophageal echocardiography views: (A) The normal atrial septum as viewed from the right atrium. The surrounding structures that define the margins of the defect are outlined; (B) The normal atrial septum as viewed from the left atrium on 3D TEE

DIFFERENT TYPES OF ARTERIAL SEPTAL DISEASE (FIGS 2A AND B)

There are four types of atrial septal defects, although some cardiologists also classify common atrium or single atrium as an additional type.

Ostium Secundum (Figs 3 and 4)

- Most common is ostium secundum (60%) located at fossa ovalis
- High association with prolapse of mitral valve.

The **Figure 3** shows the images of a centrally situated secundum ASD. This ASD has:

- Good surrounding margins
- Ideal to understand the nomenclature of the margins of fossa ovalis ASD
- ASD are designated according to the structures in their vicinity
- The margin between the defect and SVC is called the SVC margin
- The margin between the defect and IVC is called the IVC margin
- The margin at the crux is called the atrioventricular (AV) septal margin
- The margin between defect and the ascending aorta is called the aortic margin
- The margin between the defect and the superior wall of atrium near the right upper pulmonary vein is called the atrial margin.

The location of these margins of the ASD has been illustrated in **Figures 3A to D**.

Ostium Primum (Table 1 and Flow chart 1)

- Ostium primum type usually part of endocardial cushion defect
- Frequently associated with cleft mitral and tricuspid valves
- Tends to act like VSD physiologically.

Sinus venosus: It is of two types as follows:

1. *SVC type:* In the SVC type of sinus venosus ASD, there is associated partial anomalous pulmonary venous connection (PAPVC) of the right upper pulmonary veins. In these cases, a TEE is performed to verify that:
   - The ASD patch is intact and there is no turbulence to the SVC flow which should be confirmed by pressure measurements in the SVC and RA.
   - Pulmonary veins are re-routed to the LA, which should be confirmed with a pulsed wave Doppler of the pulmonary venous flow showing characteristic S and D waves.
2. *IVC type:* In the IVC type of sinus venosus ASD, there is associated PAPVC of the right lower pulmonary veins. A TEE is performed to assess the following:
   - The ASD patch is intact and the IVC is draining into the RA.
   - Pulmonary veins are re-routed to the LA and confirmed with a pulsed wave Doppler.

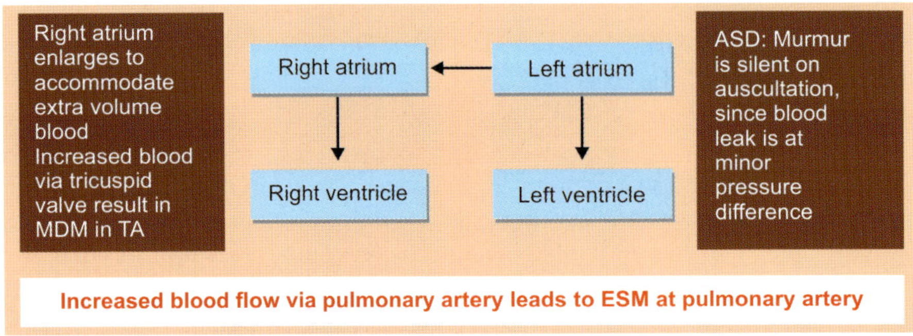

Figure 2A Pathophysiology of atrial septal defect

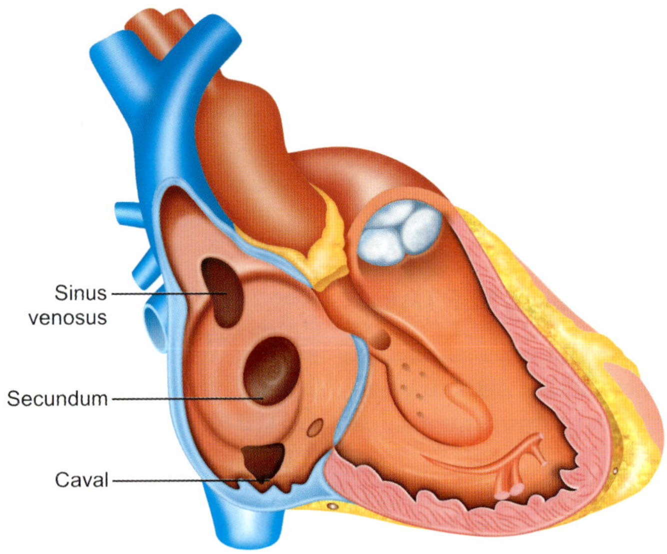

Figure 2B Position of different types of ASD

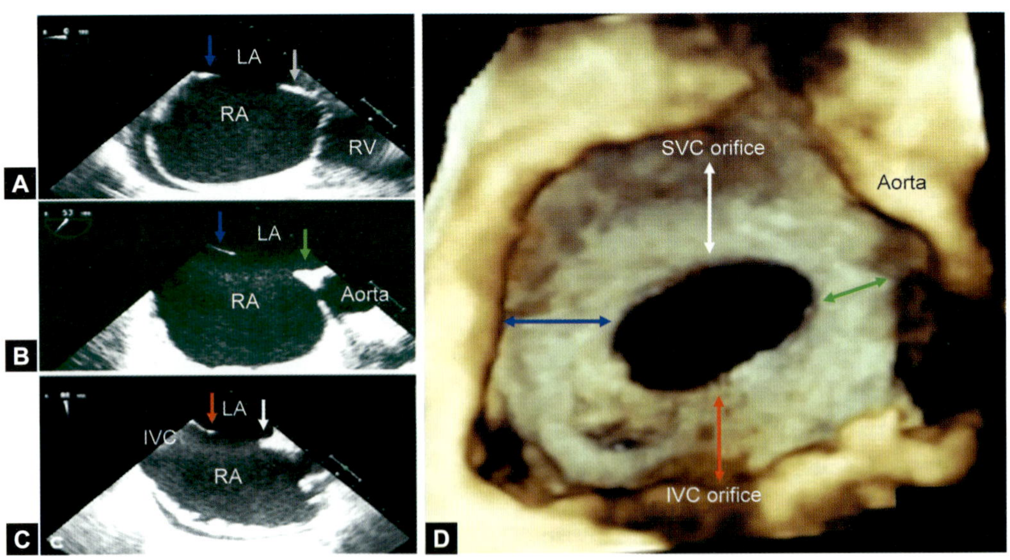

Figures 3A to D (A to C) 2D TEE images of a centrally situated secundum type ASD: (A) Four chamber view and shows AV septal margin (gray arrow) and atrial margin (blue arrow); (B) Basal short axis view and shows the retroaortic margin (green arrow); (C) Basal long axis (bicaval view) and shows the SVC margin (white arrow) and IVC margin (red arrow); (D) Three dimensional en-face view of interatrial septum from RA perspective and shows all the margins of the ASD in a single image

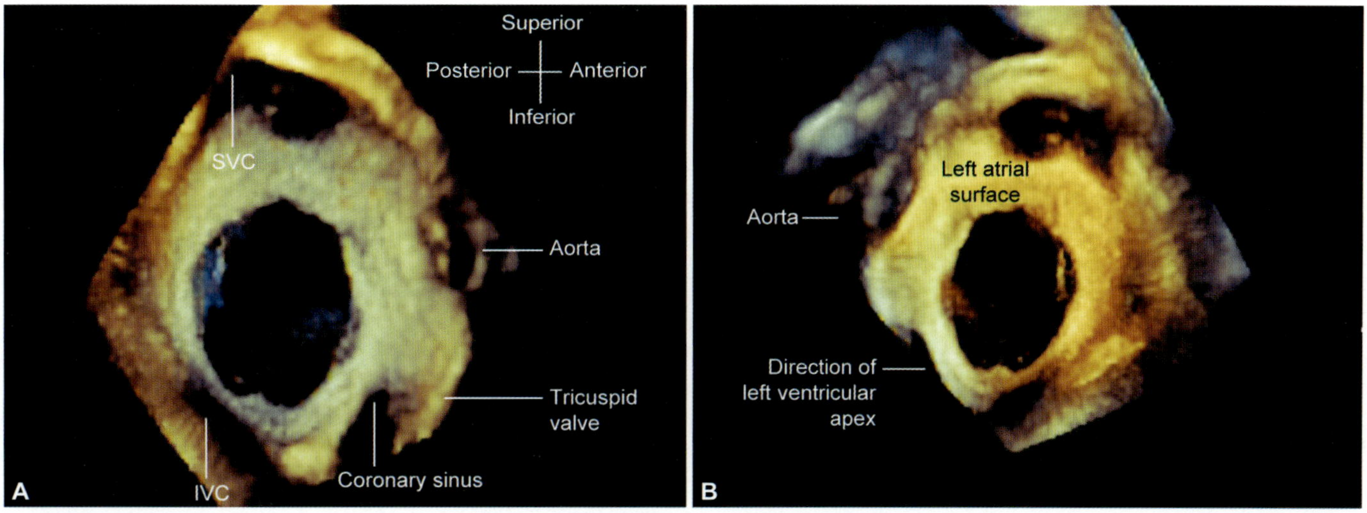

Figures 4A and B Secundum ASD—3D TEE views: (A) Right atrial view of secundum atrial septal defect (ASD). The SVC, IVC, aortic, and coronary sinus margins of the defect should be noted; (B) Left atrial view of secundum ASD

TABLE 1 Comparison of ostium primum and ostium secundum atrial septal defect

Ostium primum	*Ostium secundum*
10–15% of ASD	80–85% of ASD
Male > Female	Female > Male
Associated with MR/TR	Associated with MVPS
Increased L → R shunt	Mild
PHT: Early	Late
Poor prognosis	Good
ECG-LAD (30°)	RAD (Right axis deviation)

Flow chart 1 Margins of an atrial septal defect

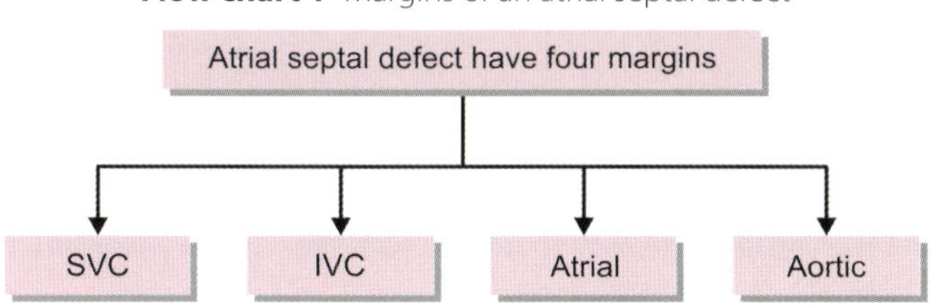

- Sinus venosus type located high in inter-atrial septum.
- 90% association of anomalous drainage of R upper pulmonary vein with SVC or right atrium.

- Partial anomalous pulmonary venous return.

Coronary Sinus (Unroofed) (Figs 5 and 6)

Coronary sinus is a rare congenital heart disease. It occurs when there is lack of septation between the back wall of the left atrium and the coronary sinus due to abnormal cell death during embryologic development, resulting in drainage of venous blood into the left atrium. The defect can be either partial or complete unroofing, which happens if superior wall is absent. It is often associated with persistent LSVC and other forms of complex congenital heart diseases, such as cor triatriatum, pulmonary atresia and anomalous pulmonary venous drainage **(Figs 6 and 7)**.

CLINICAL SYMPTOMS OF ATRIAL SEPTAL DEFECT

- Asymptomatic
- Mild effort intolerance
- Frequent chest infections
- *G/E:* No cyanosis/no clubbing
- *Signs:* BP: N/low systolic

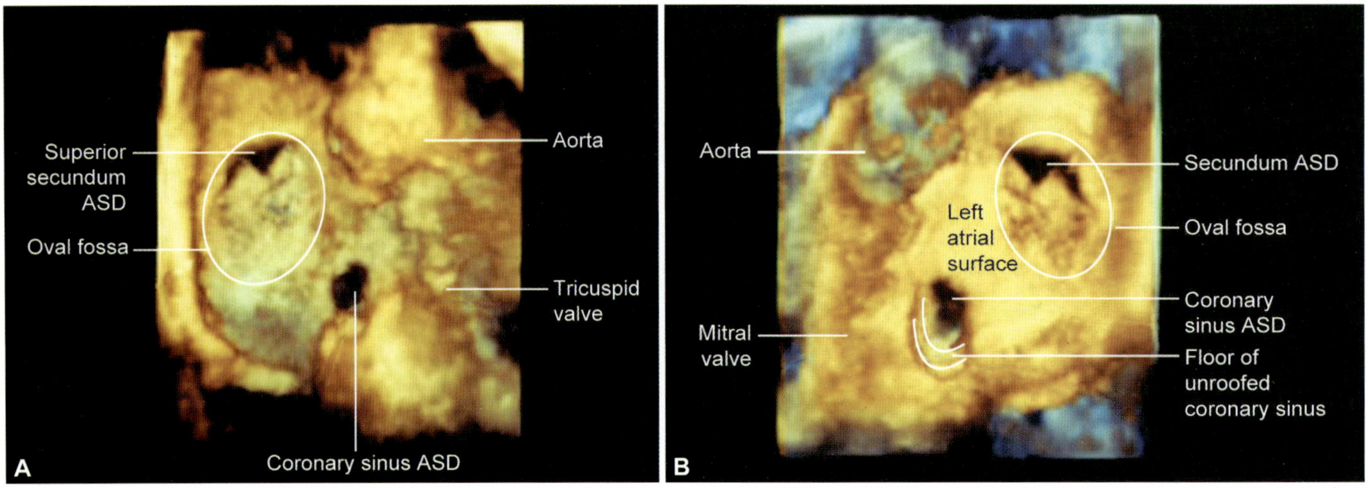

Figures 5A and B Coronary sinus ASD—3D TEE views: (A) Right atrial view of coronary sinus ASD with an additional secundum ASD at superior margin of the oval fossa; (B) Left atrial view of the coronary sinus defect. The floor of the unroofed coronary sinus can also be seen

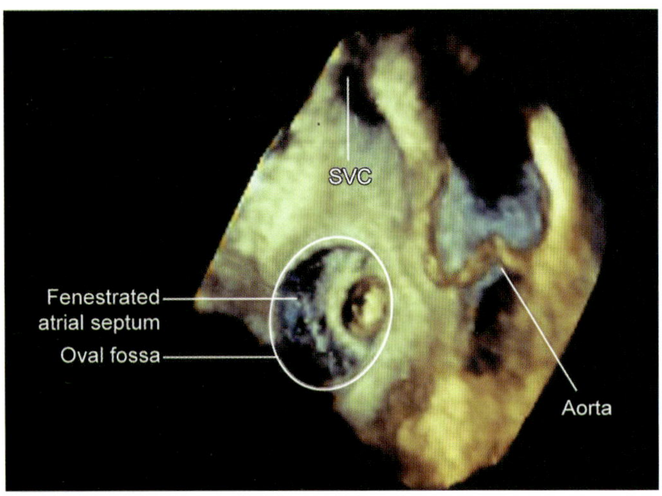

Figure 6 Fenestrated ASD—3D TEE views: Right atrial view of Fenestrated ASD. The margins of the true oval fossa are marked by an ellipse

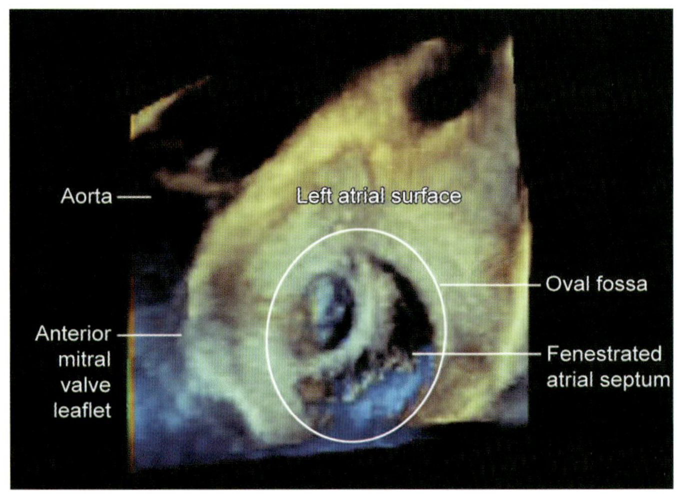

Figure 7 Left atrial view of Fenestrated ASD

- *Pulse:* N/Low volume
- *JVP:* Increase.

Inspection

Epigastric pulsation + } Due to RVH
Parasternal pulsation + }

- Pulmonary pulsation + → Dilatation of pulmonary artery
- *Palpation:* Thrill in ASD → Associated PS very large shunt
- *Auscultation:* S_1 attenuated (loud T_1)
- RV replaces LV at apex
- Increased blood flow across the tricuspid valve pushes it downwards
- Volume overload of right ventricle results in increased force of contraction
  ↓
- Forceful valve closure.

P_2 Loud

- Increased pressure in PA
- Dilatation of PA
- Wide split fixed.

Why There is a Click in Atrial Septal Defect?

- *Pulmonary vascular click:* Due to PA dilatation
- Valvular click due to pulmonary stenosis
- MVPS.

CLINICAL INVESTIGATIONS

X-ray Chest in Atrial Septal Defect (Figs 8A and B)

Apex is upwards, suggesting a right ventricular configuration **(Figs 8A and B)**. All features suggest a large secundum atrial septal defect with a large left to right shunt producing severe pulmonary hypertension. Cardiomegaly on chest X-ray is suggestive of atrial septal defect in Eisenmenger syndrome, while it is unlikely in ventricular septal defect and patent ductus arteriosus. Cardiomegaly is mainly due to the grossly dilated right atrium in atrial septal defect. The right atrium is not enlarged in the other two varieties of Eisenmenger syndrome. In ventricular septal defect with large left to right shunt, the cardiac size comes down as pulmonary hypertension develops and the shunt decreases.

- Increased RA, RV size
- *Enlarged pulmonary vessels:* Prominent main PA segment "jughandle appearance" **(Fig. 8A)**
- Mild to moderate cardiomegaly
- Normal-sized left atrium
- Normal to small aorta
- Plethoric lung fields.

ATRIAL SEPTAL DEFECT ECHOCARDIOGRAM

The echocardiogram (ECG) findings in atrial septal defect vary with the type of defect the individual has. Individuals with atrial septal defects may have **(Fig. 9)**:

- A prolonged PR interval (a first degree heart block)
- The enlargement of the atria that is common in ASDs
- Increased distance due to the defect itself
- An increased distance of internodal conduction from the SA node to the AV node
- RBBB with **rsIIr**[1].

In addition to the PR prolongation, individuals with a primum ASD have a left axis deviation of the QRS complex while those with a secundum ASD have a right axis deviation of the QRS complex. Individuals with a sinus venosus ASD exhibit a left axis deviation of the P wave (not the QRS complex).

The ECG of a patient with an atrial septal defect (ASD) should also show a right bundle branch block (sometimes incomplete) partially due to the right ventricular volume and pressure overload that occurs. When an ostium primum atrial defect is present, the ECG reveals left axis deviation. When an ostium secundum atrial septal defect is present, the ECG reveals right axis deviation.

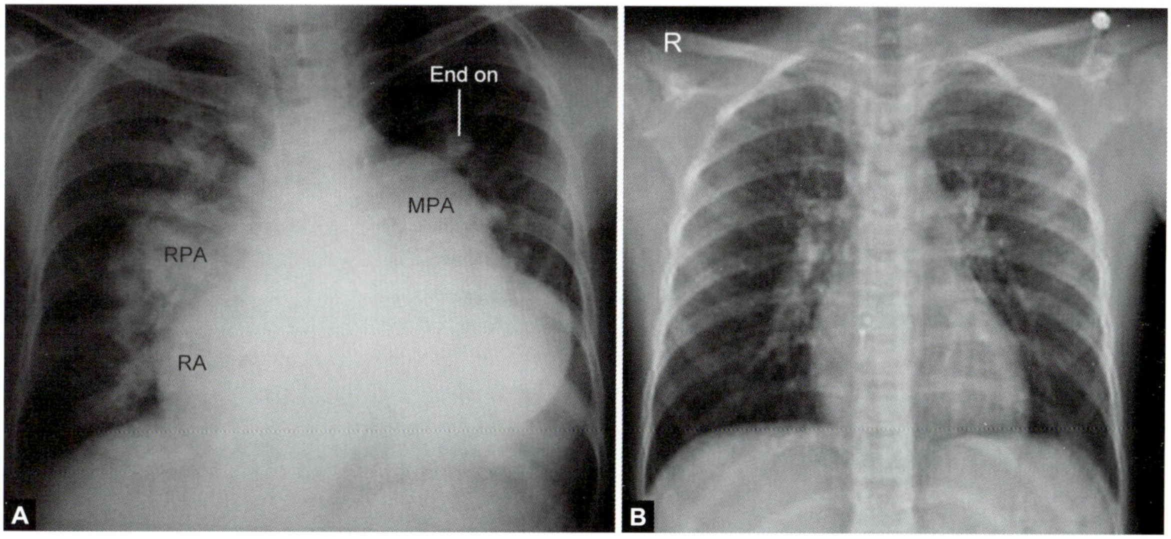

Figures 8A and B (A) Jughandle appearance in ASD due to increase PA size; (B) ASD with enlarged pulmonary vessels

CHAPTER 4

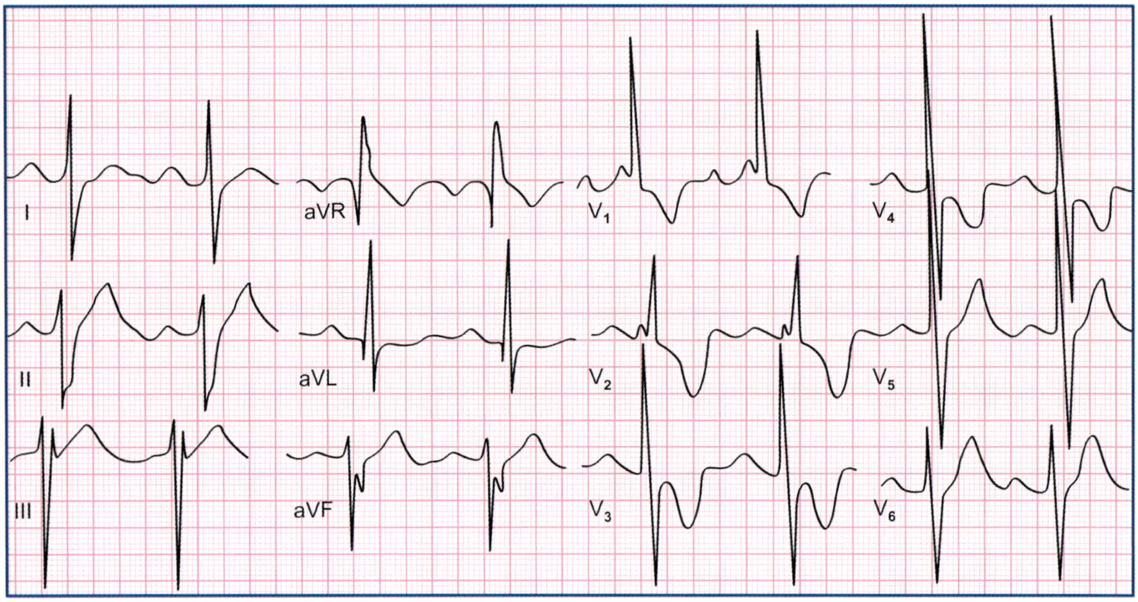

Figure 9 ECG in ASD with prolonged PR interval and RBBB and RAD

GUIDELINES WHERE PREOPERATIVE TRANSESOPHAGEAL ECHOCARDIOGRAPHY FOR ATRIAL SEPTAL DEFECT IS MUST

- Repair of a mitral or tricuspid valve, whether for stenosis, regurgitation, or both
- Primary repair of an atrioventricular septal defect (AVSD) with significant AV valve regurgitation
- Repair of a left or right AV valve post-previous AVSD repair
- Repair of an aortic valve
- Complex left ventricular outflow tract (LVOT) obstruction
- Hypertrophic obstructive cardiomyopathy
- Surgery for bacterial endocarditis
- Multiple muscular ventricular septal defects (VSD)
- Atrial septal defect (ASD) size pre-Fontan for hypoplastic left heart syndrome
- Surgery for recurrent or congenital pulmonary vein stenosis
- Other issues where the preoperative anatomy is unclear on prior investigations.

PREOPERATIVE ASSESSMENT OF TEE (FIGS 10 TO 20)

Two-dimensional TEE and 3D TEE along with Doppler echocardiography was compared with cardiac catheterization and angiography in the preoperative evaluation of ostium primum atrial septal defect. Preoperative echocardiography results in no false positive or false negative primary diagnoses when compared with the diagnoses obtained at preoperative angiography or surgery.

- Size, site, number
- Shunting (left to right, right to left or bidirectional)
- Right atrium and right ventricle dilatation
- Paradoxical motion and flattening of interventricular septum
- Mitral stenosis (Lutembacher syndrome), mitral regurgitation (mitral valve prolapse/cleft mitral valve)
- *Tricuspid regurgitation:* Pulmonary artery systolic pressure if tricuspid regurgitation present
- Pulmonary venous drainage
- Pulmonary stenosis
- Ventricular septal defect

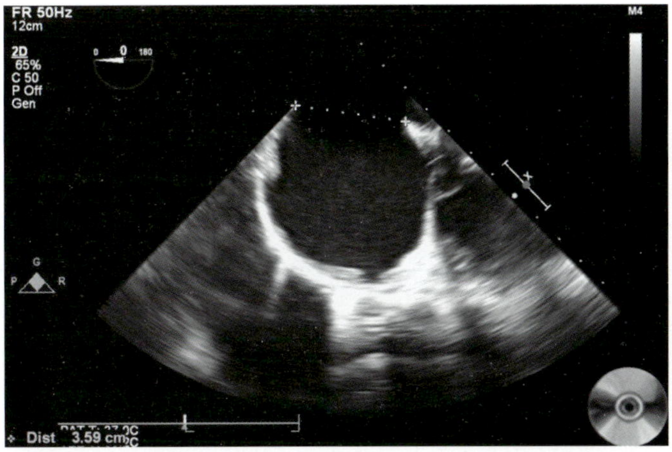

Figure 10 (Video 1) 2D assessment of atrial septal defect. Midesophageal 4 chamber view (probe rotated to right) showing interatrial septal aneurysm and an ostium secundum atrial septal defect. The repair of the defect in such a scenario is done by excising the interatrial septum aneurysm and closing the atrial septal defect with a prosthetic or pericardial (in case of associated mitral regurgitation) patch. Also seen is the tricuspid value and superior vena cava

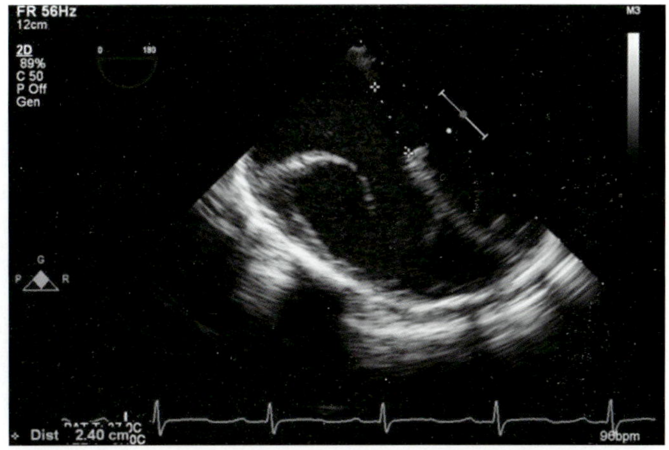

Figure 12 2D assessment of atrial septal defect. Midesophageal 4 chamber view showing a large ostium primum atrial septal defect in relation to tricuspid valve (anterior tricuspid leaflet is seen). Also seen is the intact interventricular septum (in comparison to partial atrioventricular septal defect where the inlet portion of the interventricular septum is deficient)

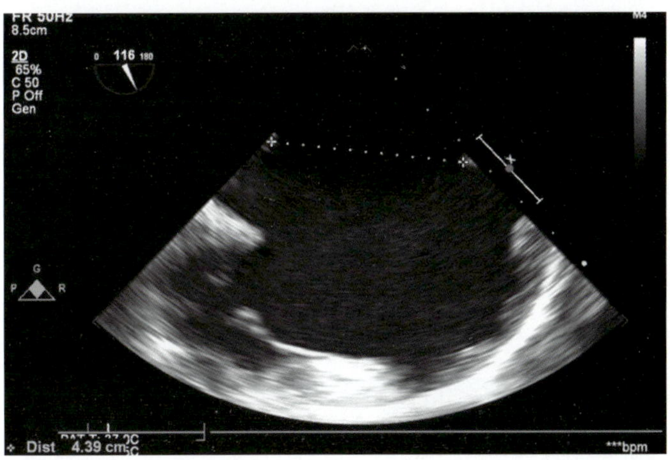

Figure 11 2D assessment of atrial septal defect. Midesophageal bicaval view showing ostium secundum atrial septal defect with superior and inferior vena cava seen. The defect measured in this view depicts the superior-inferior dimension, superior and inferior vena cava rim of the atrial septal defect

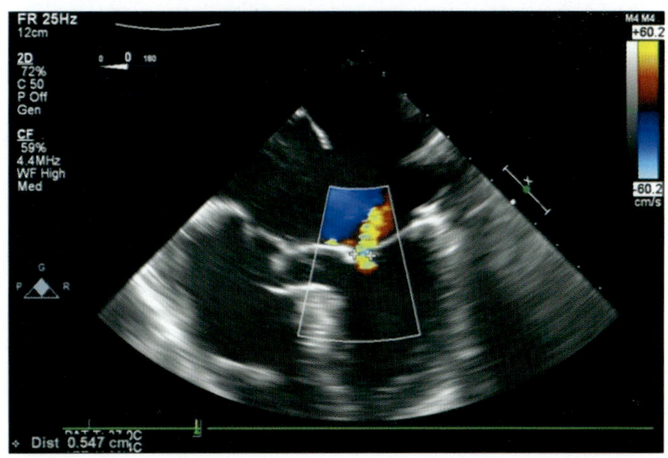

Figure 13 2D assessment of atrial septal defect. Midesophageal 4 chamber view showing a large ostium primum atrial septal defect with moderate mitral regurgitation. Note the small ventricular septal defect in the inlet portion which is being closed by septal leaflet of tricuspid valve

- Patent ductus arteriosus
- Coarctation of aorta
- Left superior vena cava
- Interatrial septum aneurysm
- Qp/Qs = Stroke volume$_{PV}$/stroke volume$_{AoV}$ = pulmonary valve area × velocity time integral$_{PV}$/ aortic valve area × velocity time integral$_{AV}$

- Does the interatrial septum appear normal or is there any aneurysm formation?
- Is there any echo dropout in the septum to indicate a defect? In the apical view, it is not unusual to see areas of 'apparent' dropout in the interatrial septum, which is quite a long way from the probe, so be careful not to report dropout as an ASD unless you

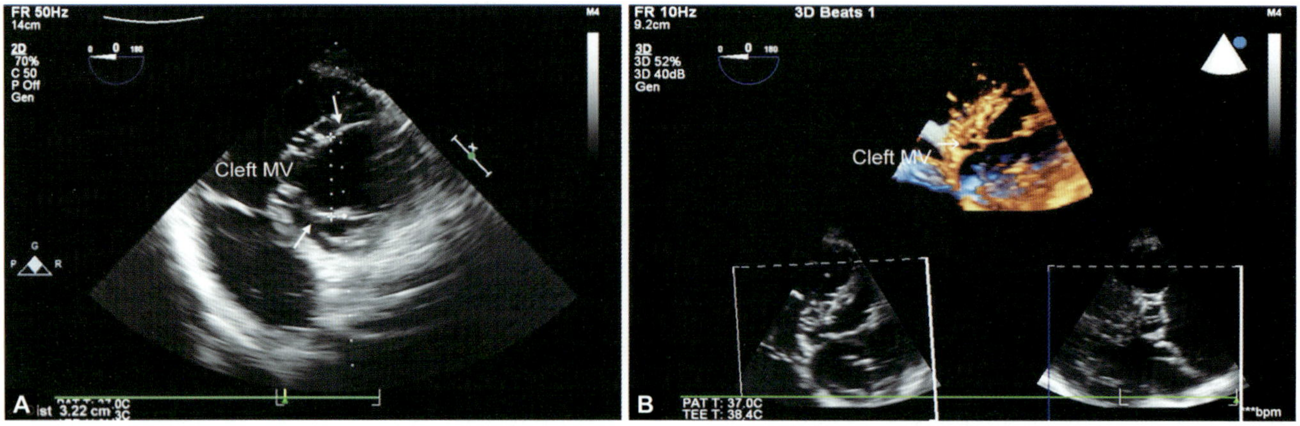

Figures 14A and B 2D assessment of mitral valve in atrial septal defect. Transgastric basal view showing cleft in the anterior mitral leaflet in the same patient with ostium primum atrial septal defect and moderate mitral regurgitation. 3D image of the anterior mitral cleft (arrow)

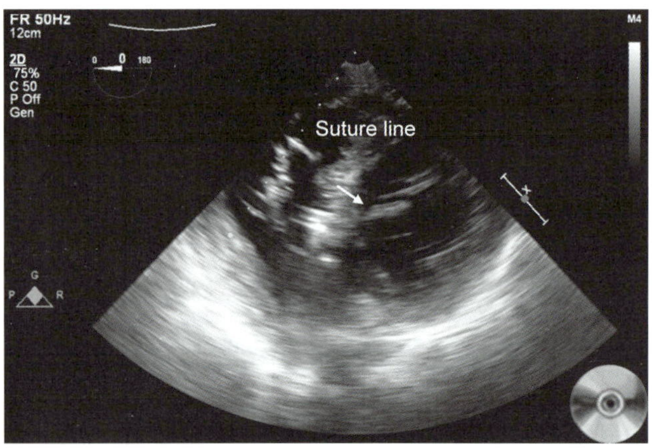

Figure 15 (Video 2) 2D assessement of mitral valve in atrial septal defect. Transgastric basal view showing the anterior mitral leaflet, postcleft repair in a patient with ostium primum atrial septal defect and moderate mitral regurgitation

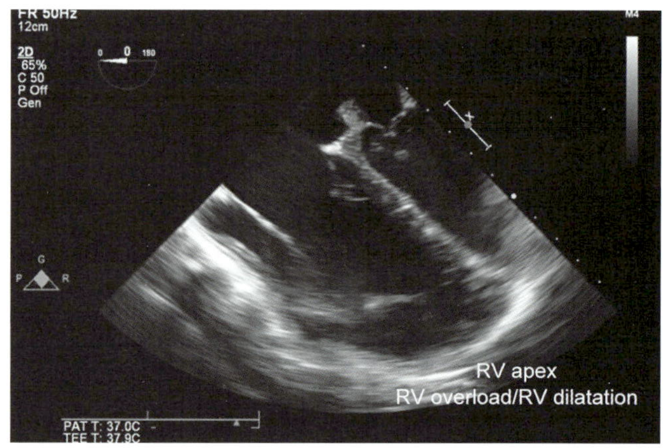

Figure 17 2D assessment of atrial septal defect. Midesophageal 4 chamber view showing RV dilatation due to volume overload and apex of heart formed by RV. Normally the free wall of right ventricle extends to 2/3rd of the interventricular septum, if the free wall extends till the apex then right ventricle is said to be dilated

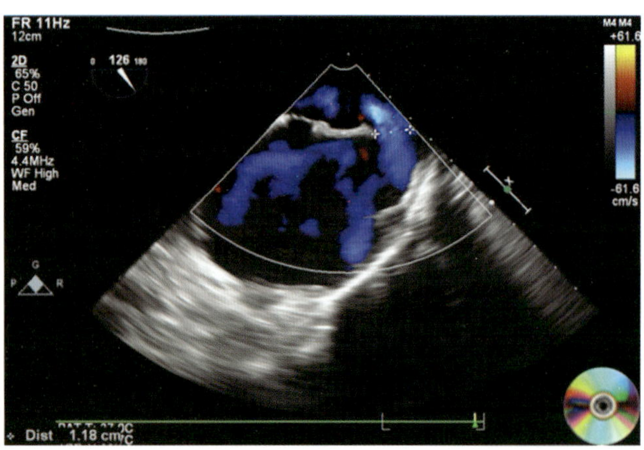

Figure 16 (Video 3) Color Doppler assessment of atrial septal defect. Midesophageal bicaval view showing superior vena cava type sinus venosus atrial septal defect shunting from left to right

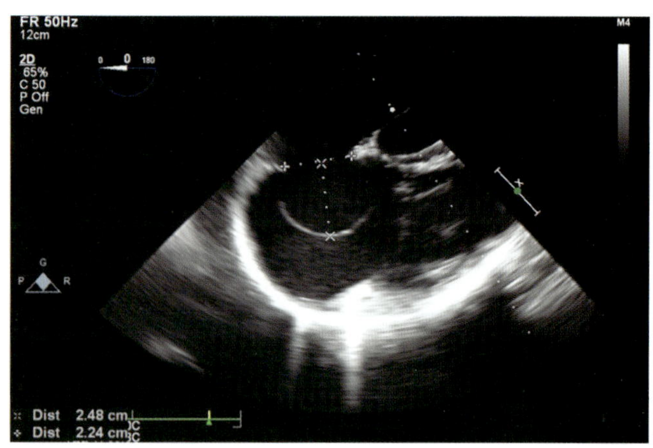

Figure 18 2D assessment of atrial septal defect. Midesophageal 4 chamber view (probe rotated to right showing interatrial septal aneurysm and an ostium secundum atrial septal defect. The repair of the defect in such a scenario is done by excising the interatrial septum aneurysm and closing the atrial septal defect with a prosthetic or pericardial (in case of associated mitral regurgitation) patch

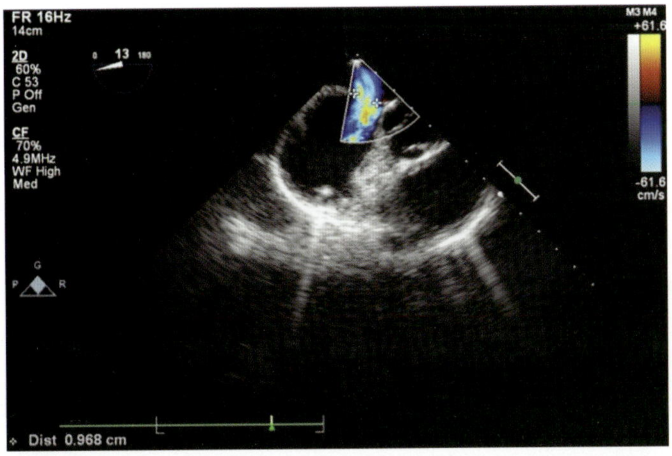

Figure 19 Color Doppler assessment of atrial septal defect. Mid-esophageal 4 chamber view showing a single ostium secundum atrial septal defect

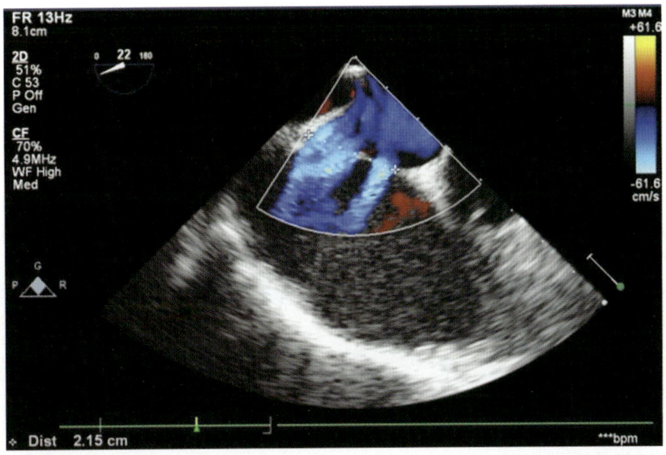

Figure 20 Color Doppler assessment of atrial septal defect. Mid-esophageal 4 chamber view showing a 2 defects in the interatrial septum. For placement of occlusion device in such a patient the intervening septum is torn off by using a balloon and a single amplatzer ductal occluder is placed according to the larger defect

can also see it in other views and/or you also have further supporting evidence.

- Assess right atrial and ventricular size/function—are they dilated as a consequence of a left-to-right shunt? Is there evidence of right, heart volume overload RVOT (paradoxical motion of the interventricular septum).

If there is doubt about the presence of an ASD, it may be necessary to perform an 'agitated' saline contrast study as for patent foramen ovale (PFO). Although transthoracic echo (TTE) can often detect evidence of an ASD, transesophageal echo (TOE) will usually be required to assess an ASD in detail (or to rule out an ASD if clinical suspicion remains after a normal TTE). Sinus venosus defects can be very difficult to visualize on TTE.

ATRIAL SEPTAL ANEURYSMS

Atrial septal aneurysms are thought to have a prevalence of around 1%. They are defined as a bulge or deformation of the interatrial septum protruding at least 10 mm into the right or left atrium (or, if mobile, swinging at least 10 mm from side to side) and with a diameter across their base of at least 15 mm. They have been reported to be associated with ASD and PFO (and also with mitral valve prolapsed) and are also thought to be a potential cardiac source of emboli.

ROBOTIC ATRIAL SEPTAL DEFECT CLOSURE

For robotic atrial septal defect closure percutaneous cannulation of the superior vena cava, inferior vena cava and femoral artery (preferably right) is done. Transesophageal echocardiography is used for confirmation of guidewires and exact position of the cannulae.

TEE FOR ASD DEVICE CLOSURE (FIGS 21 TO 24)

Precatheter Assessment

- Define the defect location and size.
- Determine the defect rims (5 mm ideal). Anterosuperior rim-ME AV SAX, posterior rim-ME4CH, inferoanterior rim-ME4CH, superopost rim-ME bicaval, inferoposterior rim-ME
- Assess mitral valve anatomy
- Evaluate the pulmonary venous drainage
- Examine the right sided structures and IVS motion
- Evaluate the RV thickness for PAH.

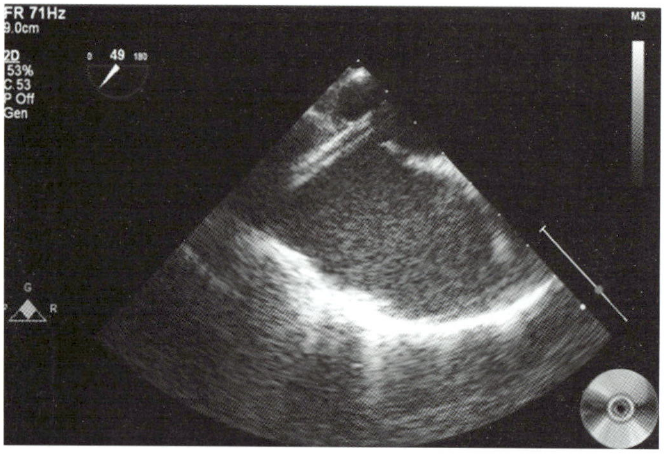

Figure 21 (Video 4) 2D echo showing percutaneous closure of an ostium secundum atrial septal defect. The catheter containing the amplatzer ductal occluder device is seen traversing the atrial septal defect

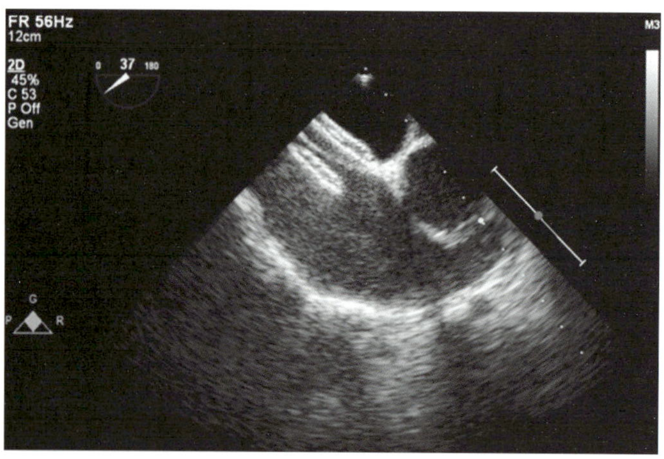

Figure 22 2D echo showing percutaneous closure of an ostium secundum atrial septal defect. Amplatzer septal occluder device is deployed in the atrial septal defect with the left atrial rim resting well above aorta

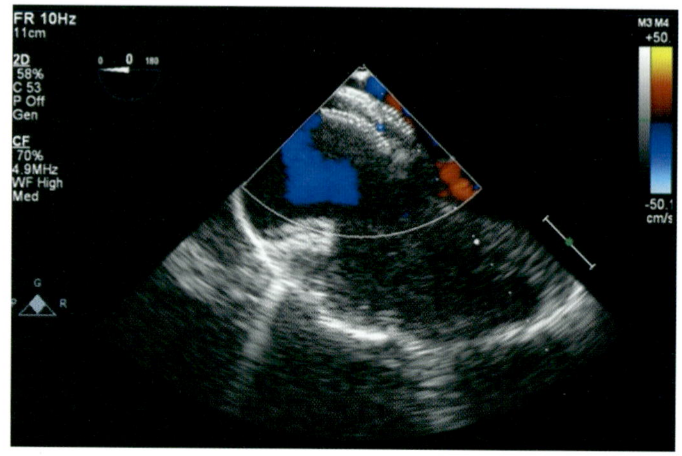

Figure 23 Color Doppler in midesophageal 4 chamber view showing percutaneous closure of an ostium secundum atrial septal defect. No residual shunt across the septal defect is visible. Both the rims of the device are fully approximated

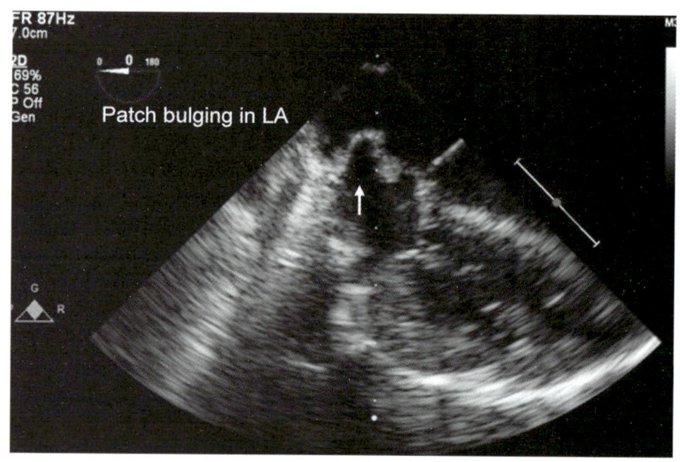

Figure 24 2D echo showing a large size prosthetic patch used to close the atrial septal defect bulging into the left atrium

During Catheter Insertion

- Determine tissue rims (lack of inferior or posterior rims are unfavorable)
- Assess relation of ASD to surrounding structures
- Assess the maximal defect diameter (balloon stretch sizing)
- Detect leaks around the balloon
- Guidance for device deployment/device stability
- Assess residual shunting.

After Device Deployment

- Detect residual shunting
- Evaluate AV valve incompetence
- Evaluate proper positioning of device (unobstructed low in systemic and adjacent pulmonary veins)
- Exclude embolization or erosion of catheter.

3D TEE

- Enhances spatial details of the defect size
- Facilitates continuous visualization of 3D relations while monitoring device deployment
- Evaluates for appropriate ASD device position and entrapment of septal rims around the occluder
- In patients destined to undergo device closure of atrial septal defect the depiction of the borders of the atrial septal defect is important. A slight deficiency in any of the rims may lead to dislodgement of

device. Therefore the atrial septal defect shall have an adequate size (> 2 mm) superior vena cava, inferior vena cava, aortic and mitral rim.

- If Robotic atrial septal defect closure is to be undertaken following things should be looked for:
  - Left superior vena cava present or not
  - Superior and inferior vena cava diameter
  - Superior and inferior vena cava cannula position
  - Guidewire for DTA cannulation.

TEE FOR MINIMALLY INVASIVE ASD CLOSURE (FIGS 25 TO 28)

- Modifications—SVC cannulation
- Modifications—IVC and aortic cannulation
- Anterolateral thoracotomy.

Right Thoracotomy (Fig. 29)

- ASD closure.
- Post-thoracoscopic minimally invasive cardiac surgery with right thoracotomy **(Fig. 29)**
- Evaluation of coronary sinus on TEE
- TOE showing coronary sinus **(Figs 30A to C).**

During Catheter/Cannula Placement (Table 2)

- Communication between TOE operator and person advancing the catheter, move TEE probe of
- 0° view for coronary sinus
- 110° view for opening of SVC and IVC
- CS opens near IVC **(Figs 30 and 31)**
- IVC can be followed by clockwise rotation
- CS can be followed by anticlockwise rotation.

SVC Cannulation

Femoral Arterial Cannulation (Figs 32A and B)

- Only guidewire—visualized.
- Cannula—not visualized.

Transfemoral IVC Cannulation (Figs 33A to C)

- Right femoral vein—direct path
- TOE operator images the guidewire as it enters RA from IVC
- Slow passage of cannula.

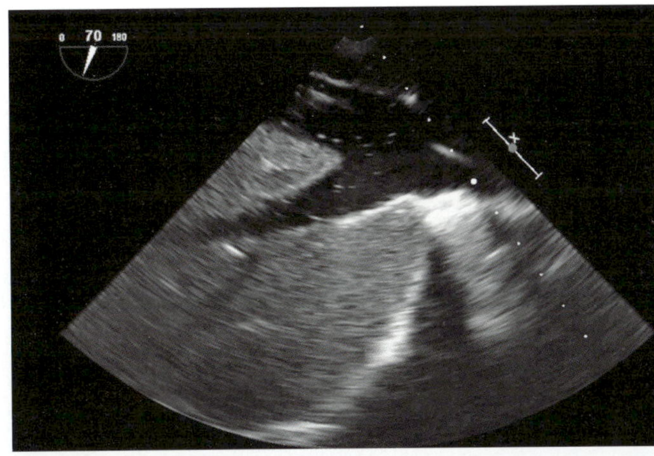

Figure 25 2D echo for percutaneous inferior vena cava cannulation. Modified hepatic vein view showing guidewire placement for the placement of inferior vena cava cannula. The cannula should be 1 cm proximal to the inferior vena cava right atrial junction

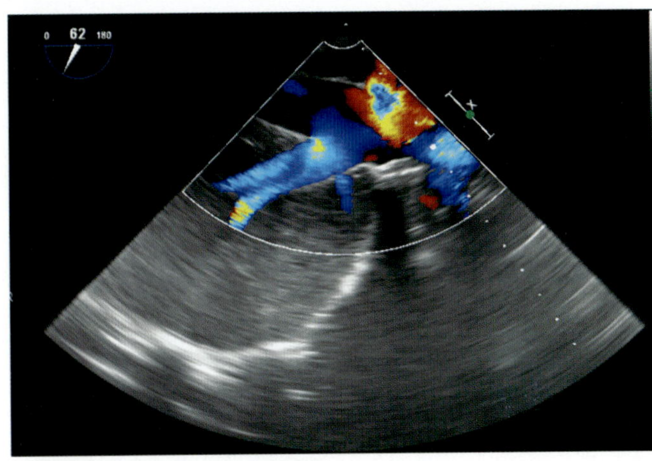

Figure 26 Color Doppler in modified hepatic vein view showing the confluence of hepatic and portal vein to form the inferior vena cava

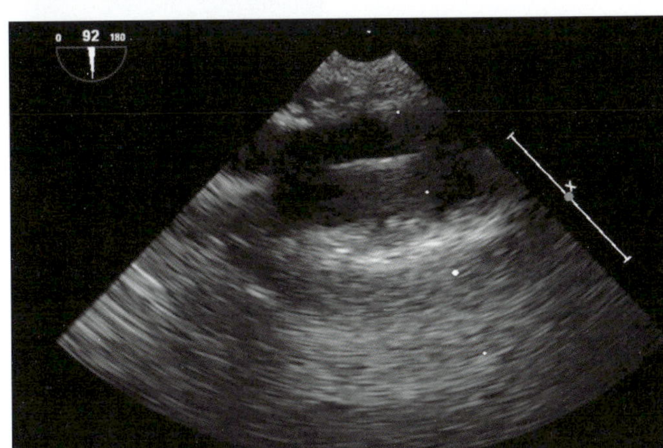

Figure 27 2D echo showing the placement of guidewire in descending thoracic aorta for cannulation of the femoral artery. The arterial cannula is not visible because it rarely traverses the abdominal aorta

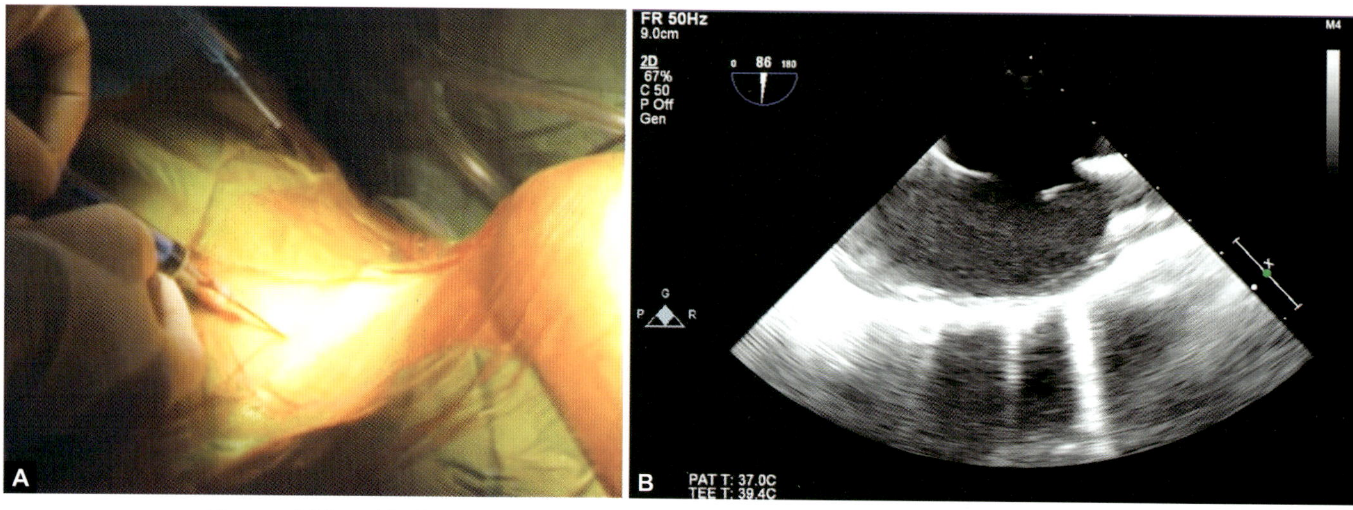

Figures 28A and B Superior vena cava cannulation and other is bicaval view for SVC cannulation

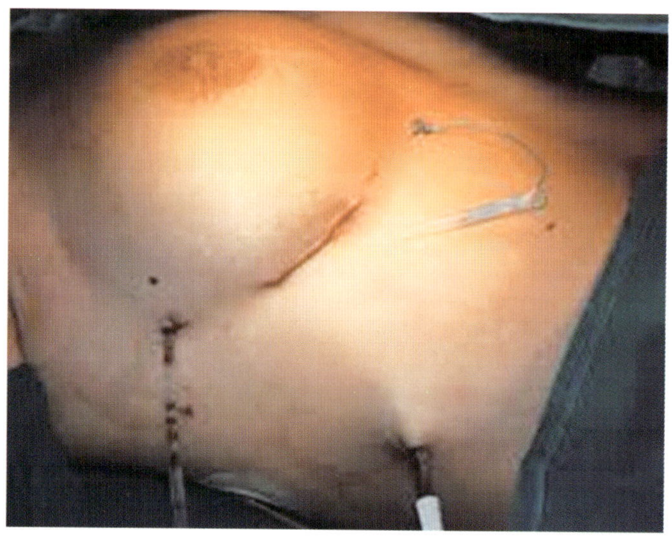

Figure 29 Thoracotomy incision for minimally invasive atrial septal defect closure

TABLE 2 Transesophageal echo (TOE)

Commonly used TOE view	*Purpose*
Midesophageal bicaval view or modified bicaval view	Confirmation of percutaneous venous cannula placement
Esophageal four chamber view	Coronary sinus
Transgastric mid short axis papillary view	Ventricular systolic dysfunction or regional movement abnormalities
All standards view	Surgical defect and adequacy of repair

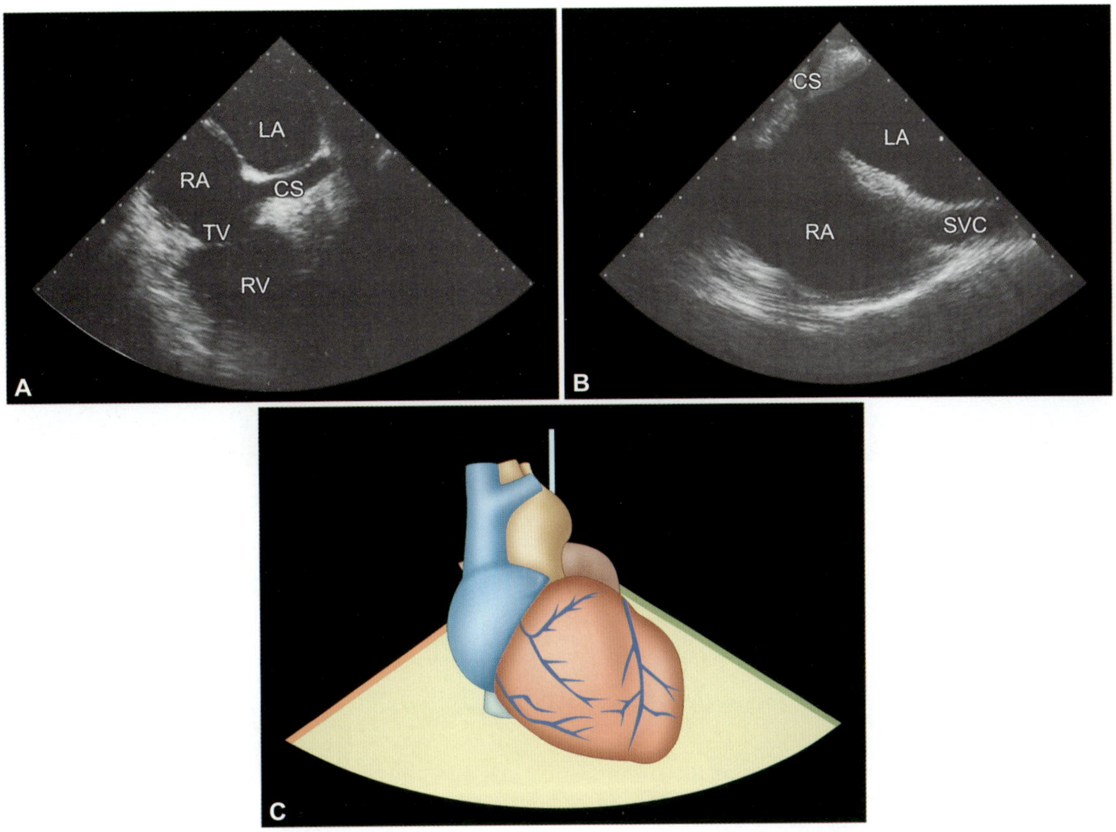

Figures 30A to C TOE showing coronary sinus (animation) and TEE views near the lower end of the IAS. CS is just behind the LA

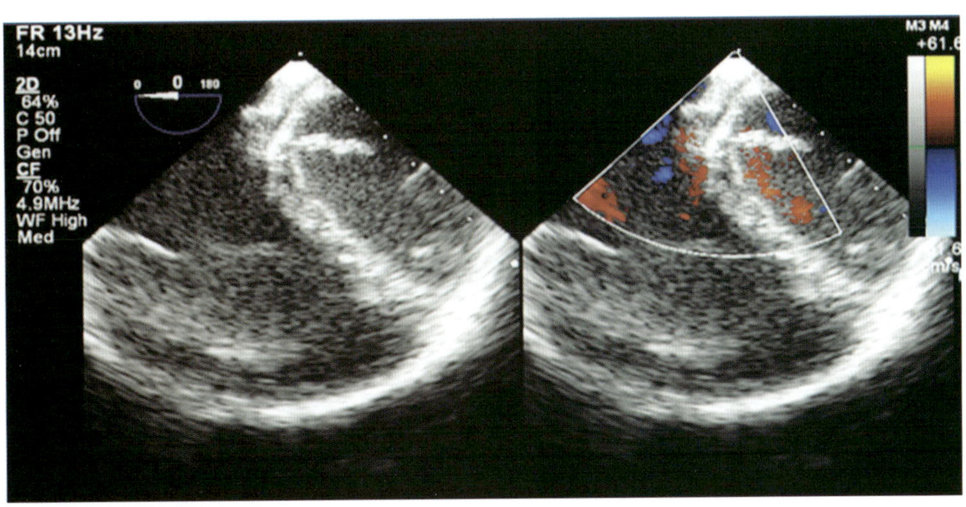

Figure 31 Evaluation of coronary sinus on transesophageal echocardiography. 7–15 mm—Normal, > 15 mm – s/o LSVC

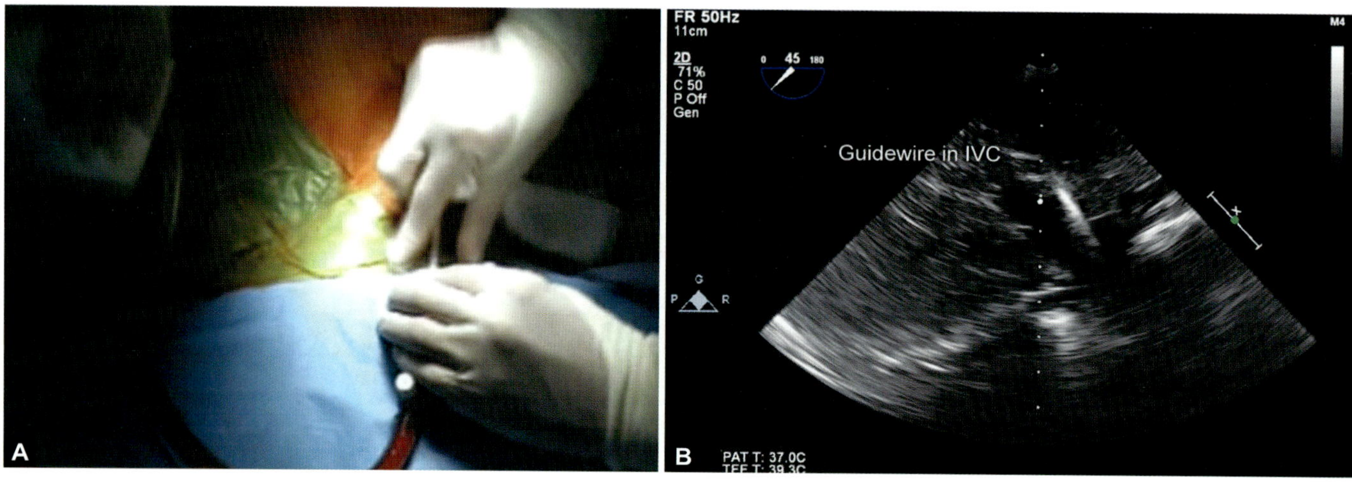

Figures 32A and B Inferior vena cava cannulation and other is TEE to show guidewire in IVC in ME lowes hepatic view

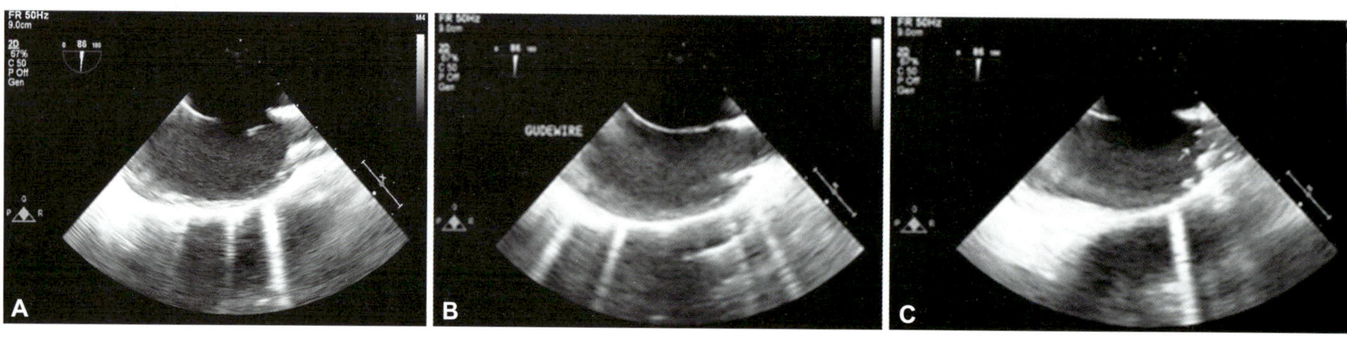

Figures 33A to C Midesophageal bicaval view at 90° for superior vena cava (SVC) cannulation showing also interventricular septum (IVS) and interatrial septum (IAS) and beginning of IVC. The whole of RA is well-visualized

Monitoring during MICS ASD with TEE

- Initiate CPB gradually
- Imaging of descending aorta
- Imaging of cardiac chambers
- During cardioplegia delivery keep an eye on long axis view
- LV distention/aortic insufficiency.

TEE for Deairing and Weaning (Figs 33 to 36)

- Lack of direct access to the heart
- Patient position
  - Retention of intracardiac air
  - CO_2 insufflation into the hemi-thorax.
- Active ventilation—deairing pulmonary veins
- TEE guided weaning of to come off CPB.

Check ECHO for ASD Repair in ME LAX View

ME LAX view in **Figure 37**.

POSTDEVICE CLOSURE ASSESSMENT

TEE plays an important role in following patient's post-ASD/PFO closure device implantation. Although 2D echocardiography is a valuable tool for minimizing the occurrence of a complication, more recently developed RT3DE adds a valuable imaging perspective and supplements the information obtainable by 2D imaging.

- Residual shunt
- Mitral regurgitation
- Aortic regurgitation
- Dislodgement of device.

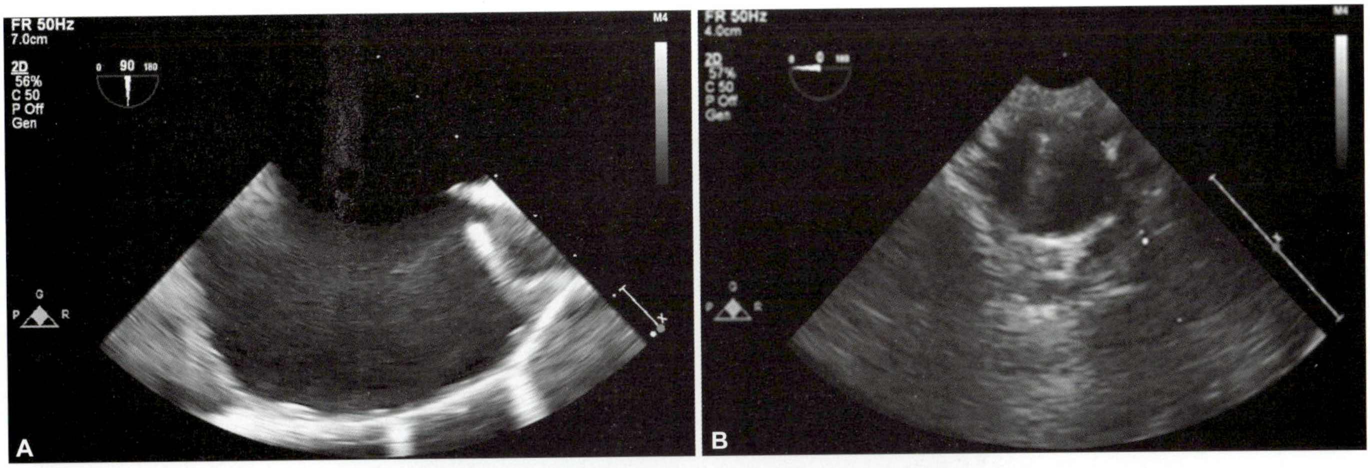

Figures 34A and B (A) ME bicaval view for SVC cannulation; (B) UE aorta SAX view for aortic cannulation

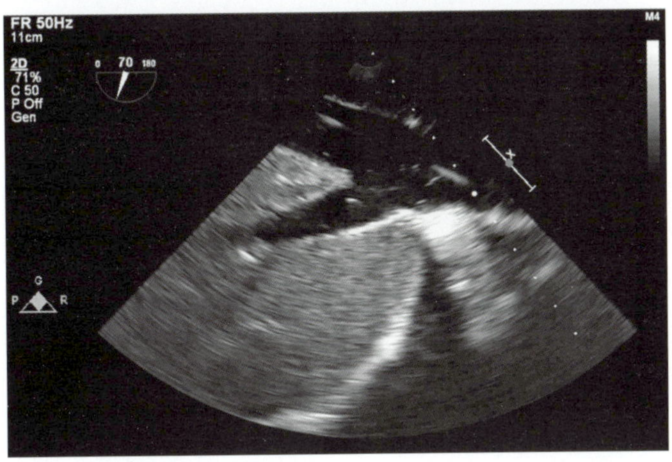

Figure 35 LE hepatic venous view for IVC cannula
Note the confluence of the hepatic veins, which form the IVC

POSTOPERATIVE TEE ASSESSMENT

Postoperative management after atrial septal defect (ASD) repair is usually standard. Patients are expected to be awake and often extubated shortly after the operation. Drainage tubes are removed from the chest the first morning after surgery, and, except when rhythm problems occur, the pacing wires are removed shortly thereafter. Most patients can eat and ambulate without difficulty on the first or second postoperative day, and most are discharged by the third or fourth postoperative day. After transcatheter occlusion, patients are generally discharged the next day. Six months of treatment with aspirin with or without clopidogrel is recommended to prevent thrombus formation.

- Residual shunting (size, gradient and direction)
- Assessment of mitral valve repair
- Drainage of superior and inferior vena cava (IVC draining into left atrium has been reported after repair of inferior vena cava type of sinus venosus ASD)
- For Robotic closure–in addition to above findings air in the chambers. Deairing is difficult with Robotic cardiac surgery **(*See* Figs 25 and Figs 38 to 40)**.

TYPES OF 2° ASD AND DEVICE CLOSURE

The most common type of ASD encountered in clinical practice is ostium secundum. These ASDs have deficient

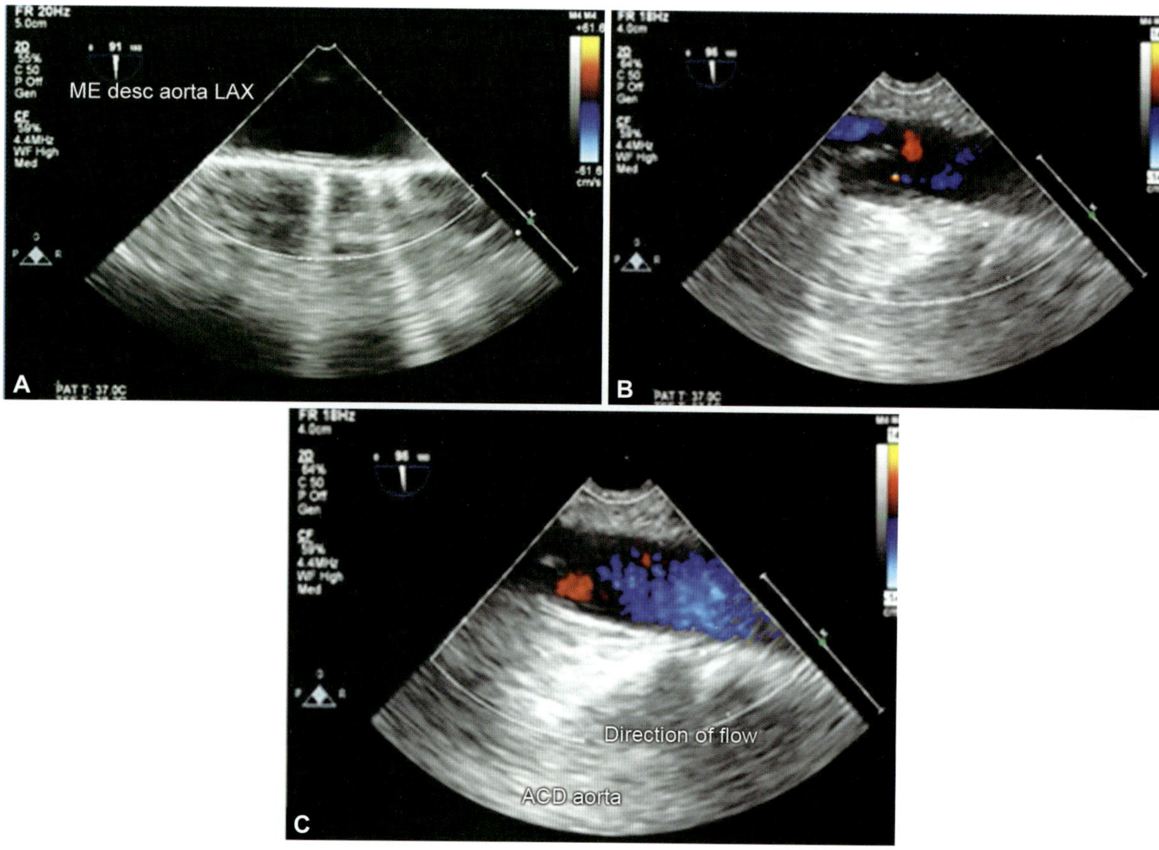

Figures 36A to C ME descending thoracic for aortic cannulation

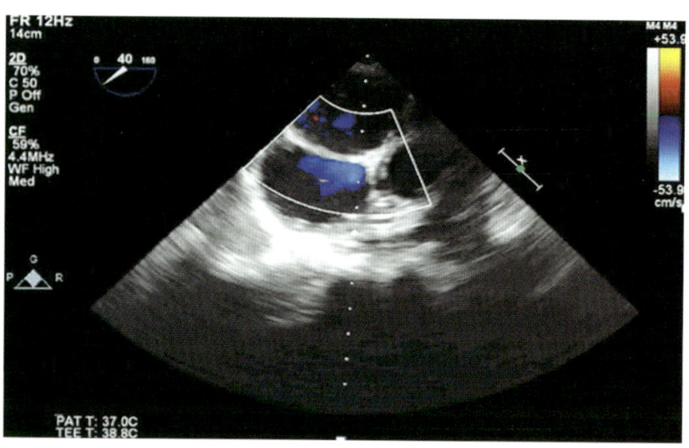

Figure 37 Echocardiography in ME LAX view

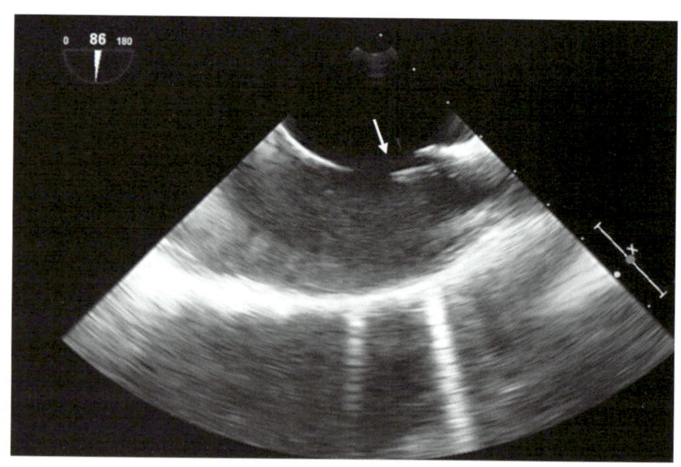

Figure 38 2D echo for percutaneous cannulation of superior vena cava. Midesophageal bicaval view showing superior vena cava cannula for robotic atrial septal defect closure. The cannula tip is in the right atrium which is the incorrect position of the cannula

aortic margins, while the other three margins, i.e. SVC, IVC and atrial margins, are big enough to grip the device. These defects can be closed with septal occlude devices but require considerably more operator experience and also carry more chances of complications, including that of device migration.

The patients with multiple ASDs require all defects to be individually evaluated to decide adequacy of their margins for device closure. Further, the margin between the two defects is also to be evaluated, to decide whether to use one device or to use two separate devices to close them. It has been suggested that the rim between the two defects should at least be 7 mm to allow the deployment of two devices.[1]

After Surgical Closure of ASD, TEE is Performed to Confirm

- ASD patch is intact and there is no residual shunt.
- Superior vena cava (SVC) and inferior vena cava (IVC) are draining into the right atrium (RA) because, very rarely, in patients with a deficient inferior rim, the IVC may get routed to the left atrium (LA).

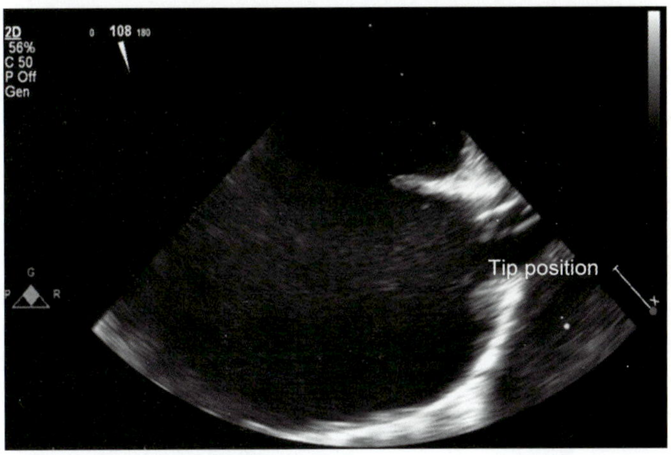

Figure 39 2D echo for percutaneous cannulation of superior vena cava. Midesophageal bicaval view showing superior vena cava cannula for robotic atrial septal defect closure. The cannula tip is at the junction of right atrium and superior vena cava which is the correct position of the cannula

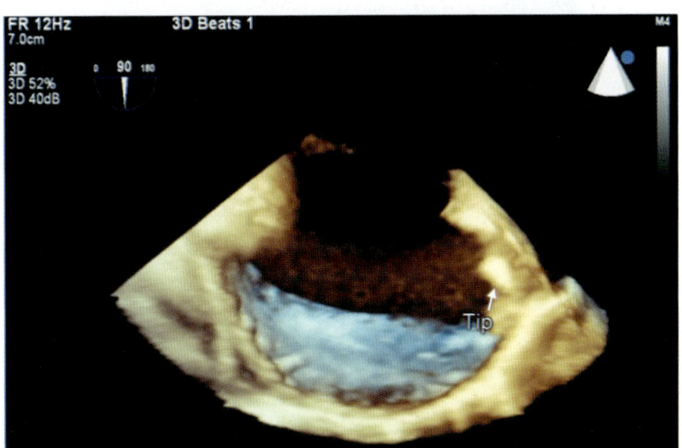

Figure 40 Real time 3D echo for percutaneous cannulation of the superior vena cava. Midesophageal bicaval view showing superior vena cava cannula tip at superior vena cava—right atrial junction

ADVANTAGES OF MINIMALLY INVASIVE CARDIAC SURGERY FOR ASD CLOSURE

Minimally invasive approaches, including limited lateral thoracotomies, partial longitudinal or transverse sternotomies and video-assisted thoracoscopic techniques:

- Limit the postoperative pain
- Limit the respiratory dysfunction
- Allow for the prompt recovery
- Reduce the cosmetic impact of scar
- Excellent cosmetic healing
- Reduced postoperative pain
- Quick functional recuperation
- Short hospital stay and cost savings
- Expediency, safety, minimal discomfort.

SPECTRUM OF MINIMALLY INVASIVE CARDIAC SURGERY

PTMC and ASD (Fig. 41)

PTMC procedures having been carried out in India in 2005 (this study included the data from only 71 centers and actual number is likely to be much higher).[2] The creation of an atrial septal defect (ASD) is inherent in the antegrade PTMC approach, and its incidence is as high as 67% at 48 hours.[3] Most of these defects are small and close spontaneously over next one year.[4] However 3–15% of patients do develop significant atrial shunts (defined as a pulmonary-to-systemic flow of > 1.3:1).[4,5] The shape of these ASDs varies, depending on the cross-sectional profile of the deflated balloon **(Figs 42A to D)**.

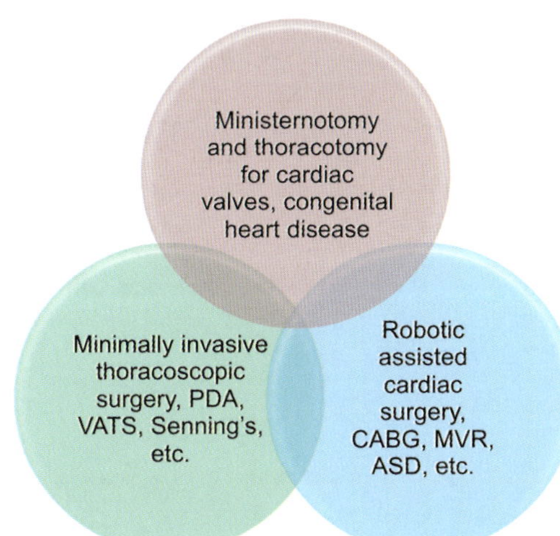

Figure 41 Indications for minimally invasive cardiac surgery

QUANTIFICATION OF 3D OVER 2D TEE (*SEE* FIGS 42 TO 65)

The 3D quantification of the ASD offers several advantages over 2D measurements. 3D imaging shows the entire defect in a single view, allowing the operator to choose the maximal diameter with certainty. The 2D imaging, on the other hand, requires a series of views to measure the defect and can miss the maximal diameter of the defect as the operator can evaluate only few of infinite number of possible 2D planes. This becomes even more important in defects which are not spherical in shape. The examples seen so far emphasize the usefulness of 3D TEE imaging in pre-device closure assessment of the size of the defect and adequacy of its margins to grip the device. However, 3D TEE also has a potentially very useful role during the procedure of device closure. The images taken during the device deployment to close a fossa ovalis defect. It rapidly confirms the proper positioning of the device across all the margins. A single 3D TEE image can provide the answer to the every question that arises before and after the deployment of the device. 3D imaging can tell whether the device is excessively mobile or whether it is encroaching onto AV valves or pulmonary veins or SVC or IVC orifices.

In Older Children

Transesophageal echocardiography needed to visualize the defect.

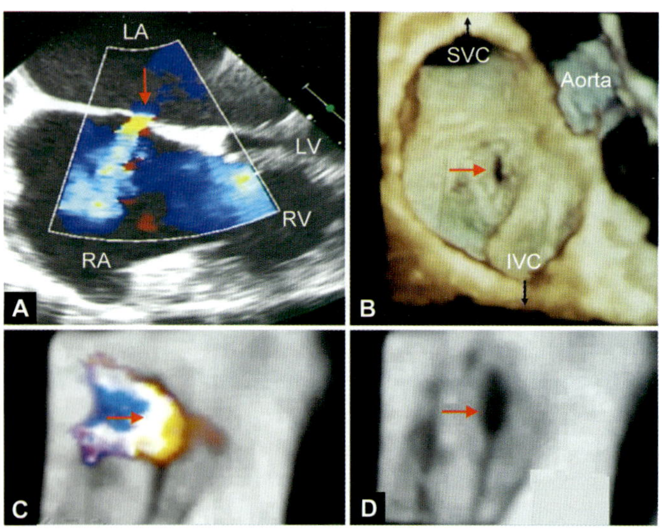

Figures 42A to D (A) 2D TEE four chamber image and shows the presence of left to right shunt across IAS; (B) 3D TEE image of the ASD and shows an atrial septal defect, situated at superior border of the fossa ovalis. The shape of the post PTMC atrial septal defects is dependent on the cross sectional profile of the balloon and the angle at which the balloon penetrates the septum. In this case the defect is elongated in shape; (C) 3D TEE color flow image of IAS from the RA perspective and confirm the presence of the atrial septal defect; (D) Same as (C) but taken after suppression of the color flow. The similarity of the shape in (B) confirms that it is actually the same defect as being seen in (B)

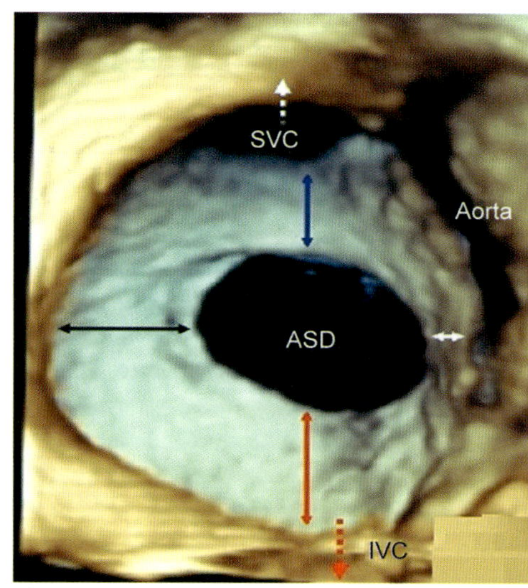

Figure 43 These margins are clockwise from top, SVC margin (white double headed arrow) aortic margin (green double headed arrow), IVC margin (red double headed arrow) and atrial margin (blue double headed arrow)

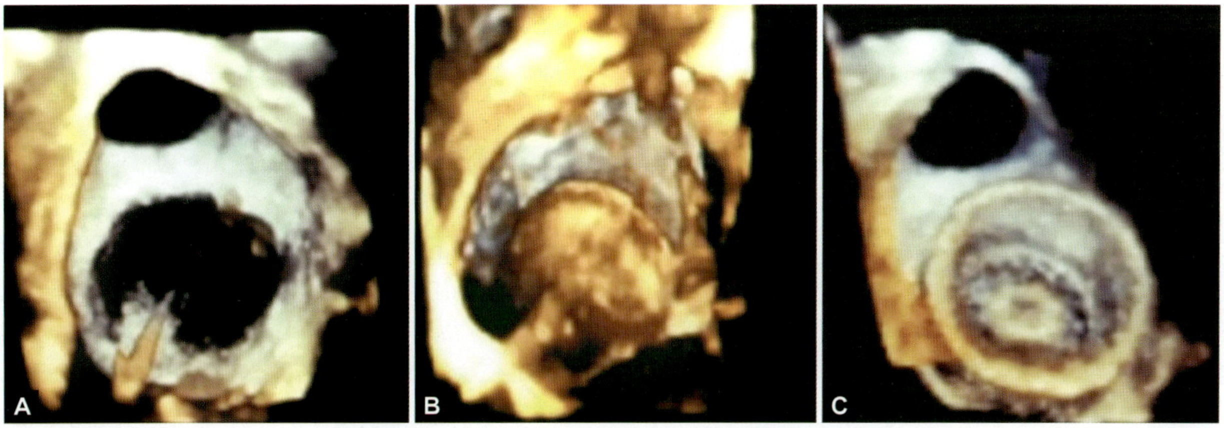

Figures 44A to C 3D TEE images of the interatrial septum form RA perspective, taken during the closure of a secundum ASD with a septal occluder device: (A) The positioning of the catheter across the defect; (B) Image of the device after it has been opened, but has not yet been released from the catheter. This image is used to evaluate the proper positioning of the device and it is relation to the surrounding margins as well as the orifices of pulmonary veins, SVC and IVC; (C) Taken after release of the device from the catheter and confirms that the device is properly positioned. A device which is properly positioned and firmly gripping all the margins of the defect should not have excess mobility

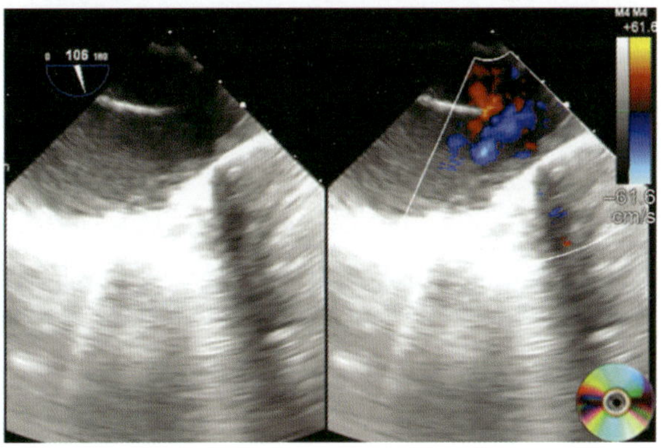

Figure 45 (Video 5) 2D and Color Doppler assessment of atrial septal defect. Midesophageal bicaval view showing superior vena cava type sinus venosus atrial septal defect shunting from left to right

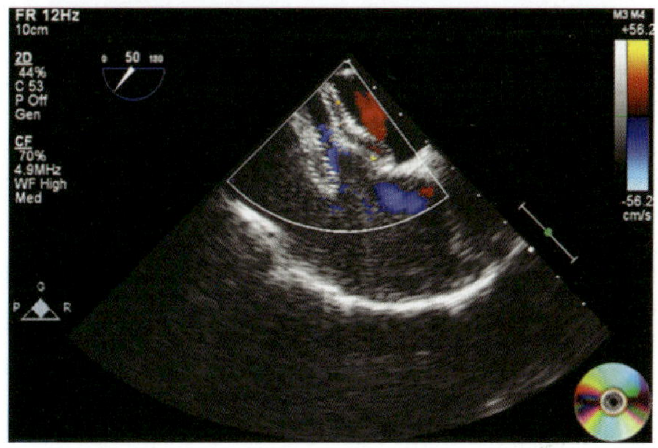

Figure 47 (Video 7) Color Doppler in midesophageal right ventricle inflow-outflow view showing the deployed amplatzer septal occlude device without any residual shunt across the atrial septal defect. In this view it may appear that the left rim of the device is resting on the aortic valve but this finding is just because of the angle at which the device is being imaged. In the midesophageal 4 chamber view it was clear that the aortic valve is free from the device

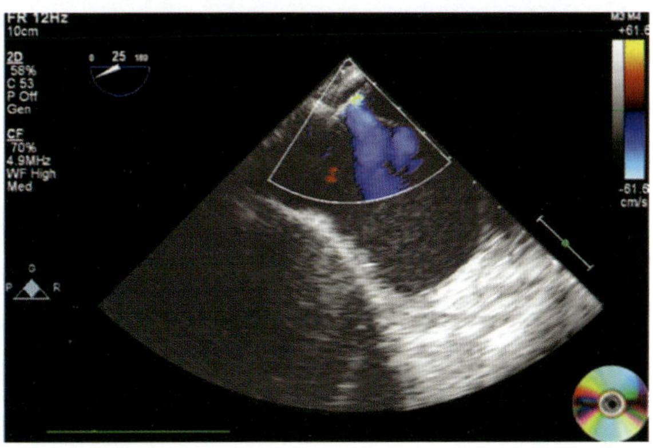

Figure 46 (Video 6) Color Doppler echocardiography in a patient for percutaneous atrial septal defect closure. The catheter containing the amplatzer septal occluder is seen traversing the atrial septal defect. A small mosaic jet is seen along the catheter

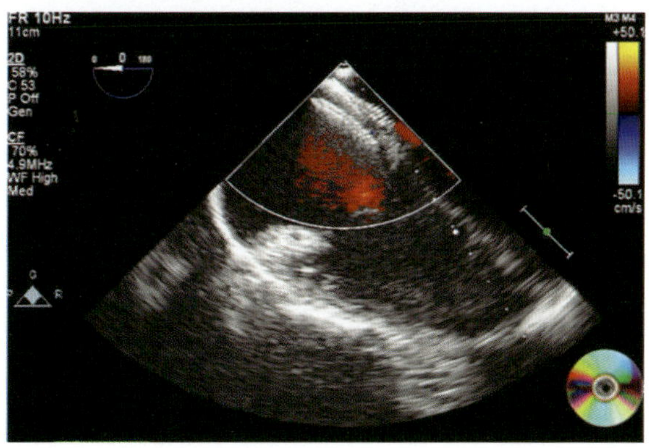

Figure 48 (Video 8) Color Doppler in midesophageal 4 chamber view showing a fully deployed and well approximated amplatzer septal occluder with no residual shunt and free of mitral valve annulus

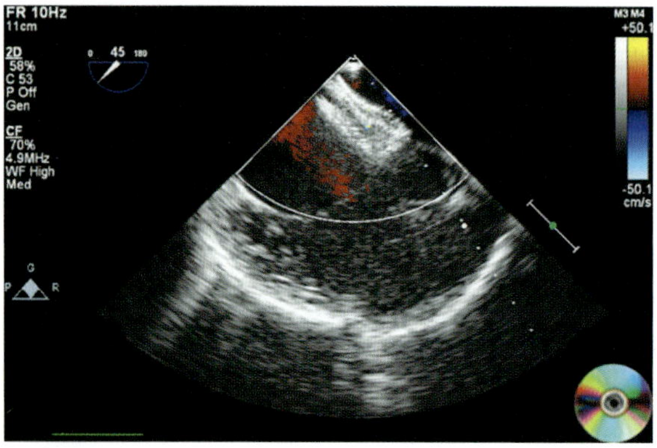

Figure 49 (Video 9) Color Doppler in midesophageal right ventricle inflow-outflow view showing a fully deployed and well approximated amplatzer septal occluder with no residual shunt and free of mitral valve annulus

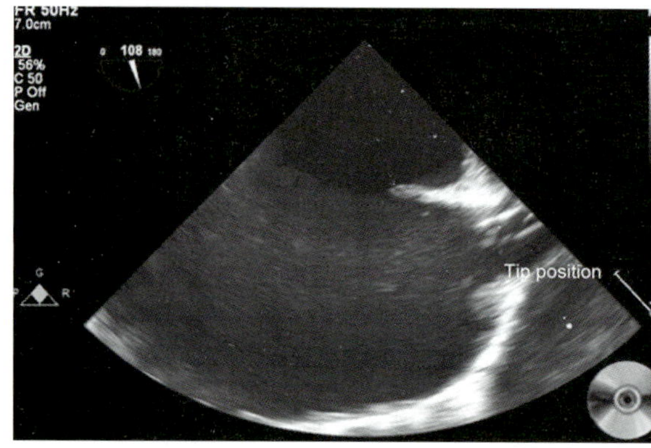

Figure 52 (Video 12) 2D echo for percutaneous cannulation of superior vena cava. Midesophageal bicaval view showing superior vena cava cannula for robotic atrial septal defect closure. The cannula tip is at the junction of right atrium and superior vena cava which is the correct position of the cannula

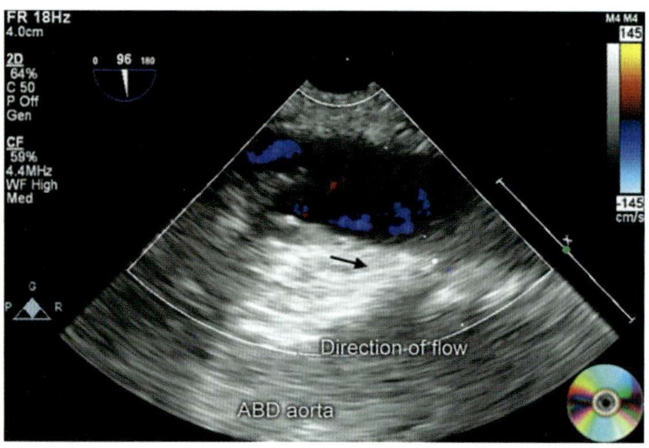

Figure 50 (Video 10) Color Doppler in midesophageal descending thoracic aortic long axis view showing blood flow through abdominal aorta on cardiopulmonary bypass when perfused via a femoral artery cannula during Robotic cardiac surgery

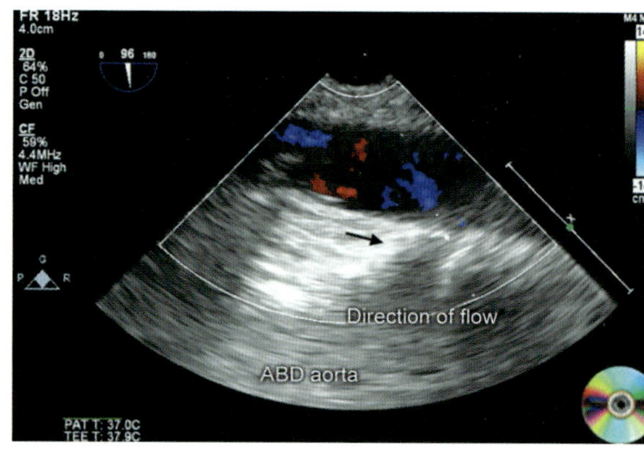

Figure 53 (Video 13) 2D echocardiography showing mid-esophageal descending thoracic aorta short axis view progressing to long axis view. This is the ideal view to visualize the retrograde guidewire insertion during cannulation of femoral artery in Redo surgeries, Robotic cardiac surgeries and placement of intra-aortic counterpulsation balloon. The tip of intra-aortic counterpulsation balloon may also be located in this view

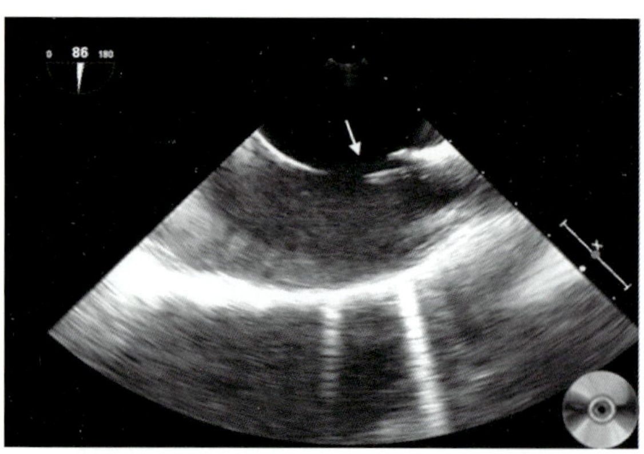

Figure 51 (Video 11) 2D echo for percutaneous cannulation of superior vena cava. Midesophageal bicaval view showing superior vena cava cannula for robotic atrial septal defect closure. The cannula tip is in the right atrium which is the incorrect position of the cannula

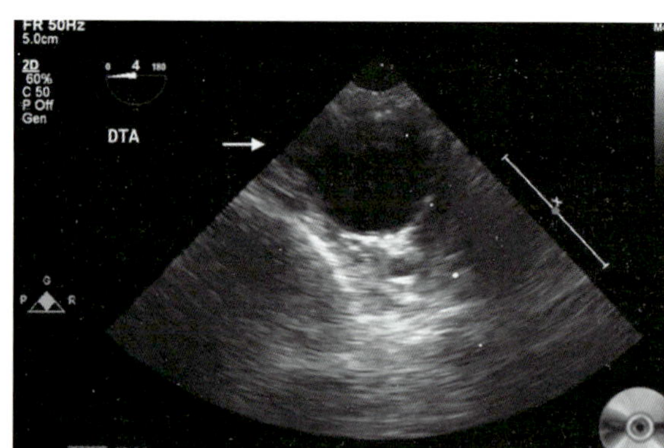

Figure 54 (Video 14) Color Doppler echocardiography showing blood flow in the midesophageal descending thoracic aorta long axis view. Note the non pulsatile nature of blood flow because the patient is on cardiopulmonary bypass. The flow is from left side of image towards right side of image

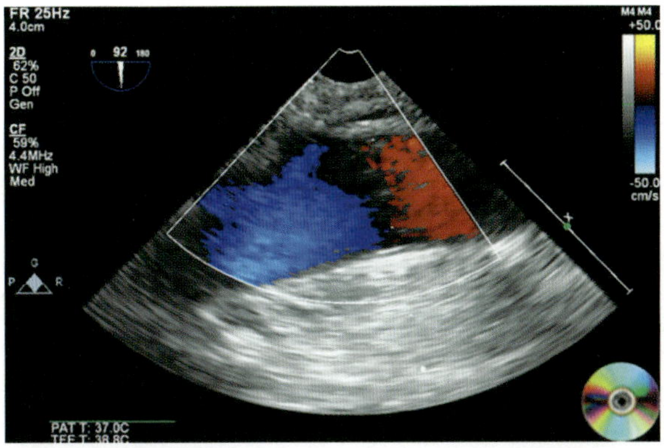

Figure 55 (Video 15) Color Doppler echocardiography showing blood flow in the midesophageal descending thoracic aorta long axis view. Note the pulsatile nature of blood flow and the flow is from right of image towards left of image

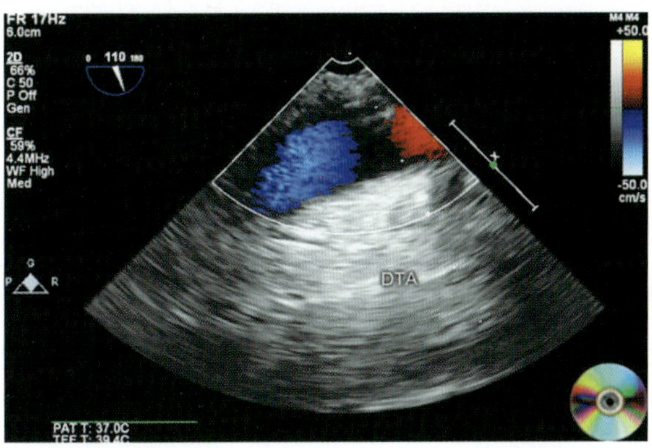

Figure 56 (Video 16) 2D echo showing the placement of guidewire in descending thoracic aorta for cannulation of the femoral artery. The arterial cannula is not visible because it rarely traverses the abdominal aorta

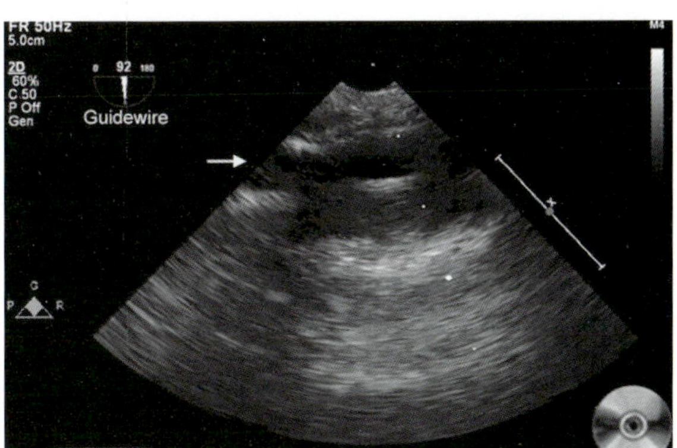

Figure 57 (Video 17) Color Doppler in midesophgeal descending thoracic aortic long axis view showing blood flow through abdominal aorta on cardiopulmonary bypass when perfused via a femoral artery cannula

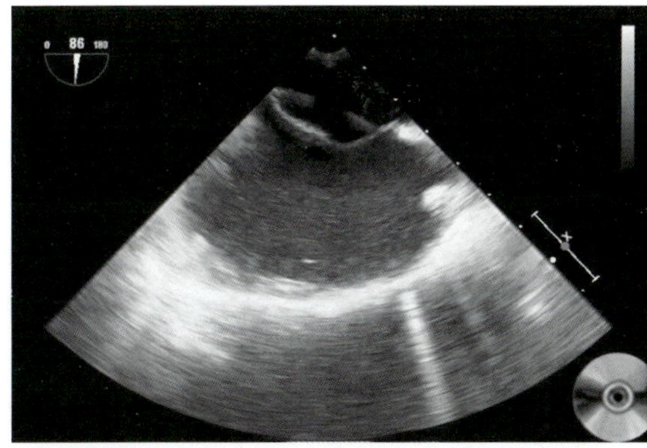

Figure 58 (Video 18) 2D echocardiography in midesophgeal bicaval view showing the placement of guidewire for percutaneous placement of superior vena cava cannula. The guidewire is hitting the interatrial septum causing arrhythmias

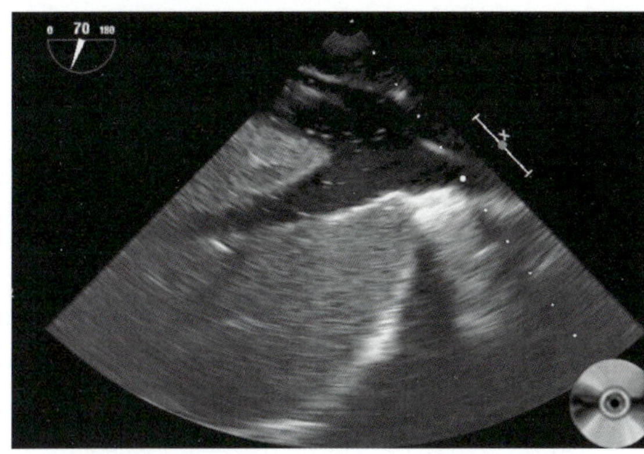

Figure 59 (Video 19) 2D echo for percutaneous inferior vena cava cannulation. Modified hepatic vein view showing guidewire placement for the placement of inferior vena cava cannula. The cannula should be 1 cm proximal to the inferior vena cava right atrial junction

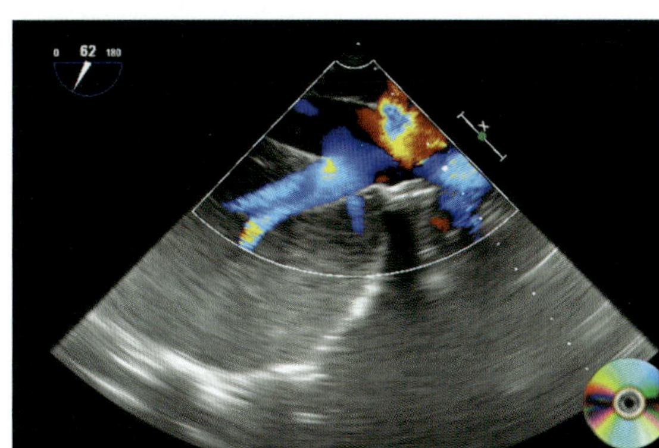

Figure 60 (Video 20) Color Doppler in modified hepatic vein view showing the confluence of hepatic and portal vein to form the inferior vena cava

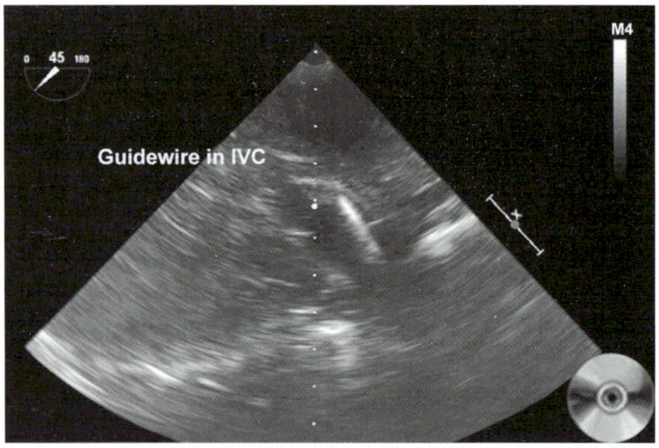

Figure 61 (Video 21) 2D echocardiography in modified hepatic vein view showing the placement of guidewire for percutaneous cannulation of inferior vena cava cannula

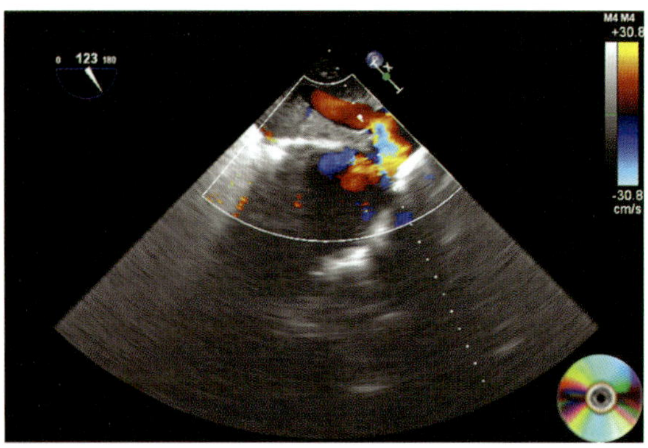

Figure 62 (Video 22) Color Doppler echocardiography showing the draining of inferior vena cava into right atrium in the modified deep transgastric view

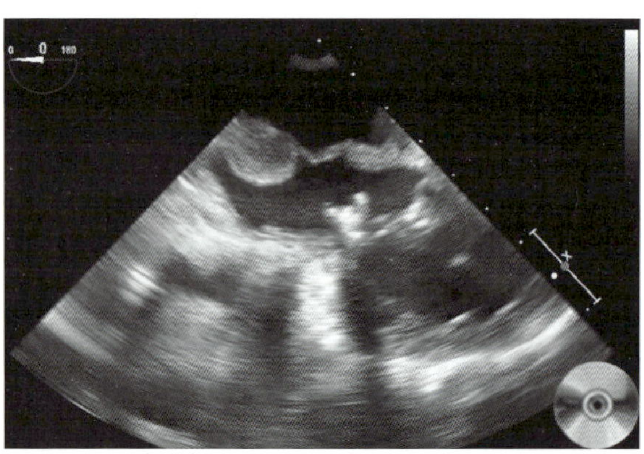

Figure 63 (Video 23) 2D echocardiography in midesophageal view showing left atrial hematoma after minimally invasive cardiac surgery

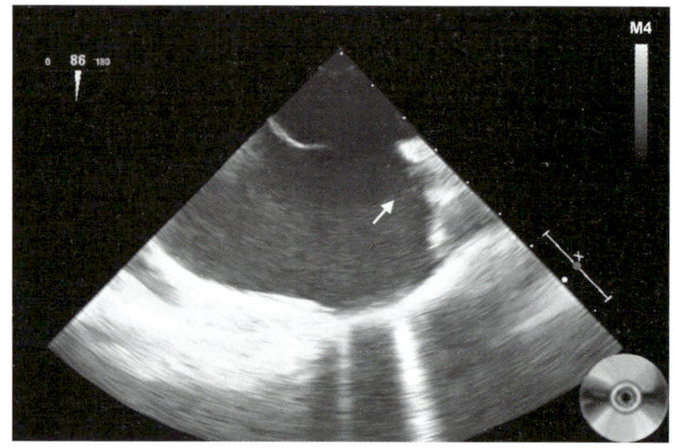

Figure 64 (Video 24) 2D echo for percutaneous cannulation of superior vena cava. Midesophageal bicaval view showing superior vena cava cannula for robotic atrial septal defect closure. The cannula tip is at the junction of right atrium and superior vena cava which is the correct position of the cannula

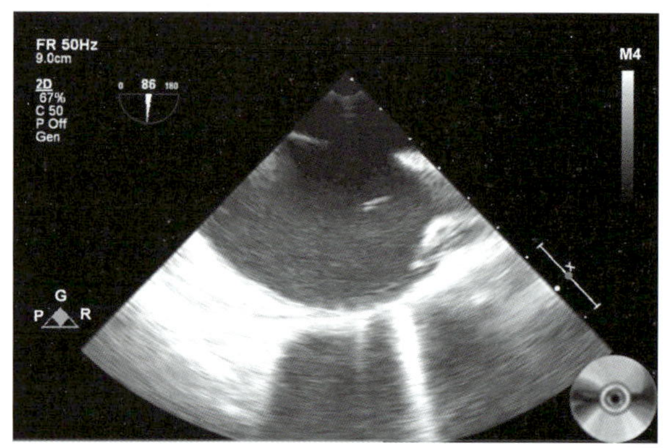

Figure 65 (Video 25) 2D echo for percutaneous cannulation of superior vena cava. Midesophageal bicaval view showing superior vena cava cannula for robotic atrial septal defect closure. The cannula tip is in the right atrium which is the incorrect position of the cannula

SUMMARY

- Two dimensional transesophageal echocardiography (2D TEE) is by far very superior to two dimensional transthoracic echocardiography (2D TTE) or three dimensional transthoracic echocardiography (3D TTE) to evaluate an ASD, as transesophageal echocardiography (TEE) is not hindered by the problem of poor echocardiographic windows.[6-8]
- In fact, an ASD is never taken up for device closure without first doing a TEE study to assess adequacy of its margins to hold the device.
- 3D TEE is further superior to 2D TEE as it provides all the needed information in a single view, which otherwise would take a series of 2D TEE views,

leading to inter- and intraobserver variation in assessment of the ASD.[9]

- The third, and probably the most important consideration in obtaining good quality 3D images, is to have optimal gain settings before the acquisition of the dataset. Low gain settings leads to echo dropouts and these parts cannot be seen in 3D images. On other hand, high gain settings lead to blurring of fine structural details.

FUTURE AND CONTROVERSIES

With increased experience over the years, transcatheter closure of suitable secundum atrial septal defects (ASDs) has now become preferable to surgical repair. Limitations currently include size and location of the defect. Perhaps the most innovative approach to surgical closure in many years was recently accomplished in the form of robotically assisted closure of ASD. Current technology allows for excellent visualization and magnification of internal anatomy, and the ability to perform surgery at a remote distance from the patient is now a reality. However, even with this amazing technology, today's devices will seem crude compared with future computer robots. Improved access and cardiopulmonary bypass technology will most likely make robotically assisted heart surgery a routine procedure in the near future.

REFERENCES

1. Cao Q, Radtke W, Berger F, et al. Transcatheter closure of multiple atrial septal defects. Initial results and value of two- and three-dimensional transesophageal echocardiography. Eur Heart J. 2000;21:941-7.
2. Chaturvedi V, Talwar S, Airan B, et al. Interventional cardiology and cardiac surgery in India. Heart. 2008;94:268-74.
3. Manjunath CN, Prabhavathi, Srinivas KH. Incidence and predictors of atrial septal defect after percutaneous transvenous mitral commissurotomy—A Transesophageal Echocardiographic Study. Indian Heart. 2009;61:113.
4. Ishikura F, Nagata S, Yasuda S, et al. Residual atrial septal perforation after percutaneous transvenous mitral commissurotomy with Inoue balloon catheter. Am Heart J. 1990;120:873-8.
5. Cequier A, Bonan R, Serra A, et al. Left-to-right atrial shunting after percutaneous mitral valvuloplasty—Incidence and long-term hemodynamic follow-up. Circulation. 1990;81:1190-7.
6. Peter H, Michael S, Burkhart AL, et al. Detection of ostium secundum atrial septal defects by transesophageal cross-sectional echocardiography. Br Heart J. 1983;49:350-8.
7. Morimoto K, Matsuzaki M, Tohma Y, et al. Diagnosis and quantitative evaluation of secundum-type atrial septal defect by transesophageal Doppler echocardiography. Am J Cardiol. 1990;66:85-91.
8. Su CH, Weng KP, Chang JK, et al. Assessment of atrial septal defect—role of real-time 3D Color Doppler echocardiography for interventional catheterization. Acta Cardiol Sin. 2005;21:146-52.
9. Sharma V, Radhakrishnan S, Shrivastava S. Transesophageal echocardiographic evaluation of atrial septal defects—How to explore the third dimension? Indian Heart J. 2009;61:328-34.

Chapter 5

TEE for Ventricular Septal Defect

Poonam Malhotra Kapoor, Parag Gharde, Sarvesh Pal Singh, Kalpana Irpachi

Chapter Outline

- Types of VSD
- Clinical Features
- Clinical Examinations
- CVS Examination
- ECG in Ventricular Septic Defect
- X-ray Findings in Ventricular Septal Defect
- Transesophageal Echocardiography in Ventricular Septal Defect
- Preoperative TEE Assessment
- Postoperative TEE Assessment: Using Same Views as for Unrepaired VSD
- TEE for VSD Device Closure
- Ventricular Septal Defect Complications
- Gerbode Ventricular Septal Defect

INTRODUCTION

Ventricular septal defect (VSD) is a deficiency in the interventricular septum—the perimembranous, inlet, outlet or muscular portion. The ventricular septal defect (VSD) is a heart malformation present at birth. A VSD, therefore, is a type of congenital heart disease (CHD). The heart with a VSD has a hole in the wall (the septum) between its two lower chambers (the ventricles).[1]

- VSD is the most common type of heart malformation present at birth (congenital heart disease).
- VSD lets blood shunt from the left ventricle to the right ventricle.
- VSD can overwork the heart.
- VSD can cause excess pressure in the blood vessels to the lungs (pulmonary hypertension).
- VSD, if small, usually needs no treatment.
- VSD, if large, needs medical management and then surgery to repair the VSD.
- VSD generally has an excellent long-term outlook.

TYPES OF VSD

Perimembranous/Infracristal/Subaortic VSD

It is the most common type, located in the membranous part of the septum below the aortic valve. It is well seen in the midesophageal (ME) four chamber view.[2]

- Membranous = Perimembranous VSD (75–80%—most common)
- *Location*: Posterior and inferior to crista supraventricular is near right and posterior (=noncoronary) aortic valve cusps
- *Associated with*: Small aneurysms of membranous septum.

Subarterial/Supracristal/ Subpulmonary VSD

It also known as supracristal, outlet or doubly committed VSD, this type is uncommon, and lies just below the aortic and pulmonary valves. It is well seen on the ME RV inflow-outflow view. This type of VSD is commonly associated with aortic regurgitation due to prolapse of the right coronary cusp of the aortic valve.

- Supracristal = conal VSD (5%—least common)
- Crista supraventricularis = inverted U-shaped muscular ridge posterior and inferior to the pulmonic valve high in interventricular septum
- *On chest X-ray*: Right aortic valve cusp may herniate → aortic insufficiency
- Best seen in ME LAX view at 120°.

Inlet VSD

It also known as canal-type or posterior VSD. This is found posterior to the tricuspid septal leaflet and may be associated with an atrioventricular canal defect. It is well seen in the deep transgastric view.

Muscular VSD

It founds in the muscular part of the septum. Muscular VSDs can be multiple (Swiss cheese septum).

- Muscular VSD (5–10%)
- Low and anterior within trabeculations of muscular septum
- May consist of multiple VSDs = Swiss cheese septum.

CLINICAL FEATURES

A large VSD may present with heart failure in infancy; small VSDs are usually asymptomatic. VSDs cause a pansystolic murmur at the lower left sternal edge, and as a general rule the smaller the defect the louder the murmur. The left-to-right shunting of blood can lead to pulmonary hypertension which can cause reversal of the shunt (Eisenmenger's syndrome). Decisions on VSD closure can be complex and should take into account symptoms, the presence of heart failure, the degree of shunting and the presence of pulmonary hypertension.

CLINICAL EXAMINATIONS

- Recurrent history of RTI
- *G/E:* built (poor weight again)
- Pallor (R/O cause of breathlessness)
- Cyanosis (Reversal of shunt)
- *Eye:* Congenital cataract, congenital rubella syndrome
- *Facies:*
  - *Elfin facies:* Supravalvular aortic stenosis
  - Down's endocardial cushion defect
  - *Mitral facies:* MS (malar flush and peripheral cyanosis)
  - Cyanotic facies
- *Ears:* Low set
- *Palate:* Cleft palate
- *Neck:* Web neck, short neck, low hair line (below C5)
  - Dyspnea
  - Tachypnea
  - Subcostal retraction
  - Acutely ill.

CVS EXAMINATION

- Pansystolic murmur at left ¾ ICS
- Ejection systolic murmur at pulmonary area
- Mid-diastolic murmur at mitral area
- Wide variable S_2
- Loud S_1.

Diagnosis

Congenital acynotic heart disease, probably VSD with left to right shunt with no signs of CCF and pulmonary hypertension patient in sinus rhythm with marasmus/ kwashiorkor.

To Summarize

- Cyanosis
- Clubbing +
- S_1S_2: Well heard
- P_2 may be single/loud
- PSM (3 – 5/6) grade

CHAPTER 5

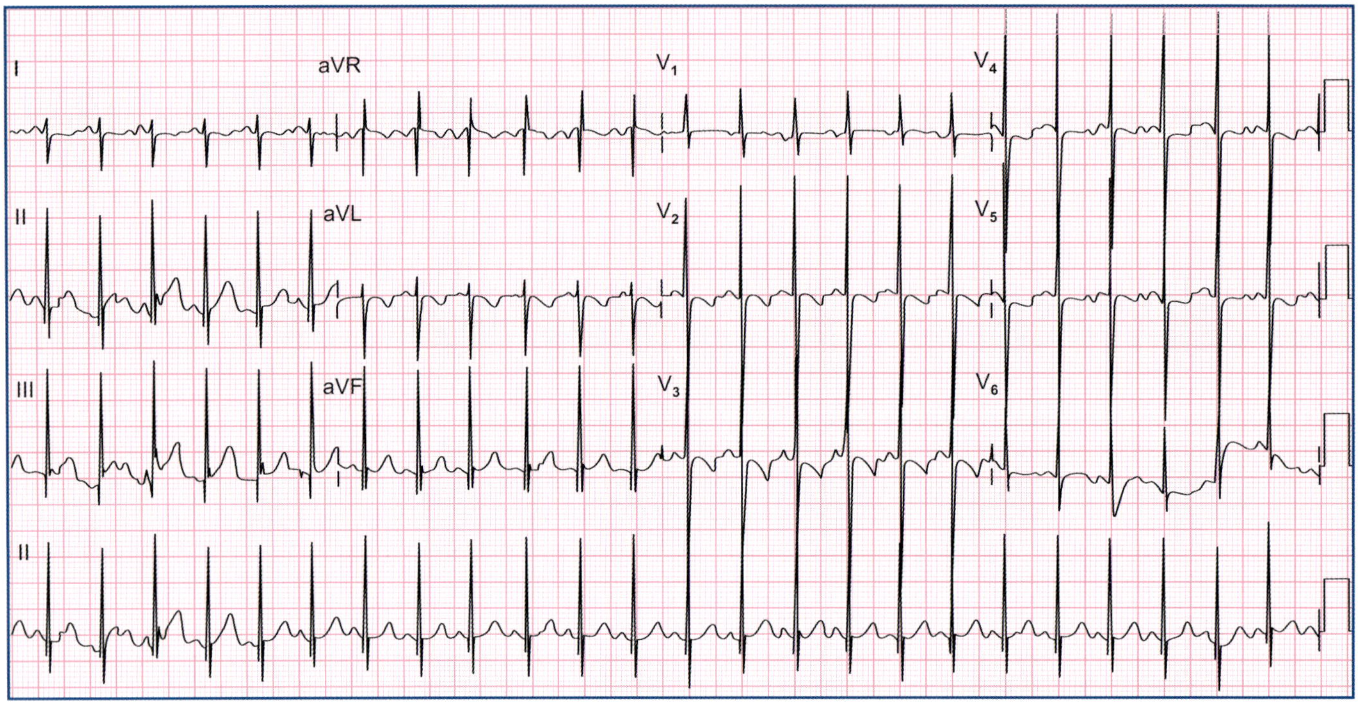

Figure 1 Katz-Wachtel phenomenon/sign on ECG in ventricular septal defect

Katz-Wachtel Phenomenon (Fig. 1)

Equiphasic R, S waves in leads V_2, V_3, V_4 showing biventricular hypertrophy.

Maladie DE Roger Syndrome

- Small VSD produces grade 5/6 PSM thrill
- Large VSD produces PSM of low intensity.

Name the Conditions where you get Precordial Bulge

- Right ventricular hypertrophy
- Left atrial hypertrophy.

Restrictive VSD

Offers high degree of restrictive at the septum.

Nonrestrictive VSD

No resistance at the septum, but present at pulmonary circulation.

Surgical Treatment

- Using a patch of woven Dacron or polytetrafluoroethylene (PTFE) as it obviates
- Approach through right atrium or right ventriculotomy.

Juxta-arterial VSD (AR + ASD)

- Absolute indication in cause where AR (aortic incompetence) has developed
- *Approach:* Transpulmonary
- Transatrial and transpulmonary (combination).

ECG IN VENTRICULAR SEPTIC DEFECT

- ECG changes in ventricular septic defect (VSD), if the defect is small the ECG may be normal while the pulmonary resistance is low the volume overload of the left ventricle produces features of left ventricular hypertrophy.
- As the pulmonary resistance increases right ventricular hypertrophy occurs as pulmonary and systemic vascular resistances become balanced and the left ventricular volume overload is lost.

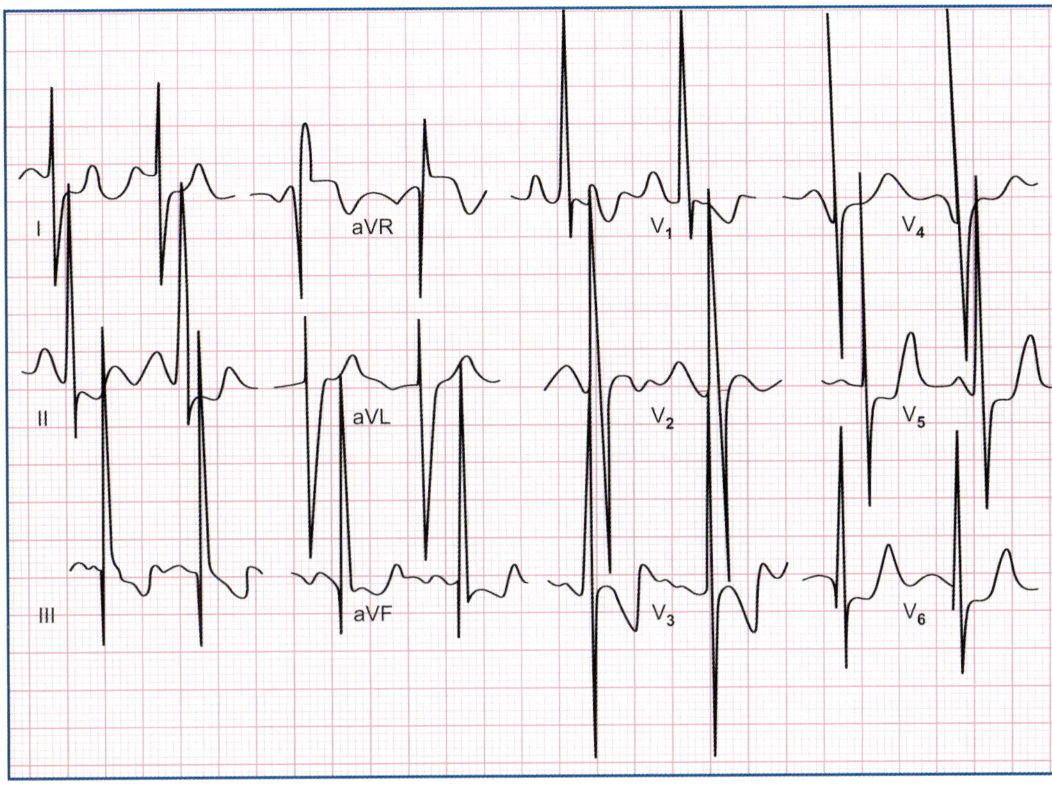

Figure 2 ECG in ventricular septal defect

- The left ventricular hypertrophy regresses leaving pure right ventricular hypertrophy to be the mainstay in large sized, chronic VSD **(Fig. 2)**.
- Right atrial abnormality (RAA).
- Left atrial abnormality (LAA).
- Right ventricular hypertrophy (RVH).
- Complete or incomplete right bundle branch block (RBBB).
- Left ventricular hypertrophy (LVH).
- If VSD is large, S_1, S_2, S_3 pattern may be observed.
- Prominent main pulmonary artery.
- Shunt vasculature (increased flow to the lungs).
- LA enlargement (80%).
- Aorta normal in size.

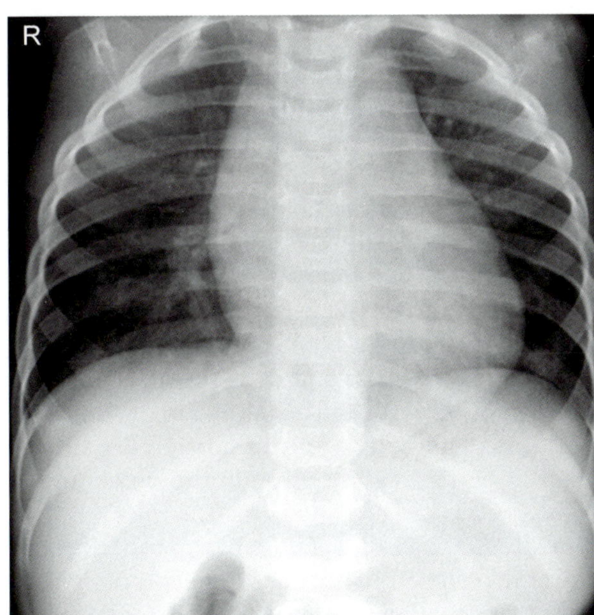

Figure 3 The right side of the heart with numerous VSDs

X-RAY FINDINGS IN VENTRICULAR SEPTAL DEFECT (FIGS 3 AND 4)

If the echocardiogram could not see all the problems, or the problems were very complex, it may be necessary to do cardiac catheterization. In this test, dye that can be seen by X-rays is put into the blood vessels. X-rays are then taken as the blood passes through the heart. This allows the doctors to see exactly where the problems are in the heart.

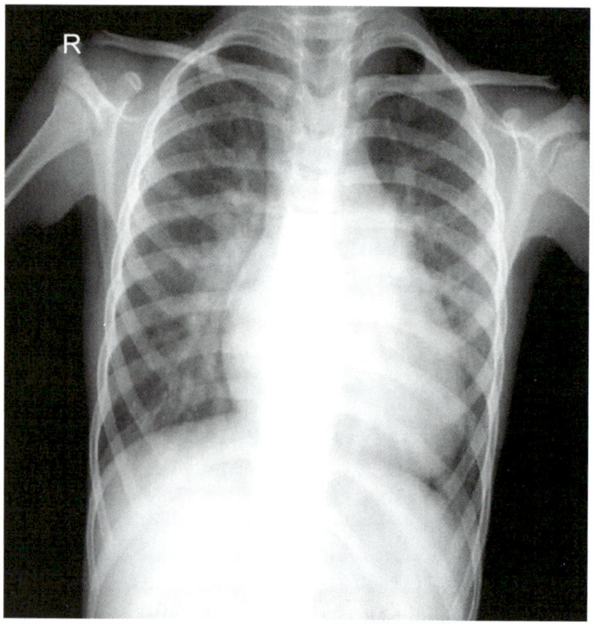

Figure 4 X-ray chest from an infant with large ventricular septal defect and pulmonary hypertension

TRANSESOPHAGEAL ECHOCARDIOGRAPHY IN VENTRICULAR SEPTAL DEFECT

- Two-dimensional (2D) and Doppler color-flow mapping may be used to identify the type of defect in the ventricular septum. Perimembranous VSDs are characterized by septal dropout in the area adjacent to the septal leaflet of the tricuspid valve and below the right border of the aortic annulus.
- The subaortic or anterior malalignment type of VSD appears just below the posterior semilunar valve cusps, entirely superior to the tricuspid valve. Subpulmonary VSD appears as echo dropout within the outflow septum and extending to the pulmonary annulus. One or two of the aortic cusps may be seen to be protruding through the defect into the right ventricular outflow tract. The inlet AV septal-type of VSD extends from the fibrous annulus of the tricuspid valve into the muscular septum; it is often entirely beneath the septal tricuspid leaflet.
- Muscular defects may appear anywhere throughout the ventricular septum. They may be either large and single or small and multiple.
- The anatomic localization of all VSDs is facilitated by coupling 2D sonograms with a Doppler system and by superimposing a color-coded direction and velocity of blood flow on the real-time images.

PREOPERATIVE TEE ASSESSMENT (FIGS 5 TO 21)

There has also been a profound change in the preoperative evaluation of patients with VSD in favor of using mainly noninvasive methodology with transesophageal echocardiogram (TEE).

- Size, site, number.
- *Size with reference to aortic annulus:* < 50% small; 50–75% moderate and >75% large.

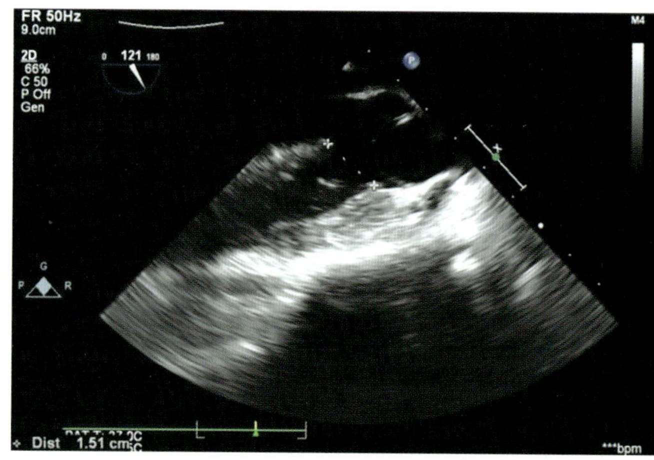

Figure 5 Midesophageal (ME) LAX view showing subaortic VSD and aortic over-ride of nearly 50%. The size of the VSD is compared to the size of the aortic annulus for routability of VSD during repair, especially in adult CHD

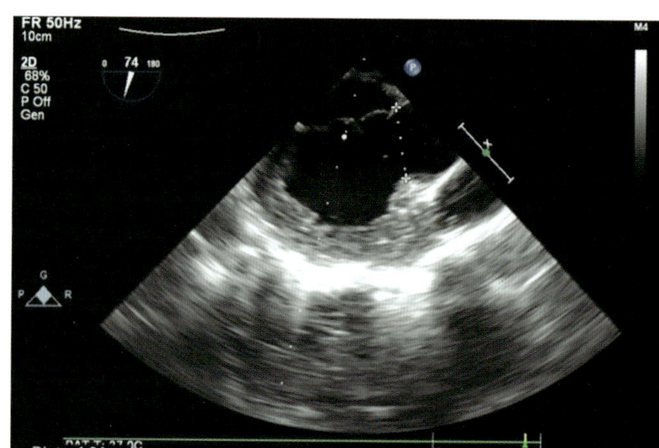

Figure 6 ME aortic valve SAX view showing subaortic VSD measuring 94 cm

- *Shunting:* Significant shunting = Qp/Qs > 1.5–2/1 and LA/Aorta > 1.2/1
- Gradient—restrictive or unrestrictive; RVSP = SBP - gr across VSD **(Table 1)**
- RV dilatation, LAE
- Prolapse of septal leaflet of TV or chordae - TR, RVSP (PASP) = gr TR + RAP
- Prolapse of right coronary cusp - AR
- Presence or absence of subaortic membrane
- Presence or absence of supramitral ring
- Rule out pulmonary stenosis
- Look for pulmonary vein stenosis
- ASD/PDA/coarctation of aorta/LSVC
- Interventricular septum or VSD aneurysm
- Gerbode defect (left ventriculo—right atrial defect).

TABLE 1 Gradients in ventricular septal defects

VSD	*Peak pressure*	*LA /LV dilatation*	*PAP*
Restrictive	>75	No	NL
Moderately restrictive	25–75	↑	↑
Nonrestrictive	<25	↑↑	↑↑

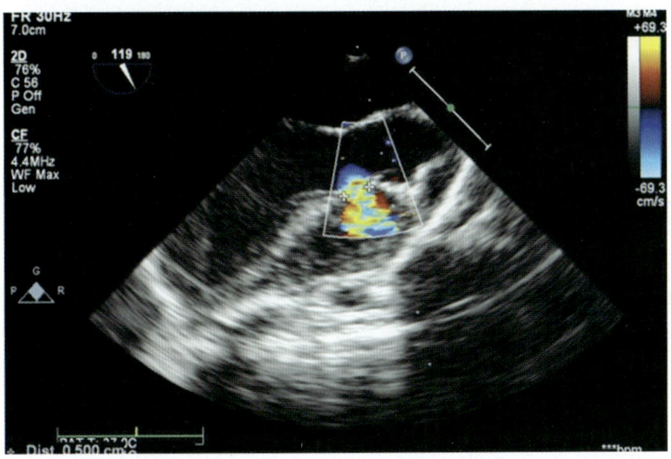

Figure 7 ME LAX view showing turbulence across VSD—suggesting restrictive flow pattern

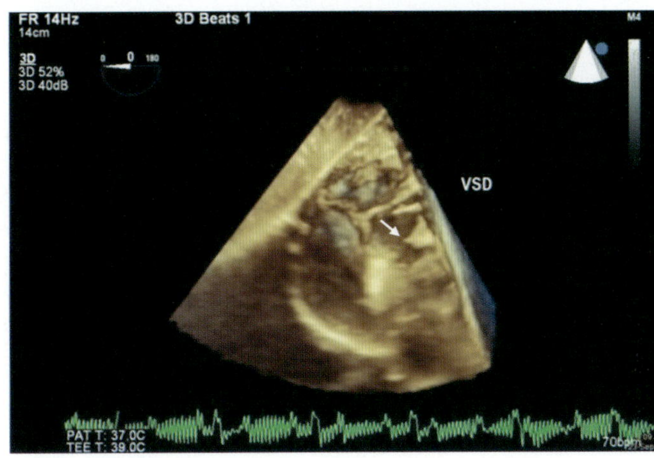

Figure 9 3D echo—transgastric view showing subaortic VSD (arrow)

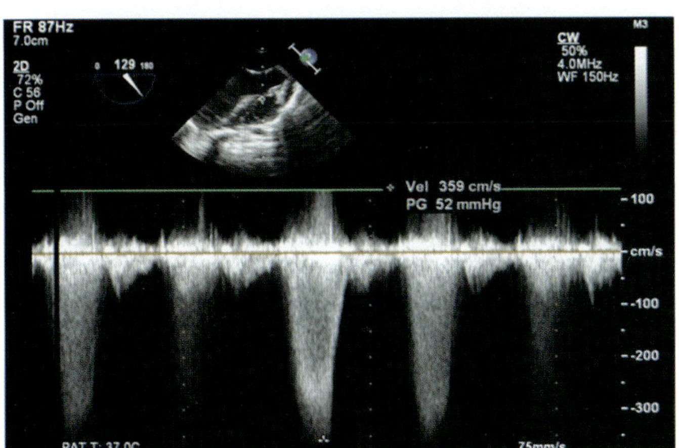

Figure 8 Continuous wave Doppler showing pressure gradient across VSD. A mean gradient of 52 mm Hg is seen in this ME LAX view across the VSD

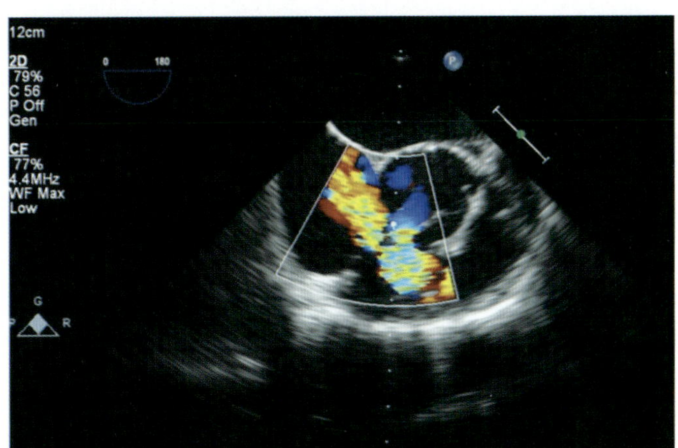

Figure 10 ME aortic valve SAX view showing prolapse of septal leaflet of TV into subaortic VSD causing tricuspid regurgitation. So a TV repair is done, along with VSD closure with a Dacron patch

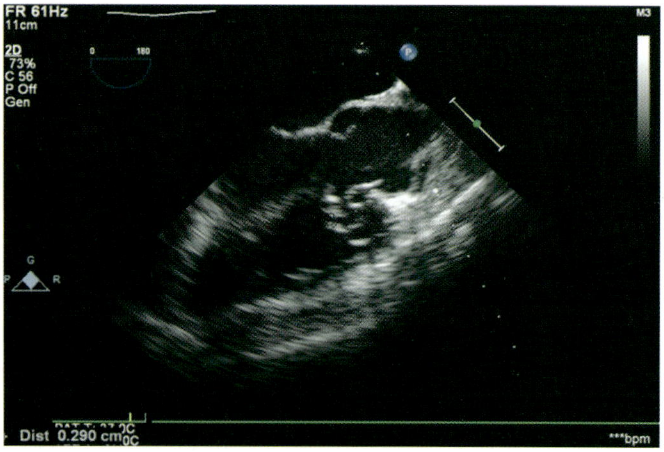

Figure 11 ME LAX view showing prolapse of right coronary cusp into subaortic VSD

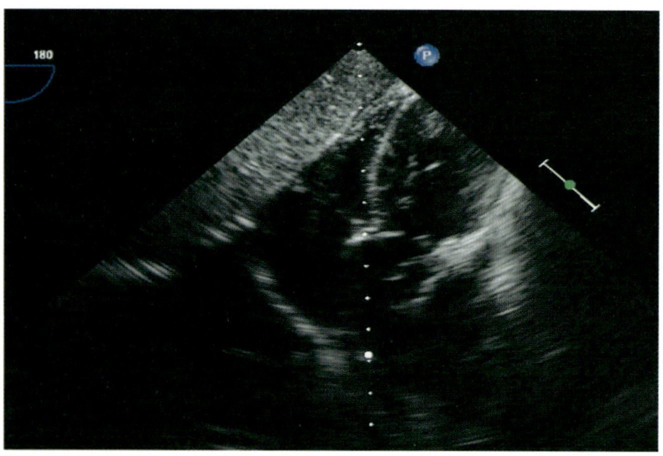

Figure 12 Deep transgastric view showing subaortic membrane (complete) just below aortic valve

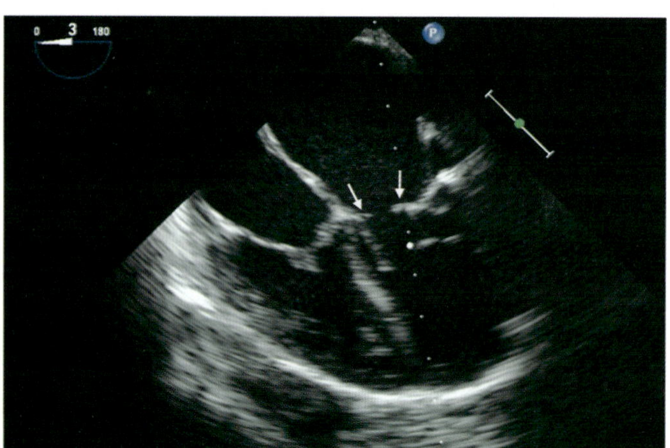

Figure 13 ME 4C view showing supramitral ring

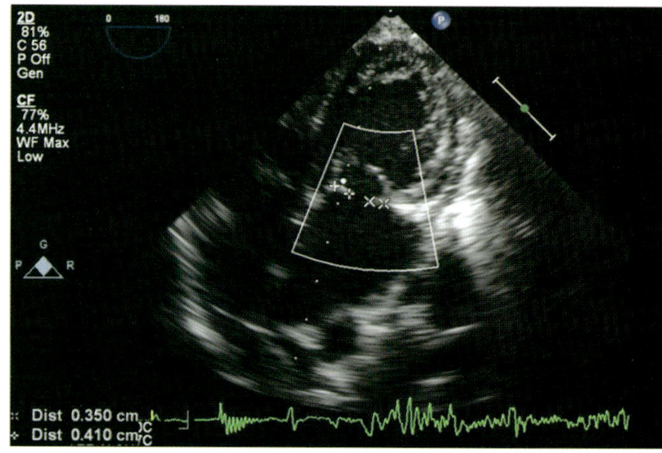

Figure 14 Deep transgastric view showing supramitral ring (complete)

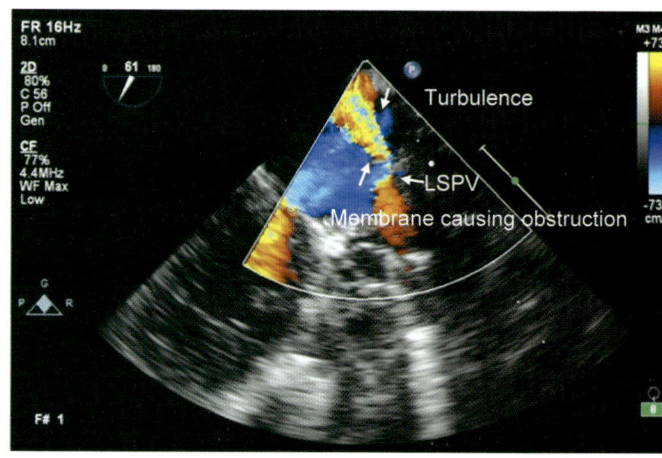

Figure 15 ME aortic valve short axis view showing left superior pulmonary vein stenosis in a patient with VSD

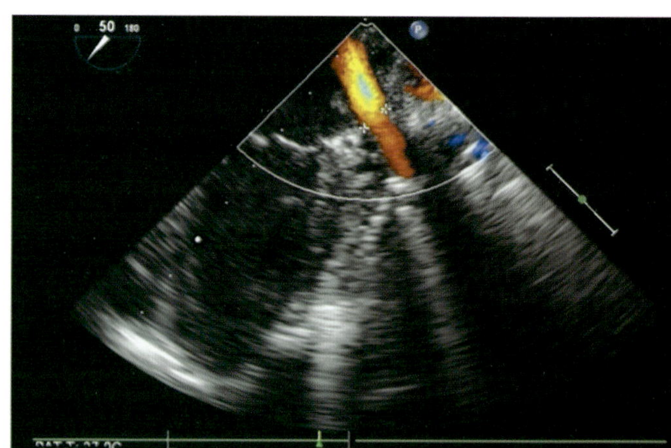

Figure 16 Modified ME aortic valve short axis view showing flow across left superior pulmonary vein after resection of membrane

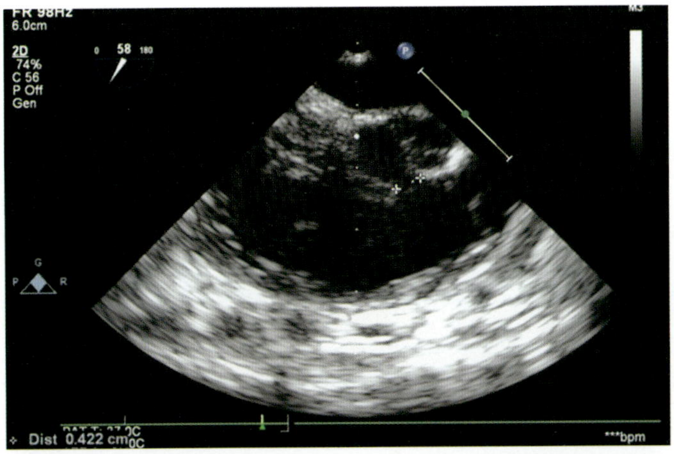

Figure 17 ME RV inflow-outflow view showing a subpulmonic VSD (note the contrast with subaortic VSD where the VSD is towards the tricuspid valve)

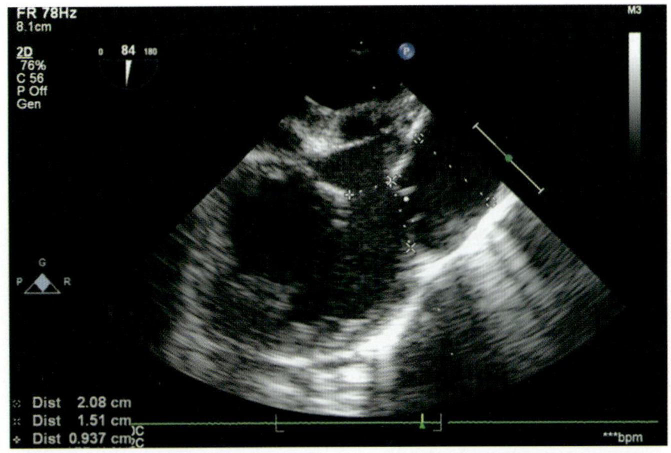

Figure 19 Doubly committed VSD—cardiac output enters equally both the pulmonary and systemic circulations

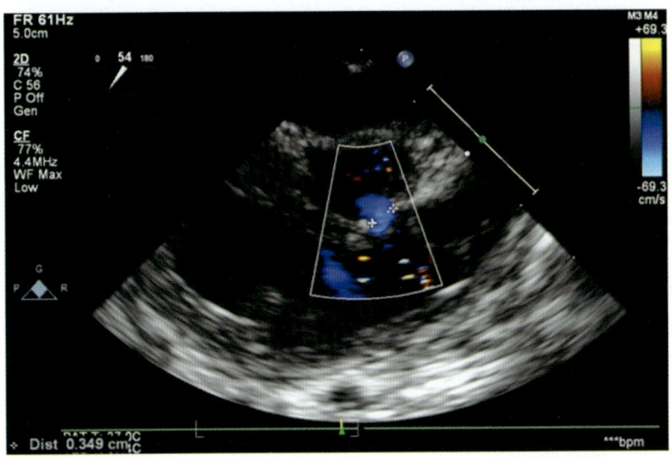

Figure 18 Color flow Doppler showing the direction of shunt from left to right side

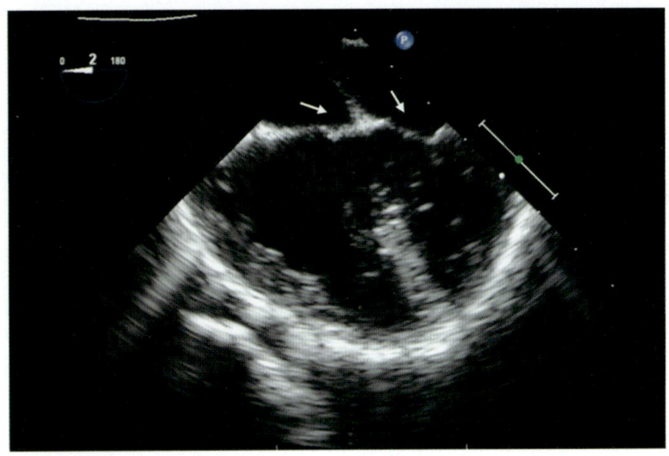

Figure 20 ME 4C view showing inlet VSD with both the tricuspid and mitral valves closed. Inlet VSDs are frequently associated with muscular extensions

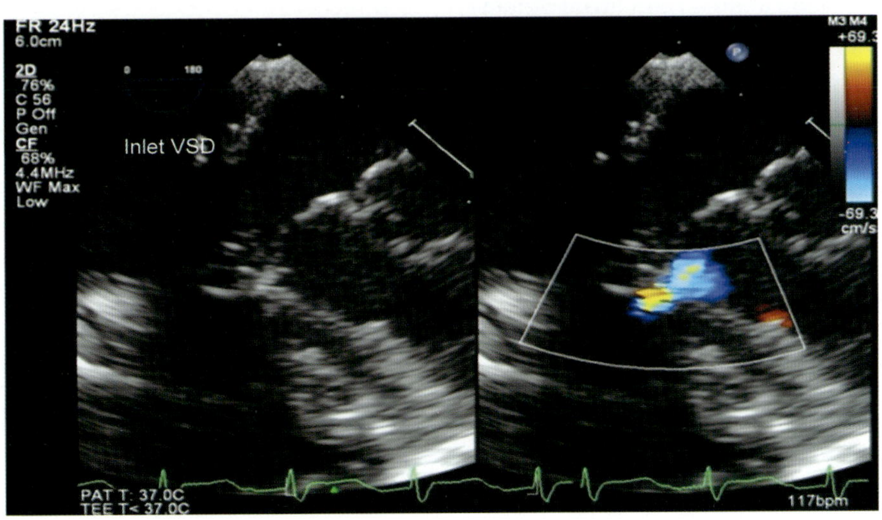

Figure 21 Color Doppler showing left to right flow across VSD

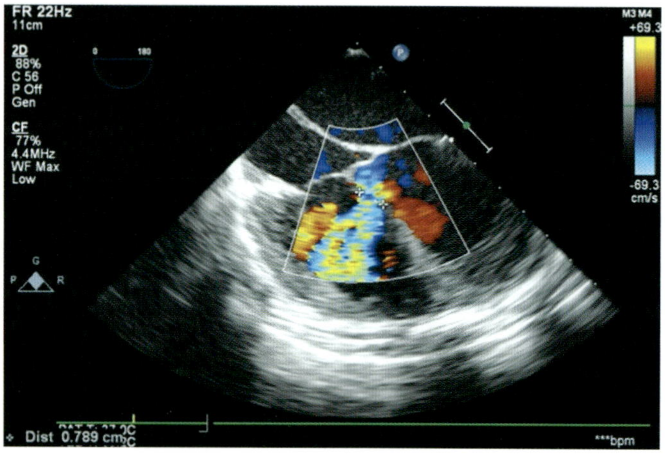

Figure 22 ME 4C view showing a muscular VSD. Note that there is a small amount of septum, the membranous part below which the muscular septum is deficient

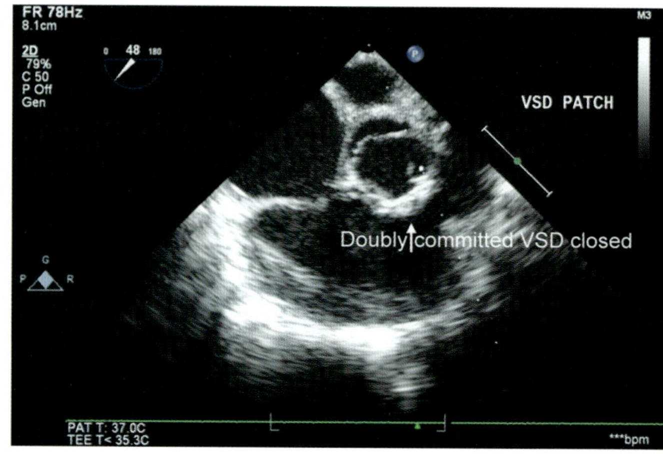

Figure 23 Post-VSD repair—Dacron patch is seen

POSTOPERATIVE TEE ASSESSMENT: USING SAME VIEWS AS FOR UNREPAIRED VSD (FIG. 22)

- Comment on the presence of a septal patch
- Residual shunt (size, direction of shunting and gradient); a high gradient signifies small shunt
- Additional small VSDs may be seen after closure of a large VSD especially in the muscular region
- Tricuspid regurgitation; if present severity and PASP
- Residual gradient across pulmonary valve or pulmonary vein
- Left ventricular function (LV stroke volume, wall stress and stroke work all increase after VSD closure)
- Post repair AR
- Gerbode defect (left ventriculo—right atrial defect)
- Assess pulmonary artery pressure
- Assess right and left heart size and function.

TEE FOR VSD DEVICE CLOSURE (FIGS 23 TO 34)

Pre-catheter Assessment[2]

- Define the defect location and size
- Determine the associated abnormalities like septal aneurysms
- Assess aortic valve anatomy for herniation or prolapse
- Examine the left sided structures and IVS motion
- Evaluate the RV thickness for PAH.

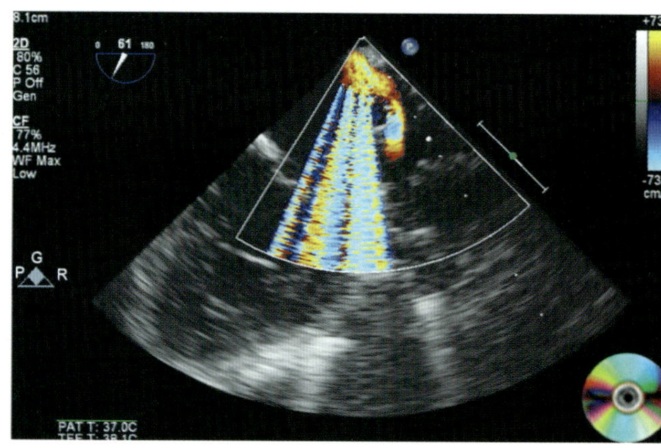

Figure 24 (Video 1) Color Doppler midesophageal aortic valve short axis view showing left superior pulmonary vein stenosis in a patient with VSD

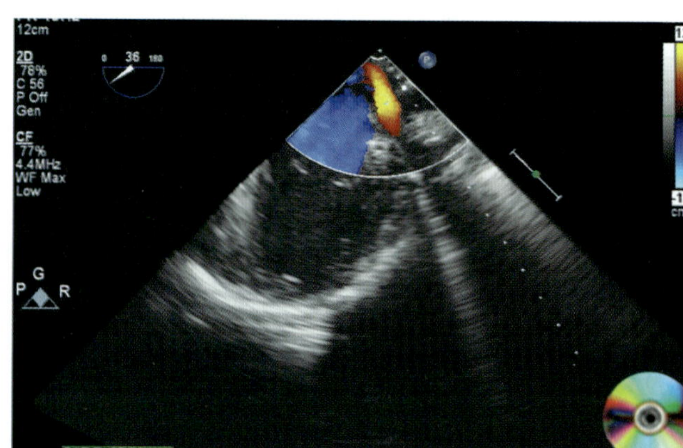

Figure 25 (Video 2) Color Doppler modified midesophageal aortic valve short axis view showing flow across left superior pulmonary vein after resection of membrane

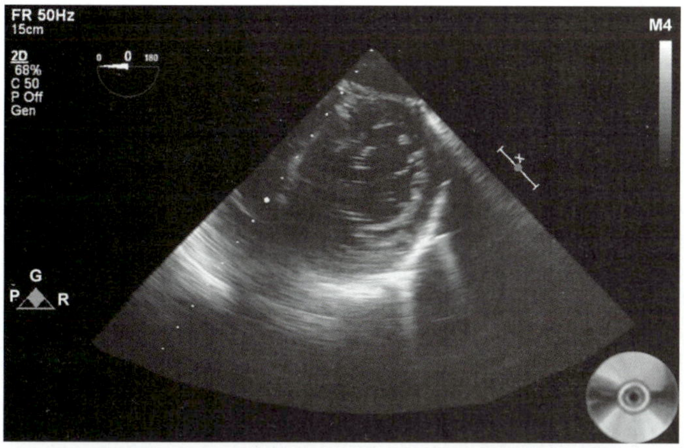

Figure 26 (Video 3) 2D assessement of mitral valve in atrial septal defect. Transgastric basal view showing the anterior mitral leaflet postcleft repair in the same patient with ostium primum atrial septal defect and moderate mitral regurgitation

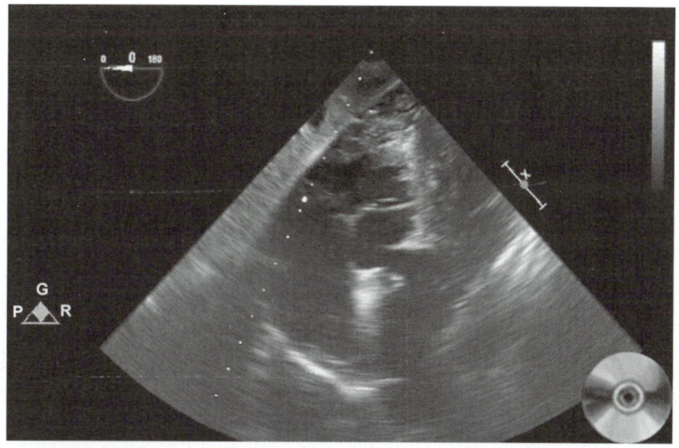

Figure 29 (Video 6) 2D echocardiography in deep transgastric view showing a subaortic ventricular septal defect just adjoining the septal leaflet of tricuspid valve

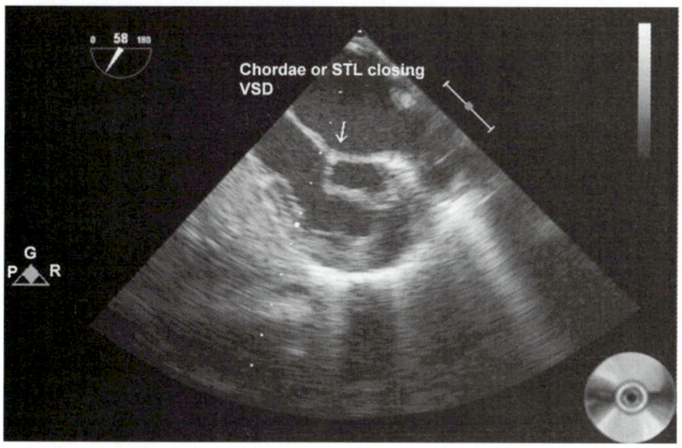

Figure 27 (Video 4) 2D echocardiography in midesophageal aortic valve short axis view showing prolapse of septal leaflet of TV into subaortic VSD causing closure of ventricular septal defect

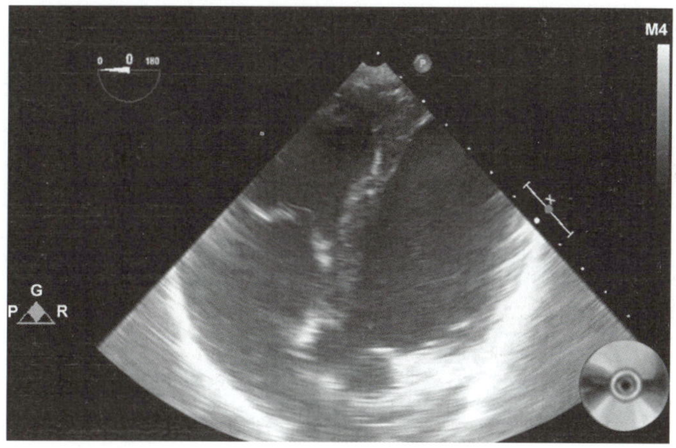

Figure 30 (Video 7) 2D echocardiography in deep transgastric view showing a subaortic ventricular septal defect just adjoining the septal leaflet of tricuspid valve and beneath the aortic valve

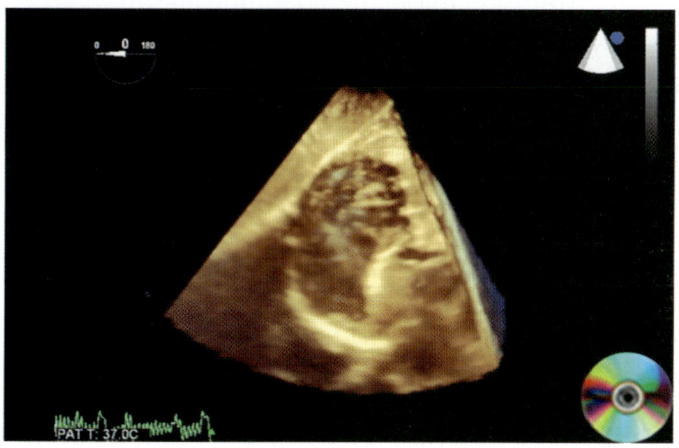

Figure 28 (Video 5) 3D echocardiography in deep transgastric view showing a subaortic ventricular septal defect just adjoining the septal leaflet of tricuspid valve

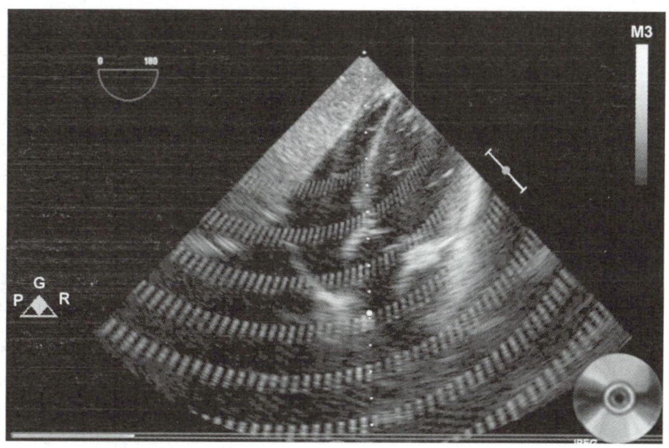

Figure 31 (Video 8) 2D echocardiography in deep transgastric view showing subaortic membrane (complete) just below aortic valve

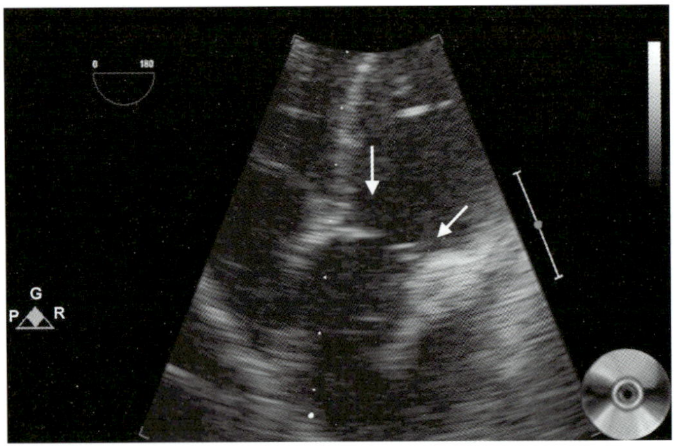

Figure 32 (Video 9) 2D echocardiography in deep transgastric view showing (closer look) subaortic membrane (complete) just below aortic valve

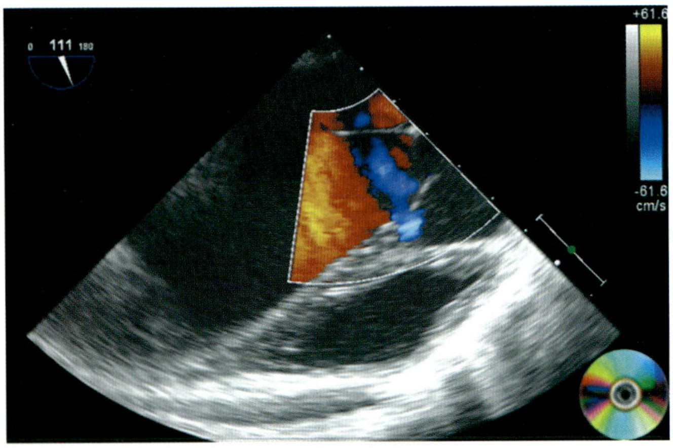

Figure 33 (Video 10) Color Doppler in midesophageal long axis view showing subaortic membrane (partial) just below aortic valve

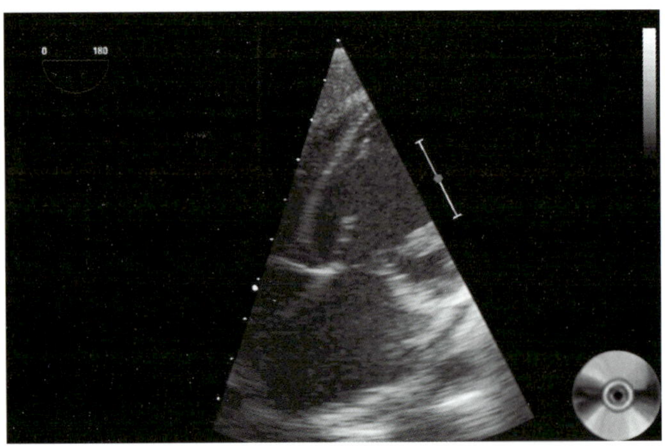

Figure 34 (Video 11) 2D echocardiography in deep transgastric view showing a supramitral ring (complete)

During Catheter Insertion

- Determine VSD anatomy and size
- Assess relation of VSD to ventricular inflows and outflows
- Assess the maximal defect diameter (balloon stretch sizing)
- Detect leaks around the balloon
- Guidance for device deployment/device stability
- Assess residual shunting.

After VSD Device Deployment

- Detect residual shunting
- Evaluate aortic valve incompetence
- Evaluate proper positioning of device
- Exclude embolization or erosion of catheter
- Assessment of ventricular function.

VENTRICULAR SEPTAL DEFECT COMPLICATIONS

Over time, if a VSD is not repaired, it may cause heart problems. A moderate to large VSD can cause:

- *Heart failure:* Infants who have large VSDs may develop heart failure because the left side of the heart pumps blood into the right ventricle in addition to its normal work of pumping blood to the body. The increased workload on the heart also increases the heart rate and the body's demand for energy.
- *Growth failure:* Especially in infancy. A baby may not be able to eat enough to keep up with his or her body's increased energy demands. As a result, the baby may lose weight or not grow and develop normally.
- *Arrhythmias:* The extra blood flowing through the heart can cause areas of the heart to stretch and enlarge. This can disturb the heart's normal electrical activity, leading to arrhythmias.
- *Pulmonary artery hypertension:* The high pressure and high volume of extra blood pumped through a large VSD into the right ventricle and lungs can scar the lung's delicate arteries. Today, PH rarely develops because most large VSDs are repaired in infancy.

GERBODE VENTRICULAR SEPTAL DEFECT (FIGS 35 AND 36)

A Gerbode defect is a ventricular septal defect communicating directly between the left ventricle and

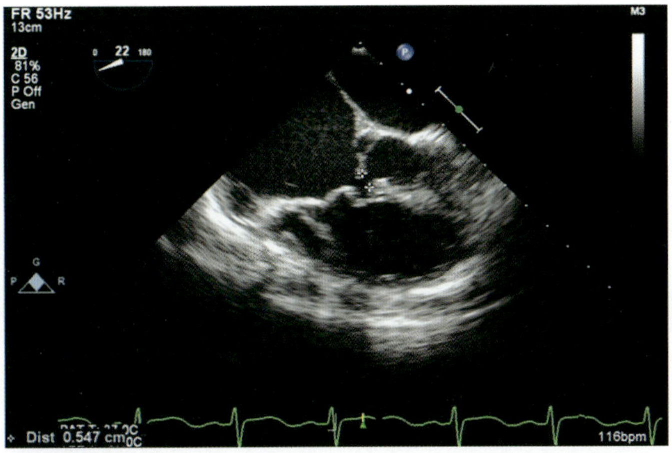

Figure 35 Gerbode defect (left ventricle to right atrial shunt)—2D in ME aortic valve short axis view

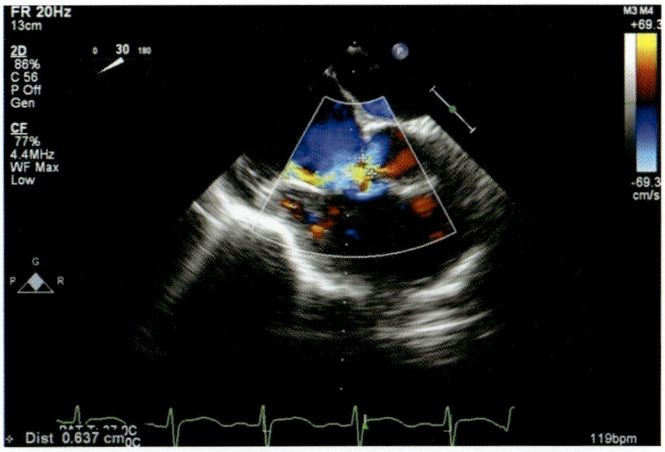

Figure 36 Gerbode defect (left ventricle to right atrial shunt)—color Doppler in ME aortic valve short axis view. Gerbode defect can be present initially or can be a result of a perimembranous VSD closure

right atrium. This is anatomically possible because the normal tricuspid valve is more apically displaced than the mitral valve. The large systolic pressure gradient between the left ventricle and the right atrium would expectedly result in an unmistakeable high velocity systolic Doppler flow signal. Yet, the diagnosis is rarely reported in the literature. One diagnostic echocardiographic pitfall is the mistaken diagnosis of Gerbode defect in a patient with a membranous ventricular septal defect. The flow from left ventricle to right ventricle can continue into the right atrium as a regurgitant jet.[3]

The **Gerbode ventriculo-atrial defect** is a very rare congenital anomaly. A Gerbode defect should be suspected on echocardiogram when there is an unusually dilated right atrium. The other sine qua non of the Gerbode defect is the high Doppler gradient between the left ventricle and the right atrium. The mean gradient is as high (95 mm Hg) as it is recommended closure of all as the spontaneous closure of these defects is very rare. The left ventricular-to-right atrial shunts cause these patients to have significant symptoms of either congestive heart failure, failure to thrive, or exercise intolerance. The operation to close these defects is quite safe. The defect is away from the conduction system and postoperatively, most of the patients revert to sinus rhythm with residual defects, no reoperations, and no significant tricuspid valve insufficiency. The Gerbode ventriculo-atrial defect is a rare defect with excellent surgical results.

CONCLUSION

Number, site, size and type of VSD is well visualised on TEE and this is a mandatory tool in VSD closure surgery and its outcome.

Outcome in well-selected patients with a small VSD is good. Surgical closure does not appear to be required during childhood as long as left-to-right shunt is <50% and signs of LV volume overload are absent, when PAP is not elevated, and no VSD-related AR or symptoms are present.

REFERENCES

1. Serraf A, Lacour-Gayet F, Bruniaux J, Ouaknine R, Losay J, Petit J, Binet JP, et al. Isolated management of isolated multiple ventricular septal defects. J Thorac Cardiovasc Surg. 1992;103:437-43.
2. Dua JS, Carminati M, Lucente M, Piazza L, Chessa M, Negura D, et al. Transcatheter closure of postsurgical residual ventricular septal defects: early and mid-term results. Catheter Cardiovasc Interv. 2010;75(2):246-55.
3. Faramarz T, Mohammad-Reza M. How to prevent echocardiographic misinterpretation of Gerbode type defect as pulmonary arterial hypertension. Eur J Echocardiogr. 2007;8(6):494-7.

Chapter 6

TEE for Atrioventricular Septal Defect

Sarvesh Pal Singh, Poonam Malhotra Kapoor, Arin Choudhury, Arun Subramaniam

Chapter Outline

- Chest X-ray: PAV
- ECG
- Transesophageal Echocardiography Views
- Preoperative Transesophageal Echocardiography
- Postoperative TEE Assessment
- Fetal Echocardiogram in AVSD
- Complications
- Long-term Outcome

INTRODUCTION

The ontogenesis of the apical portion of the atrial septum, of the basal portion of the interventricular septum and of the atrioventricular valves depends on development of mesenchymal masses (endocardial cushions).

There is a spectrum of size of the atrial and ventricular components of the defect which may range from very small to very large and altered formation of the atrioventricular valves.[1,2] In the *complete form* of this malformation there is an inferior interatrial communication or ostium primum defect, an interventricular communication at the superior aspect of the inlet or posterior muscular septum and a common atrioventricular valve. In the ***partial form***, an ostium primum atrial septal defect (ASD) is accompanied by a cleft or commissure in the left-sided atrioventricular valve and two functionally distinct atrioventricular valvular orifices are generally identified. The prevalence of these defects is frequent among patients with Down syndrome **(Figs 1A and B)**.

Complete atrioventricular septal defects (AVSDs) are typically associated with:

- Nonrestrictive intracardiac shunting
- Excessive pulmonary blood flow
- Excessive systemic pressures in the right ventricle and pulmonary artery.

Without intervention this may result in early pulmonary vascular changes and the development of fixed pulmonary vascular obstructive disease. The severity of atrioventricular valve regurgitation also influences the clinical presentation. Partial AVSDs are less likely to be associated with pulmonary overcirculation severe enough to cause significant heart failure symptoms.

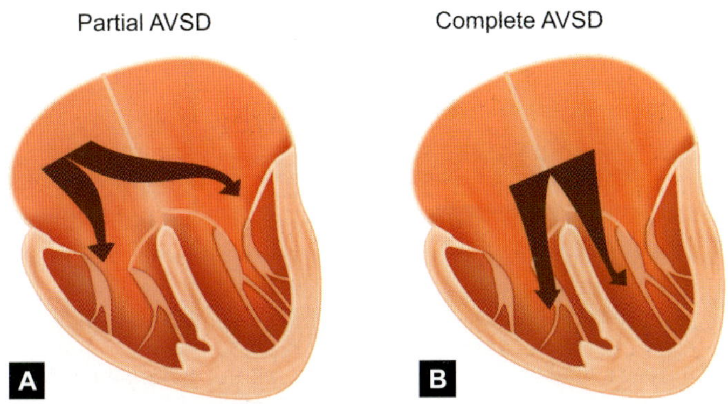

Figures 1A and B Diagrammatic representation of types of AVSD: (A) Partial and (B) complete

CHEST X-RAY: PAV

Chest X-ray (CXR) will vary depending on the extent of the AVSD. In those with a partial AVSD defect, CXR may resemble a secundum atrial septal defect **(Fig. 2)**.

Partial Atrioventricular Septal Defect

Cardiomegaly and increased pulmonary vascularity, both of which become more prominent with increasing mitral regurgitation.

Complete Atrioventricular Septal Defect

- The CXR will reveal cardiomegaly in most cases and there will be pulmonary vasculature congestion.
- Include prominent shunt vascularity markings toward the lung apices.

On lateral film, the posterior aspect of the heart may be enlarged, projecting into the airways and esophagus.

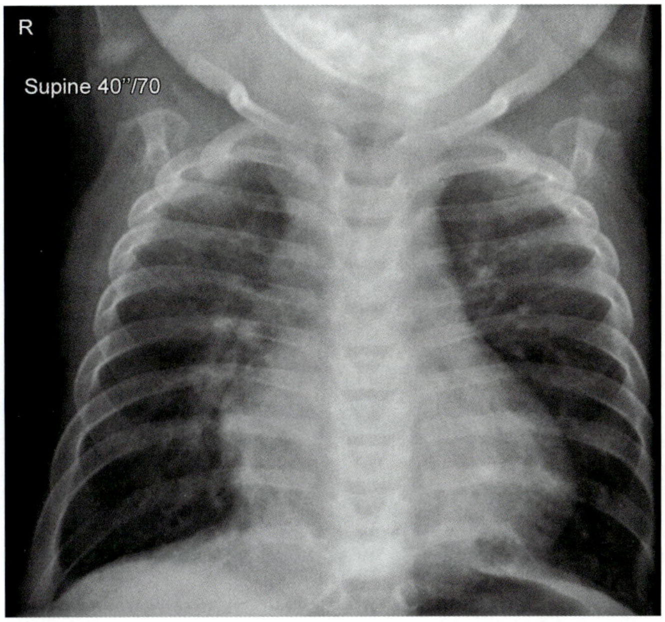

Figure 2 Chest X-ray of a patient with AVSD showing cardiomegaly and pulmonary, vascular congestion

ECG (Fig. 3)

As a result of the location of the AVSD defect the *normal* course of the conduction system is affected. The AV node is displaced inferiorly and the bundle branches are also abnormal. This results in a typical pattern of the electrocardiogram seen in almost all patients with an atrioventricular septal defect. The electrocardiogram (ECG) typically reveals:

- Leftward and superior frontal QRS axis as the ventricles are depolarized from a right inferior position to a left superior position

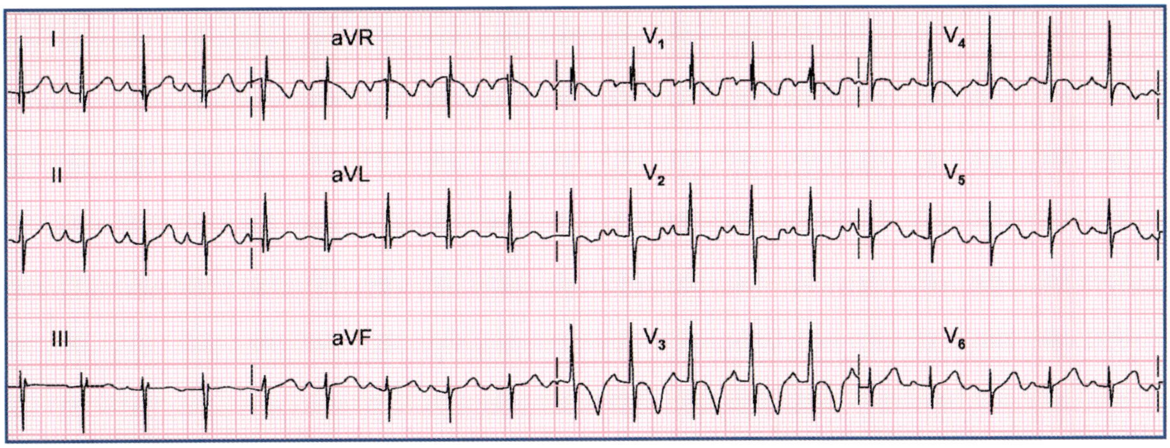

Figure 3 Electrocardiogram seen an atrioventricular septal defect

- A superior rightward axis may also be seen
- Usually sinus rhythm, but an associated first-degree heart block may be present
- Often an *rSr* pattern seen in the anterior precordial leads
- Evidence of right ventricular—or combined ventricular—hypertrophy present **(Fig. 3)**.

TRANSESOPHAGEAL ECHOCARDIOGRAPHY VIEWS

Transesophageal echocardiograph is most useful for diagnosis and management of AVSD and is usually best achieved from the:

- **Midesophageal (ME) four-chamber view**
- **Transgastric basal view**.

Together, these two views provide excellent visualization of:

- Atrial septum
- Ventricular septum
- Atrioventricular valve structure
- The degree of atrioventricular valve regurgitation
- Left-sided component of the atrioventricular valve
- Chordal insertions of the valve
- Patency of the outflow tracts
- Relative ventricular sizes.

With the addition of color flow Doppler, the assessment of atrial level and ventricular level shunting can be made.

PREOPERATIVE TRANSESOPHAGEAL ECHOCARDIOGRAPHY

Transesophageal echocardiography (TEE) provides outstanding imaging of the posterior cardiac structures such as the atrial and ventricular septa and the atrioventricular valves. However, because of its relative semi-invasive nature, it is utility in the young patient with an atrioventricular septal defect is greatest in the operating room. When performed prior to the operative repair, TEE can provide important information about:

- Insertion of the atrioventricular valve apparatus
- How the components of the valve are distributed to the ventricles
- The degree of atrioventricular (AV) valve regurgitation and the nature of the cleft off cardiopulmonary bypass, TEE can provide useful information to

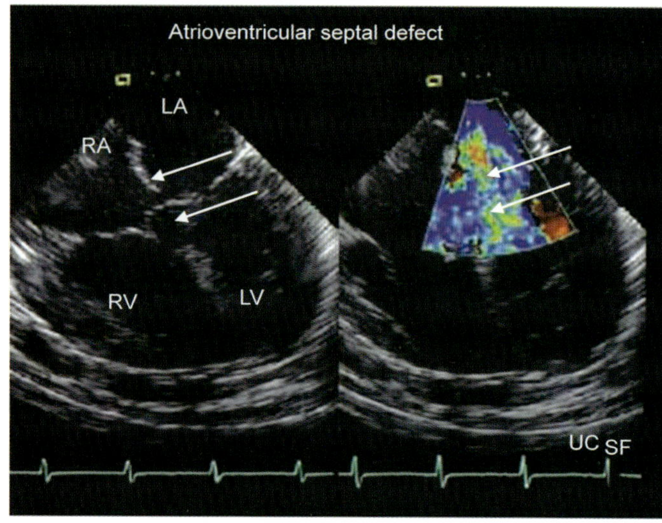

Figure 4 Complete atrioventricular septal defect. *Left:* Mid-esophageal four-chamber view demonstrating a complete atrioventricular septal defect, a primum atrial septal defect at the inferior aspect of the interatrial septum (upper arrow) and the posteriorly located, inlet-type ventricular septal defect (indicated by the lower arrow)

surgical and medical teams regarding the status of the repair and identify residual pathology.

- In patients with AVSDs, TEE is useful in confirming the anatomy and defining the type and extension of the septal defects.[3] Two- and three-dimensional TEE imaging has been shown to be of benefit preoperatively, not only during the initial repair but also when reinterventions have been necessary.[4,5] The deficiency in the atrial and ventricular septa and the large common atrioventricular valve can be readily identified in the mid-esophageal four-chamber view **(Fig. 4)**. The ventricular component of the defect is best defined during systole when the atrioventricular valves are closed.
- If there are dense chordal attachments to the crest the ventricular component may be delineated with color flow imaging. Characterization of the "bridging leaflets," which span the common orifice, assists in the classification of these defects into types A, B, or C as proposed by Rastelli et al.[1] according to the anterosuperior bridging leaflet morphology **(Fig. 5)**.
- The posteroinferior leaflet almost invariably has chordal attachments to the crest of the septum. Other information of interest that is well outlined by TEE includes atrioventricular valve competency,

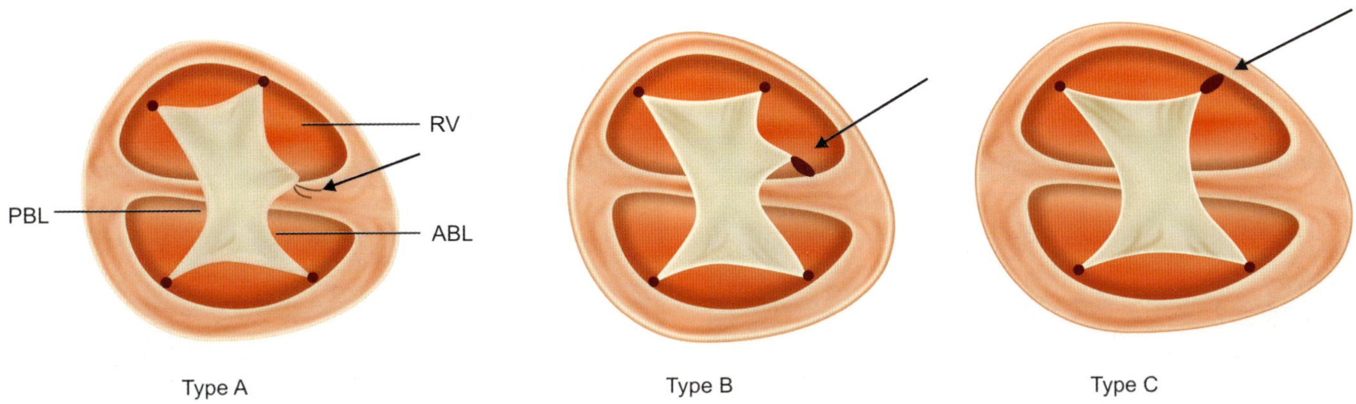

Figure 5 Schematic demonstration of the three different types of atrioventricular septal defects according to Rastelli et al.[1] (Type A) The anterior bridging leaflet (ABL) is attached to the crest of the ventricular septum (arrow), characteristic of a type A defect. (Type B) The anterior bridging leaflet is attached to a papillary muscle on the right side of the ventricular septum (arrow), characteristic of the type B defect. (Type C) The anterior bridging leaflet is unattached to the septum but is attached to a large anterior papillary muscle in the right ventricle (arrow), characteristic of a type C defect. (From Higgins C, Silverman NH, Kersting Sommerhoff B, Schmidt KG. Congenital heart disease: Echocardiography and magnetic resonance imaging. New York: Raven Press, 1990)

associated ventricular outflow obstruction, and noninvasive assessment of pulmonary artery pressures. Additional muscular VSDs can be found in 10% of the patients. Other lesions less frequently encountered include tetralogy of Fallot (3.5%), valvar pulmonar stenosis, double outlet right ventricule, truncus arteriosus and ventriculoarterial discordance.

- One of the most frequent associated lesions is left ventricular outflow obstruction, including subaortic stenosis either due to chordal attachments to the crest of the septum or due to a subaortic fibrous ridge (4%), valvar stenosis and aortic subaortic coarctation. Presence of a patent ductus arteriosus is common, particularly in Down's syndrome and can create an additional risk of pulmonary hypertension.
- In the postoperative patient, TEE can assist in the determination of residual defects, status of the atrioventricular valves, and evaluation of ventricular function. TEE is also helpful in the situation of assessing ventricular size, in unbalanced AVSD's where one ventricle is smaller an alternative surgical approach is pulmonary artery banding which allows the diminutive ventricle to grow.

Partial Atrioventricular Septal Defect (Figs 6A and B)

- OP atrial septal defect (ASD)
- 2 atria, 2 ventricles, 2 atrioventricular valves
- Tricuspid valve (TV) commissure between anterior tricuspid leaflet (ATL) and septal tricuspid leaflet (STL) and presence of a TR
- Cleft mitral valve (MV) with mitral regurgitation
- Inlet VSD—restrictive or no shunting.

Complete Atrioventricular Septal Defect: Associated Commonly with Down's Syndrome (Figs 7 to 10)

- Large ASD—common atrium
- Large VSD—inlet extending to muscular septum
- Single atrioventricular valve—4 cusps or 6 cusps (intermediate)
- Common AV valve or left or right AV valve regurgitation
- *Size:* LVOT and left and right AV valve annuli diameters (intermediate)
- *Balanced or unbalanced:* Either the flow from RA to RV and LA to LV is equal or one of the flows is more, i.e. one side is more dominant than other. Surgical options need to be decided accordingly. On TEE the IVS can be extrapolated and the intersection of IVS and the common AV valve will decide the dominance of left or right inflow.

Other Features

- Pulmonary artery—main and branch pulmonary arteries

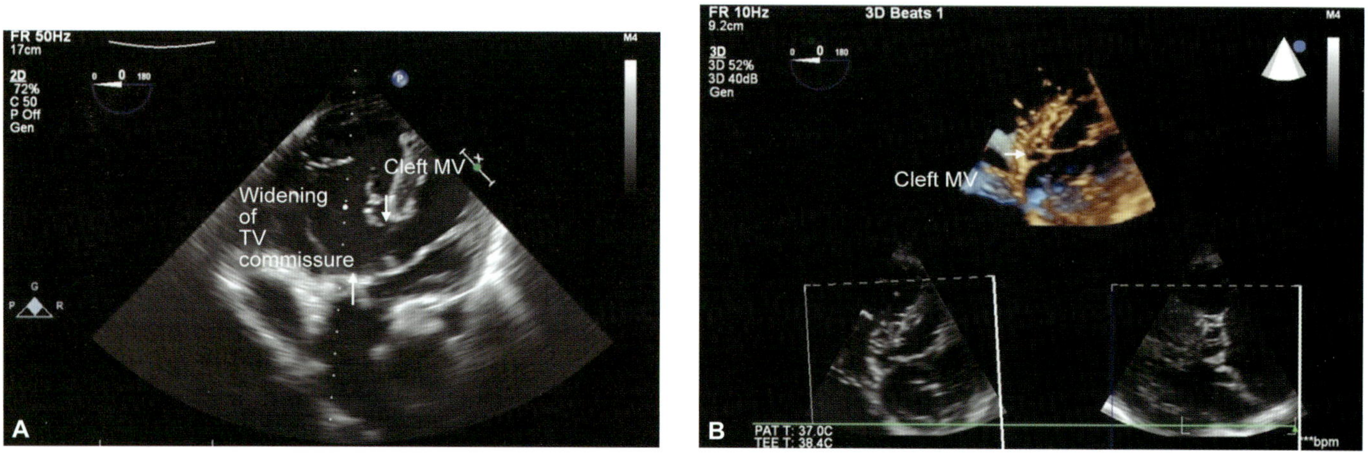

Figures 6A and B Partial AVSD: Deep transgastric view showing OP-ASD, inlet VS cleft mitral valve and widening of TV commissure; 2D and 3D images

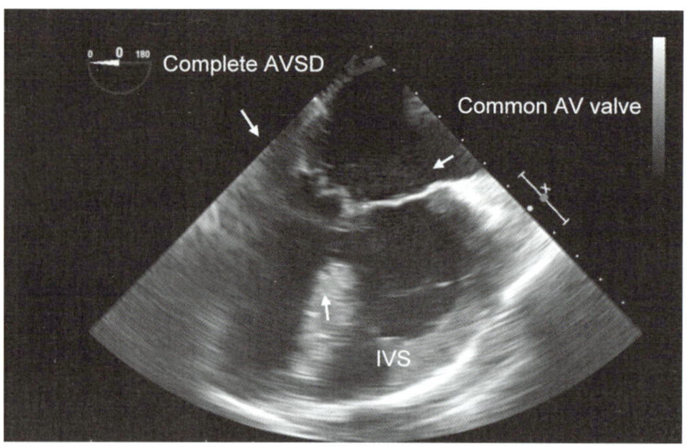

Figure 7 Complete AVSD: ME 4C view showing absence of interatrial septum, inlet VSD and a common atrioventricular valve

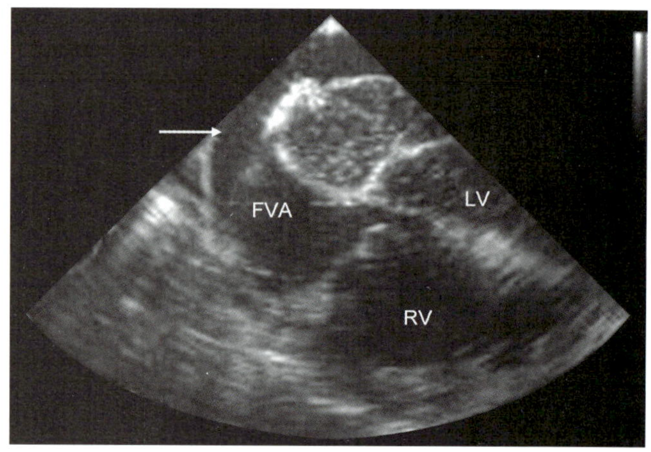

Figure 9 Mid-esophageal four chamber view of postoperative Senning showing contrast in the SVA to check baffle leak

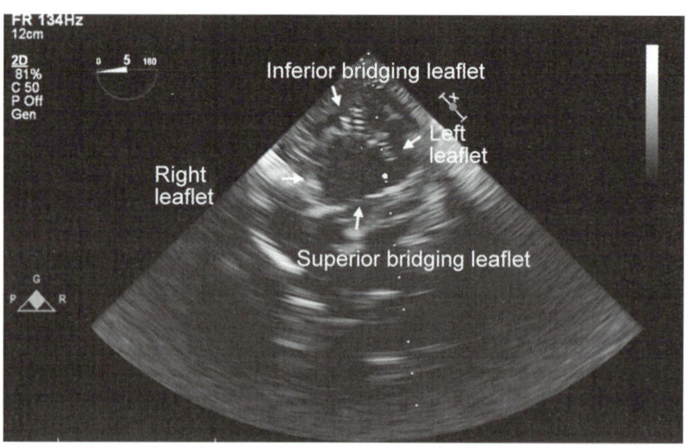

Figure 8 2D ECHO: Deep transgastric view showing a common atrioventricular valve in complete atrioventricular septal defect. The valve is in diastole and the right, left, superior and inferior bridging leaflet are seen. In case of intermediate atrioventricular septal defect, there are two distinct valves and two separate openings may be seen

- Pulmonary venous drainage
- Patent ductus arteriosis (PDA)/Coarctation of the Aorta (CoA)
- Tetralogy of Fallot (TOF)/Transposition of the great arteries (TGA).

POSTOPERATIVE TEE ASSESSMENT

- Size of both the ventricular inflow (AV valves) and any systolic anterior motion of anterior leaflet of left AV valve
- Function of both ventricles
- Residual shunting
- Regurgitation across both AV valves
- PA pressures.

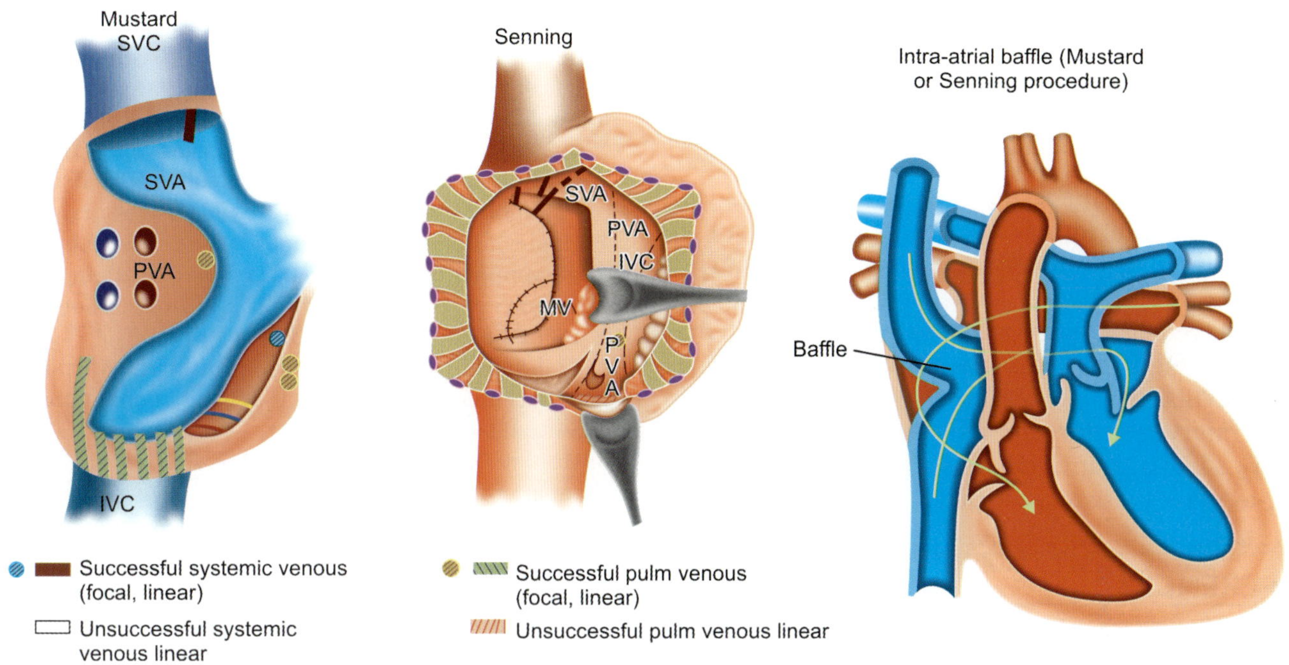

Figure 10 Baffle in Mustard and Senning procedure

FETAL ECHOCARDIOGRAM IN AVSD

Prenatally, fetal echo can accurately diagnose the presence of an atrioventricular septal defect. Characteristic findings can be seen as early as 12–16 weeks of gestation. The typical four-chamber view is distinctly abnormal in these cases as there is a deficiency in the central portion or *crux* of the heart. In addition, an assessment of ventricular size, AV valve regurgitation and associated defects can be ascertained. Because of the association of atrioventricular septal defects with genetic abnormalities and syndromes, a thorough fetal examination should be performed when such cardiac abnormalities are identified.

COMPLICATIONS

Most repeat surgeries following repair of atrioventricular septal defect (AVSD) are because of left atrioventricular (AV) valve regurgitation. According to Puga, Minich et al. and Hanley et al. significant postoperative AV valve regurgitation occurs in 10–15% of patients, necessitating additional surgery for valve repair or replacement in 7–12% of patients.[6,7]

With improved understanding of the conduction system in atrioventricular septal defects, incidence of permanent complete heart block is approximately 1%, as reported by Studer et al. and Kadoba et al.[8] Heart block encountered in the immediate postoperative period may be transient and result from edema of or trauma to the AV node or bundle of His. However, according to Kadoba et al. right bundle branch block is common (22%).[8]

Complications after repair of an AVSD include:

- Residual intracardiac shunting
- Left atrioventricular valve stenosis or regurgitation
- Subaortic obstruction.

LONG-TERM OUTCOME

Most adults with the complete form of this defect have undergone complete repair in childhood. In some patients, initial palliation may have consisted of pulmonary artery banding to restrict pulmonary blood flow, followed by subsequent definite repair. Over the last several decades, the surgical approach has evolved from a two-stage intervention to a single surgical strategy of primary repair in infancy.[9] The long-term outlook

CHAPTER 6

after repair of AVSDs is generally good. In a few patients, uncorrected defects have resulted in Eisenmenger's physiology, rendering them inoperable candidates. This is associated with significant late morbidity and early death.[10-12] Although definitive repair is usually accomplished during childhood, various publications have documented the results of surgical intervention in adults with partial forms of defects. Patients older than 40 years of age may undergo reparative surgery with low operative risk;[13] however, they may require long-term surveillance because late mitral valve dysfunction may occur. Among 50 patients who underwent surgery for partial AVSDs (mean age, 36.6 years; 39 years of them being intervened for the first time for a substantial shunt), a low operative risk was reported and excellent long-term results were achieved.[14]

REFERENCES

1. Rastelli G, Kirklin JW, Titus JL. Anatomic observations on complete form of persistent common atrioventricular canal with special reference to atrioventricular valves. Mayo Clin Proc. 1966;41:296-308.
2. Anderson RH, Baker EJ, Ho SY. The morphology and diagnosis of AVSDs. Cardiol Young. 1991;1:290.
3. Roberson DA, Muhiudeen IA, Silverman NH, et al. Intraoperative transesophageal echocardiography of atrioventricular septal defect. J Am Coll Cardiol. 1991;18:537-45.
4. Randolph GR, Hagler DJ, Connolly HM, et al. Intraoperative transesophageal echocardiography during surgery for congenital heart defects. J Thorac Cardiovasc Surg. 2002;124:1176-82.
5. Miller AP, Nanda NC, Aaluri S, et al. Three-dimensional transesophageal echocardiographic demonstration of anatomical defects in AV septal defect patients presenting for reoperation. Echocardiography. 2003;20:105-9.
6. Minich LL, Tani LY, Pagotto LT, et al. Size of ventricular structures influences surgical outcome in Down syndrome infants with atrioventricular septal defect. Am J Cardiol. 1998;81(8):1062-5.
7. Hanley FL, Fenton KN, Jonas RA, et al. Surgical repair of complete atrioventricular canal defects in infancy. Twenty-year trends. J Thorac Cardiovasc Surg. 1993;106(3):387-94; discussion 394-7.
8. Kadoba K, Jonas RA, Mayer JE, et al. Mitral valve replacement in the first year of life. J Thorac Cardiovasc Surg. 1990;100(5):762-8.
9. Hanley FL, Fenton KN, Jonas RA, et al. Surgical repair of complete atrioventricular canal defects in infancy: twenty-year trends. J Thorac Cardiovasc Surg. 1993;106:387-94.
10. Saha A, Balakrishnan KG, Jaiswal PK, et al. Prognosis for patients with Eisenmenger syndrome of various aetiology. Int J Cardiol. 1994;45:199-207.
11. Young D, Mark H. Fate of the patient with the Eisenmenger syndrome. Am J Cardiol. 1971;28:658-69.
12. Vongpatanasin W, Brickner ME, Hillis LD, et al. The Eisenmenger syndrome in adults. Ann Intern Med. 1998;128:745-55.
13. Bergin ML, Warnes CA, Tajik AJ, et al. Partial atrioventricular canal defect: long-term follow-up after initial repair in patients less than or more than 40 years old. J Am Coll Cardiol. 1995;25:1189-94.
14. Gatzoulis MA, Hechter S, Webb GD, et al. Surgery for partial atrioventricular septal defect in the adult. Ann Thorac Surg. 1999;67:504-10.

Chapter 7

TEE for Pulmonary Stenosis

Poonam Malhotra Kapoor, Sarvesh Pal Singh, Jitin Narula

Chapter Outline

INTRODUCTION

Pulmonary stenosis is most commonly a congenital heart defect, often presenting in infancy or childhood, though it can be seen from previous rheumatic fever or carcinoid disease as well.

Normal pulmonary valve area is 2 cm^2/m^2 and it is trileaflet. The congenitally stenotic valve may be trileaflet, bileaflet, or dysplastic.

PATHOPHYSIOLOGY OF PULMONARY STENOSIS

Pulmonary stenosis is a condition characterized by obstruction to blood flow from the right ventricle to the pulmonary artery. This obstruction is caused by narrowing or stenosis at one or more of several points from the right ventricle to the pulmonary artery. It includes obstruction from thickened muscle below

Calcification of the valve is relatively rare so the valve appearance does not play a huge role in decisions for balloon valvuloplasty

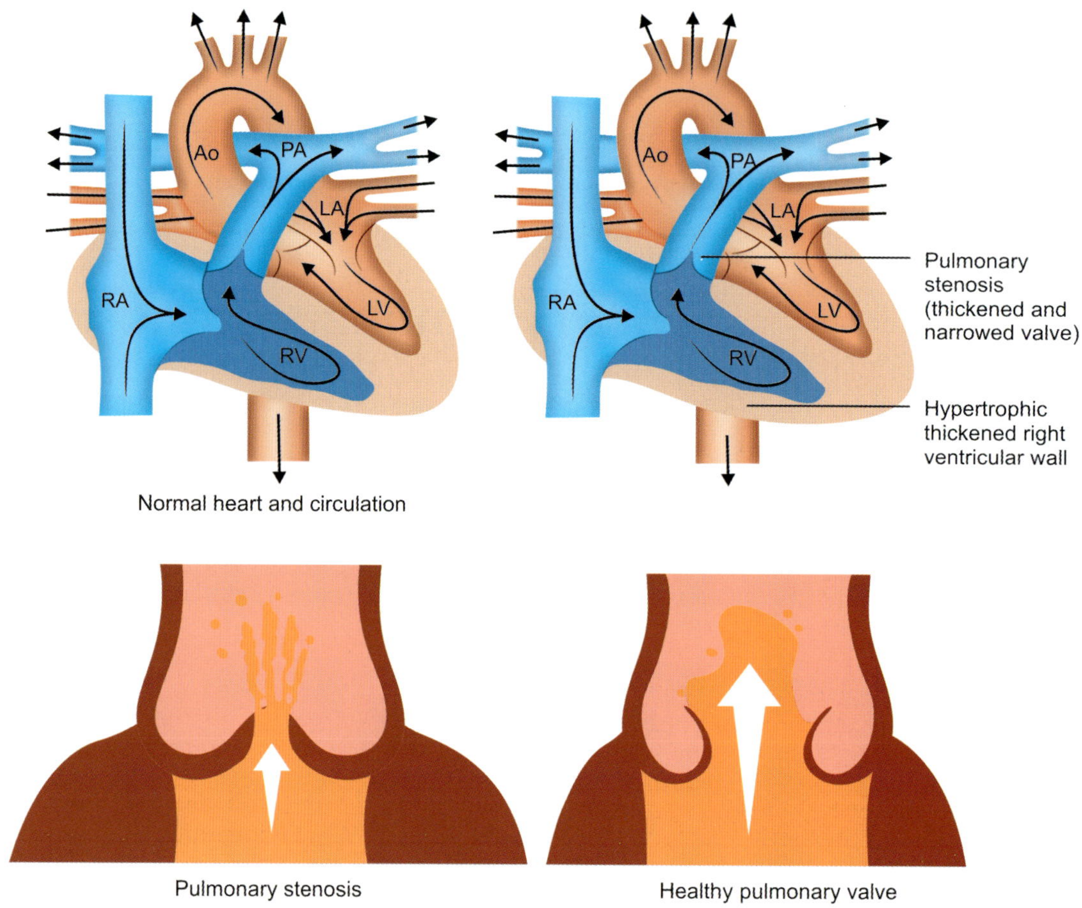

Figure 1 Diagrammatic representation of pulmonary stenosis

the pulmonary valve, narrowing of the valve itself, or narrowing of the pulmonary artery above the valve. The most common form of pulmonary stenosis is obstruction at the valve itself, referred to as pulmonary valvular stenosis. The normal pulmonary valve consists of three thin and pliable valve leaflets **(Fig. 1)**.

BRANCH PERIPHERAL PULMONIC STENOSIS

Transient pulmonary branch stenosis (PBS) in preterm and term neonates is well recognized. In preterm infants, closure of a patent ductus arteriosus (PDA) seems to be an important factor in the development of PBS but in only one of the studies reported in literature was the natural history reported. The presence of a heart murmur a few days or weeks after closure of a PDA in a preterm infant is often thought to be due to reopening of the ductus arteriosus, but the relation between a murmur and PDA is poor, and in term infants it has been shown to be more often associated with PBS than with PDA.

CAUSES AND CLINICAL PRESENTATION

Congenital pulmonary stenosis occurs due to improper development of the pulmonary valve in the first 8 weeks of fetal growth. It can be caused by a number of factors, though most of the time this heart defect occurs sporadically (by chance), with no clear reason evident for its development. Pulmonary stenosis usually does not cause symptoms in infants or small children. As the child gets older, abnormal signs and symptoms may appear, including:

- Fatigue
- A heart murmur (an extra heart sound when a doctor listens with a stethoscope)
- Chest pain
- Fainting
- Heavy or rapid breathing

- Shortness of breath
- Fatigue
- Rapid heart rate
- Swelling in the feet, ankles, face, eyelids, and/or abdomen
- Fewer wet diapers or trips to the bathroom.

Some congenital heart defects may have a genetic link, either occurring due to a defect in a gene, a chromosome abnormality, or environmental exposure, causing heart problems to occur more often in certain families. The normal pulmonary valve is trileaflet. The congenitally stenotic valve may be trileaflet, bicuspid, unicuspid, or dysplastic.[1]

Rheumatic pulmonary stenosis is rare even when the valve is affected by the rheumatic process.[2] Carcinoid disease is the most common cause of acquired pulmonary valve disease (combined stenosis and regurgitation with usually predominant regurgitation) and this may be sufficiently severe to require prosthetic replacement. Various tumors may compress the RV outflow tract leading to functional pulmonary stenosis. These tumors may arise from within the heart or associated vasculature or be external to the heart and compress from without.[3,4] Pulmonary valve stenosis may also occur as part of more complex congenital lesions such as tetralogy of Fallot **(Fig. 2)**, complete atrioventricular canal, double outlet RV, and univentricular heart. Peripheral pulmonary artery stenosis may co-exist with valvular pulmonary stenosis such as in Noonan's syndrome and Williams's syndrome as shown later.

INFUNDIBULAR PULMONARY STENOSIS

Stenosis below (proximal to) the pulmonary valve may result from a number of causes, both congenital and acquired. Congenital ventricular septal defect (VSD) may also be associated with RV outflow tract obstruction secondary to development of obstructive midcavitary or infundibular muscle bundles (double chamber RV) **(Fig. 3)** or in rare cases as a result of the jet lesion produced by the VSD in this area. Severe right ventricular hypertrophy of any cause but in some cases caused by valvular pulmonary stenosis itself may be responsible for narrowing of the infundibular area below the pulmonary valve. Iatrogenic causes include prior surgery or intervention on this area. Other causes include hypertrophic or infiltrative processes such as hypertrophic obstructive cardiomyopathy or glycogen storage disorders and compression from a tumour or vascular structure.

CLINICAL SIGNS OF PULMONARY STENOSIS

Physical signs include a widely split second heart sound and an ejection systolic murmur in the pulmonary area

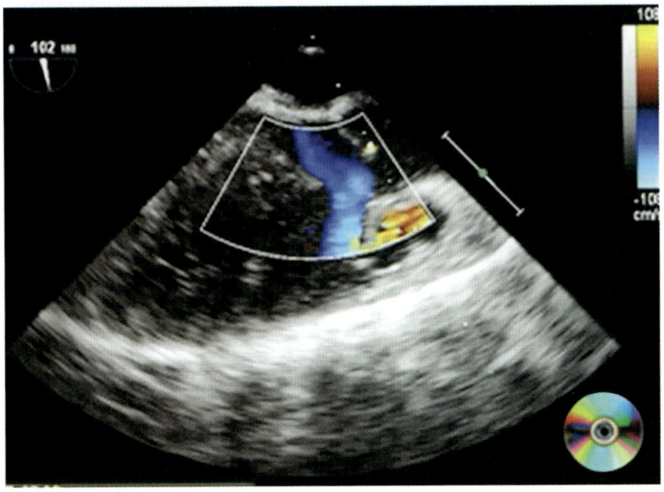

Figure 2 (Video 1) Tetralogy of Fallot in pulmonary stenosis

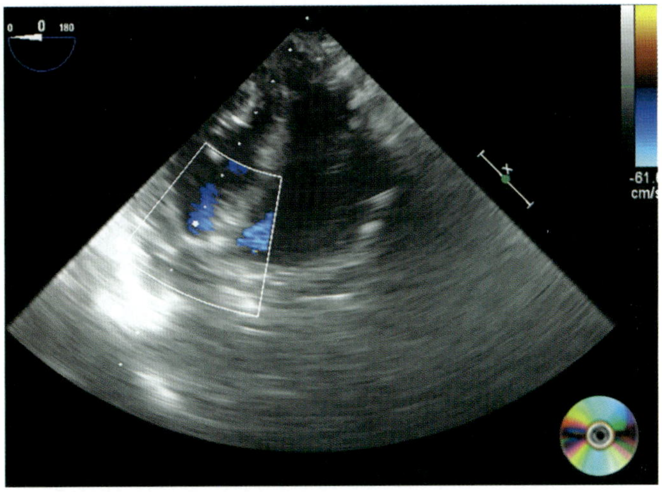

Figure 3 (Video 2) Double chamber right ventricular in pulmonary stenosis

Pulmonary stenosis is almost always congenital in origin. Acquired stenosis of the pulmonary valve is very uncommon and in very severe stenosis there may be evidence of right ventricle hypertrophy (See X-ray chest PAV and ECG for same).

PULMONARY ARTERY AND VEIN STENOSIS

Stenosis of the pulmonary artery above the valve (distal to the valve) may occur in the main pulmonary trunk at the bifurcation, or more distally in the branch vessels or in the pulmonary vein. In rare instances, a membrane just above the valve may cause stenosis. Pulmonary artery stenosis may occur as an isolated finding without other malformations.

TEE Findings in a Child with Pulmonary Vein Stenosis and Ventricular Septal Defect

A one year male child presented with history of recurrent episodes of upper respiratory tract infection since birth. On the basis of clinical examination, electrocardiography and transthoracic echocardiography (TTE) he was diagnosed as a case of perimembranous ventricular septal defect (VSD) with severe pulmonary hypertension. A VSD closure was planned and child was posted for surgery.

Intraoperatively, on transesophageal echocardiography (TEE) examination a large perimembranous VSD of 12.5 mm was seen. A further, detailed, examination revealed a membrane at the ostium of left superior pulmonary vein (LSPV) in the left atrium. A Color Doppler examination showed turbulence in the course of LSPV **(Fig. 4)**. A continuous wave Doppler examination showed a gradient of 23 mm Hg across this membrane **(Fig. 5)**. After the intracardiac repair of VSD and excision of the stenotic membrane there was no turbulence in the course of LSPV **(Fig. 6)** and the gradient across it decreased to 7 mm Hg **(Fig. 7)**. The child was extubated after 6 hours and was discharged from the hospital on the 5th postoperative day. On the first follow-up visit he was doing well with no complaints. This report reiterates the importance of TEE in the repair of congenital heart defects and the use of color Doppler in diagnosing pulmonary vein stenosis, missed on transthoracic echocardiography.

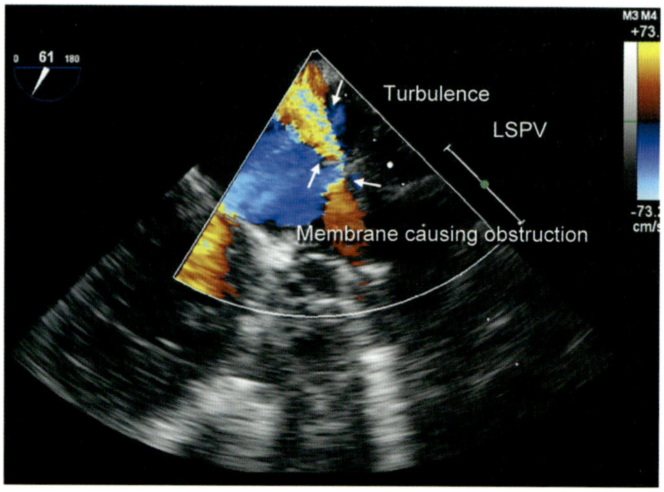

Figure 4 Color Doppler: Midesophageal modified bicommissural view showing a discrete membrane obstructing the opening of left superior pulmonary vein

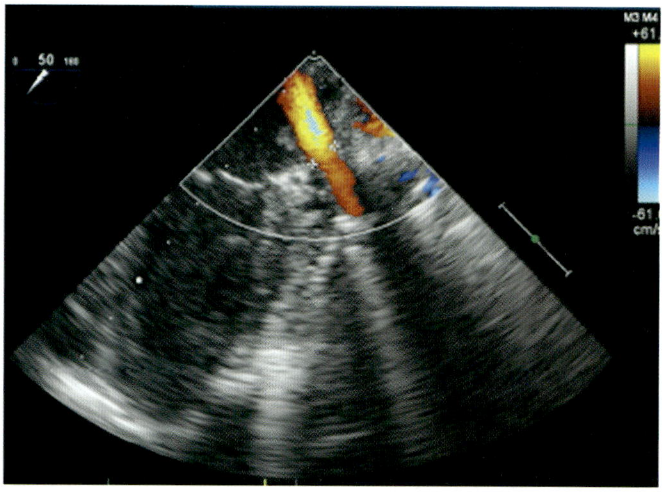

Figure 5 Color Doppler: Midesophageal modified bicommissural view showing no obstruction to blood flow from left superior pulmonary vein after resection of the membrane

WHY IS PULMONARY STENOSIS A CONCERN?

Mild pulmonary stenosis may not cause any symptoms. Problems can occur when pulmonary stenosis is moderate to severe, including the following:

The right ventricle has to work harder to try to move blood through the tight pulmonary valve. Eventually, the right ventricle is no longer able to handle the extra workload, and it fails to pump forward efficiently.

CHAPTER 7

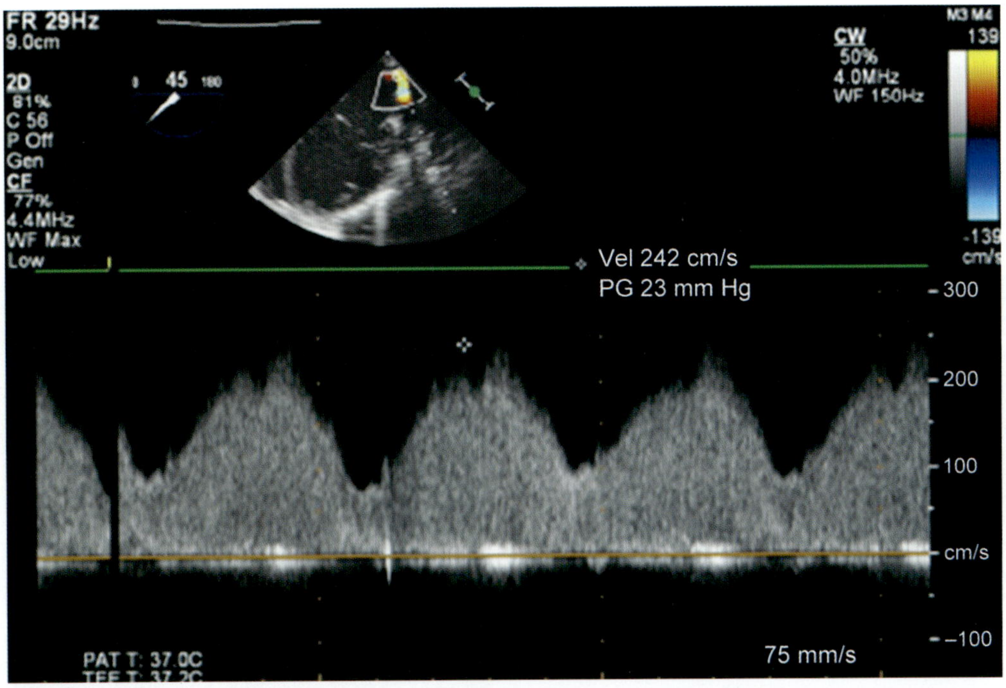

Figure 6 Continuous wave Doppler: Showing a gradient of 23 mm Hg across the obstructing membrane

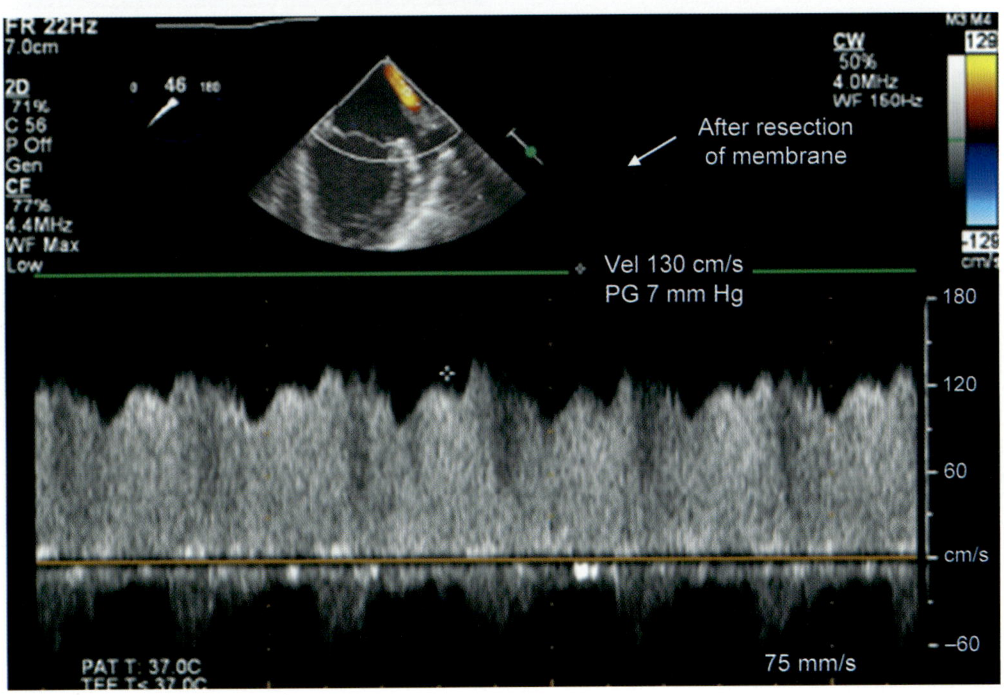

Figure 7 Continuous wave Doppler: Showing a gradient of 7 mm Hg across left superior pulmonary vein

Pressure builds up in the right atrium, and then in the veins bringing blood back to the right side of the heart. Fluid retention and swelling may occur.

There is a higher than average chance of developing an infection in the valves of the heart known as bacterial endocarditis.

TABLE 1 Grading of pulmonary stenosis

	Mild	*Moderate*	*Severe*
Peak velocity (m/s)	<3	3–4	>4
Peak gradient (mm Hg)	<36	36–64	>64

SEVERITY DEFINITIONS OF PULMONARY STENOSIS

Pulmonary stenosis is graded as mild, moderate and severe as shown in **Table 1**.

Mild stenosis: Peak jet velocity is: less than 3 m/s (peak gradient less than 36 mm Hg)

Moderate stenosis: Peak jet velocity of 3–4 m/s (peak gradient 36–64 mm Hg)

Severe stenosis: A peak jet velocity more than 4 m/s (peak gradient greater than 64 mm Hg). In determining the need for intervention, no specific Doppler gradients have been agreed upon.

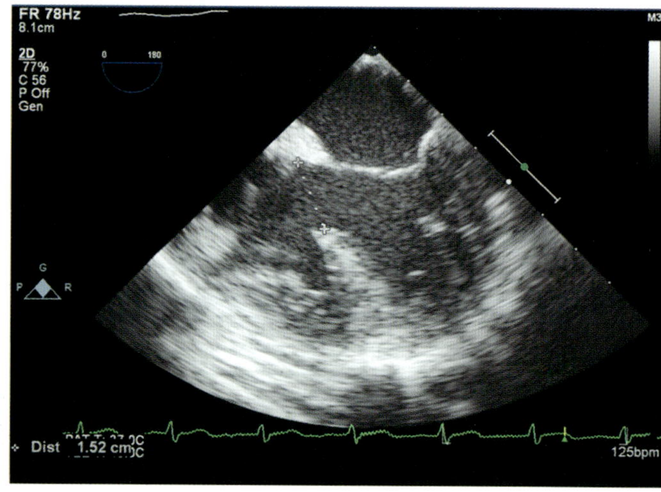

Figure 8 Midesophageal 4 chamber view showing a ventricular septal defect of 1.52 mm subaortic in position in a tetralogy of Fallot (TOF) patient

TETRALOGY OF FALLOT WITH INFECTIVE ENDOCARDITIS

Pulmonary valve stenosis can coexist with a large perimembranous ventricular septal defect of 1.52 mm, with aortic overriding of more than 50% **(Fig. 8)** and vegetation in main pulmonary artery (1.67 mm × 0.735 mm) as seen on transesophageal echocardiography **(Figs 9 to 11)**. Continuous-wave Doppler (CWD) should be done here. It shows a gradient of 40 mm Hg across the VSD **(Fig. 12)**.

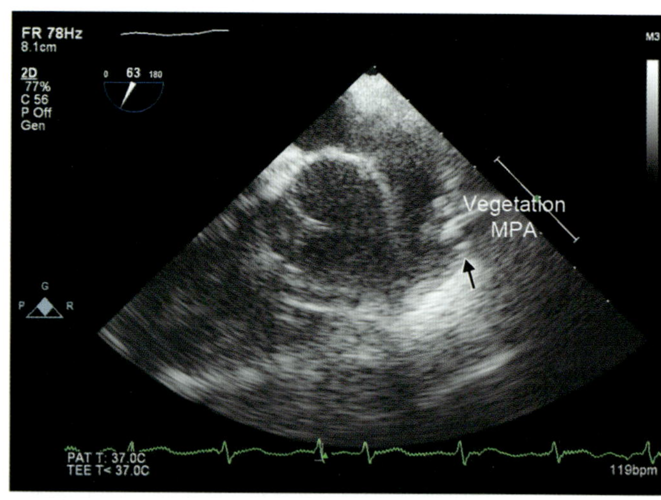

Figure 9 ME Asc aorta SAX showing vegetation in main pulmonary artery in a tetralogy of Fallot (TOF) patient

ETIOLOGY OF MPA ENDOCARDITIS

Pulmonary valve infective endocarditis is uncommon, comprising less than 2% of hospital admissions for endocarditis.[5] The low incidence of pulmonary valve infective endocarditis compared with other cardiac valves may relate to different hemodynamic pressure gradients across the valves, different frequencies of underlying congenital or acquired valvular abnormalities, lower right-sided blood oxygen content, and differences in the vascularity and endothelial lining of the valves.[6] Ramadan et al. reported only 81 cases of isolated pulmonary valve endocarditis from 1960 to 1999. The majority of these cases (55%) occurred in patients with congenital heart disease with 36 patients (44%) having isolated pulmonary valve infective endocarditis in a normal heart.[7] In a case of a 7-year-old boy at our center with TOF with vegetation in MPA (*see* **Figs 5 to 8**), we speculate that this rare nonbacterial

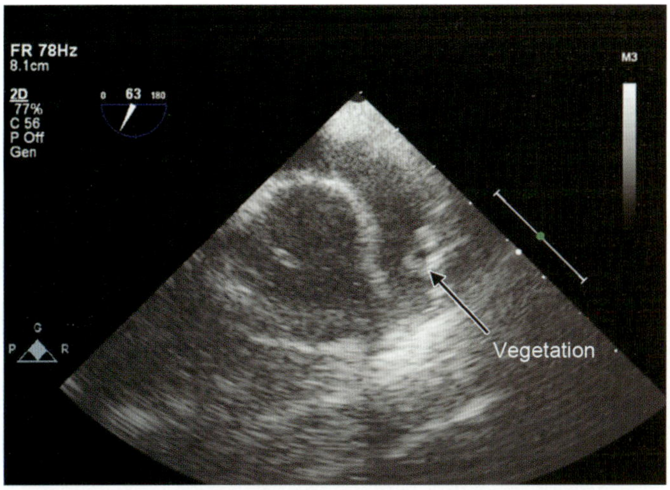

Figure 10 ME Asc aorta SAX showing vegetation in main pulmonary artery in tetralogy of Fallot (TOF). The MPA is well seen in this view and it is ideal to measure gradients here

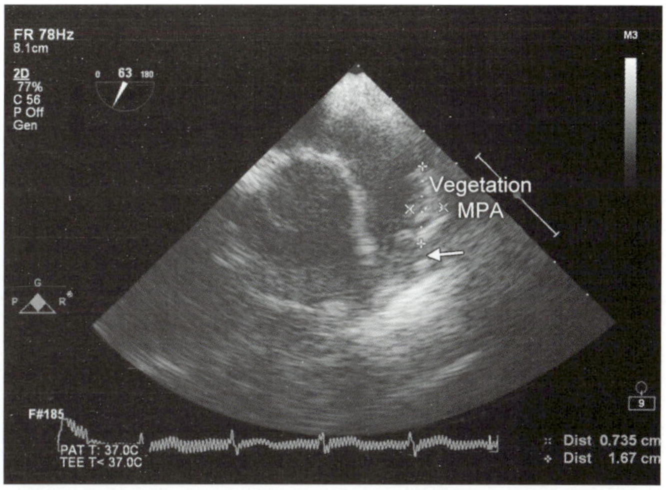

Figure 11 ME Asc aorta SAX showing vegetation in main pulmonary artery in a 7-year-old boy with tetralogy of Fallot (TOF) pathology. The vegetation measured 1.67 × 0.8 cm and was pedunculated

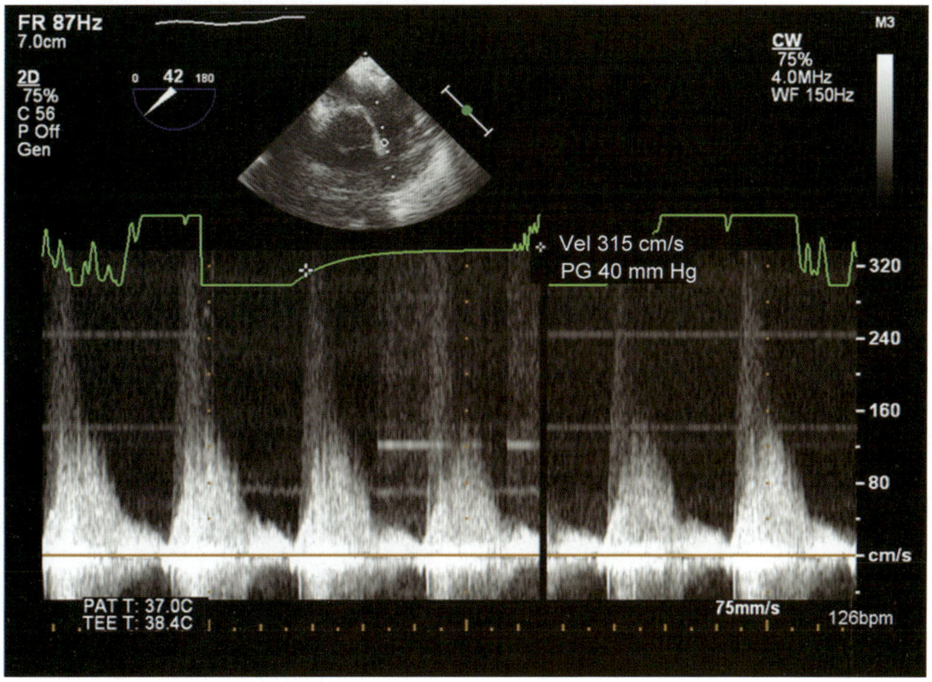

Figure 12 Continuous-wave Doppler showing a gradient of 40 mm Hg across the VSD

endocarditis involving the main pulmonary artery was thought to be initiated by the jet causing the subpulmonary ventricular septal defect causing the thrombus which is formed by the injured endocardial surface and subsequently became infected by bacteria. Theoretically, any acquired heart disease that causes turbulent blood flow can predispose to infective endocarditis.

Echocardiography has a known key role in the diagnosis of infective endocarditis, the diagnosis of complications, follow-up evaluation after therapy, and prognostic assessment as reported by Habib et al.[8] report describes a boy with tetralogy of Fallot who presented with infective endocarditis and large vegetation occluding the main pulmonary artery, thus resulting in a pulmonary stenosis. The role of echocardiography in diagnosis of postoperative residual lesion and providing hemodynamic data in time is all very making TEE a level 1a indication in diagnosis of endocarditis and pulmonary stenosis.

TEE ASSESSMENT OF PULMONARY STENOSIS

Preoperative Assessment

Important to look for:

- Site of stenosis
- *Nature of valve:* Is it tricuspid, bicuspid or dysplastic?
- Is there any thickening or calcification of leaflets? Is it diffuse or focal?
- Observe the CUSP mobility. Is it normal or reduced?
- Is there any doming of the Cusps?
- Is there any infundibular or valvular stenosis?
- Severity—gradient of stenosis, peak, mean gradients Pre-cardiopulmonary bypass (CPB)
- Presence of ASD/VSD
- Size of MPA and branch PAs size
- *Pulmonary valve:* Bicuspid/tricuspid, thickening and size of annulus
- Size of PV annulus, TV annulus; RV size (hypoplasia?)
- Are there any vegetations, thrombus or masses attached to the valve or in the main pulmonary artery (Pulmonary embolism)?

Doppler Findings

Color: Turbulent systolic flow at level of obstruction, also on pulsed wave (PW) Doppler, any pulmonary insufficiency (PI) to locate level of obstruction **(Figs 13 and 14A and B)**.

Stenosis severity (severe):

- Peak velocity > 4 m/s
- Peak gradient > 80 mm Hg
- Continuity equation for valve area less than 0.5 cm^2. *Prosthetic valve function:* Peak, mean gradients, paravalvular
- *Valve morphology:* Prosthetic failure poststenotic pulmonary artery (PA) dilatation > 20 mm Annulus size 21 ± 3 mm.

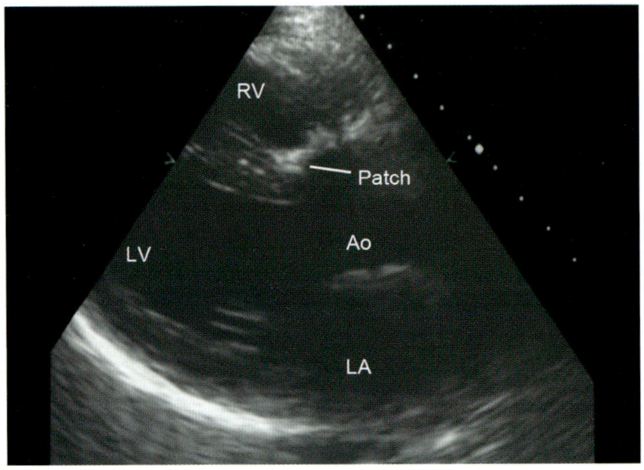

Figure 13 Color turbulent systolic flow at level of obstruction

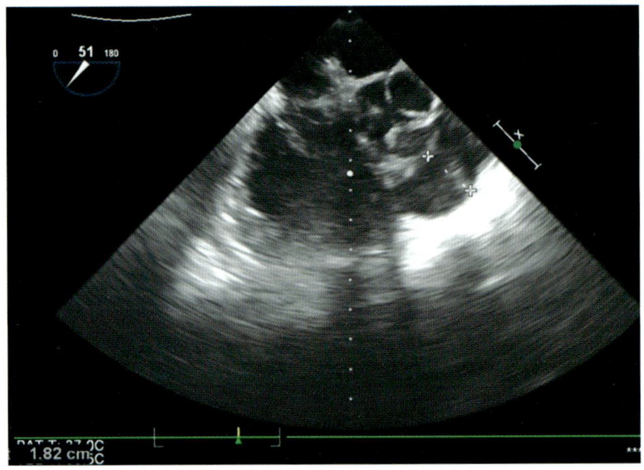

Figure 14A ME RV inflow-outflow view showing thickened and stenotic pulmonary valve

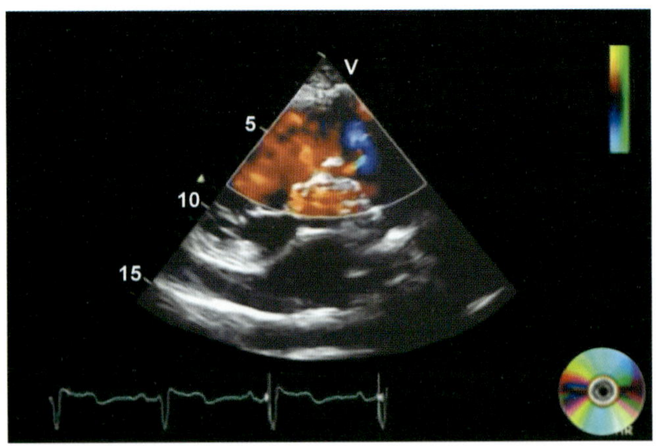

Figure 14B (Video 3) Pulmonary insufficiency

PERIOPERATIVE CARDIOPULMONARY BYPASS (2D ECHOCARDIOGRAPHY FINDINGS)

- *Uncorrected:* Ventricular septal defect (VSD), right ventricular outflow tract (RVOT) level of obstruction, override aorta, (RVH) **(Figs 15 to 19)**
- *Corrected:* VSD leak, pulmonic valve (PS/PI severity), RVOT obstruction
- RV size and function, aneurysmal RVOT if PI
- *Associated findings:* AI, LV function Post-CPB
- Residual VSD patch leak
- Pulmonic valve function (prosthetic)
- RV size and contractility

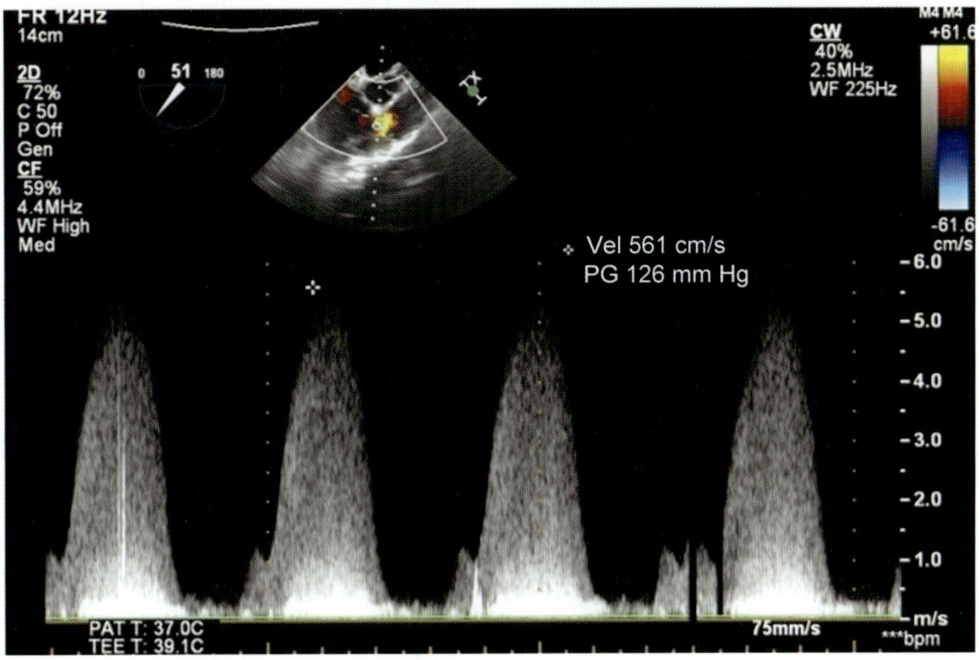

Figure 15 Continuous wave Doppler measuring gradient across pulmonary valve in a patient with isolated pulmonary stenosis

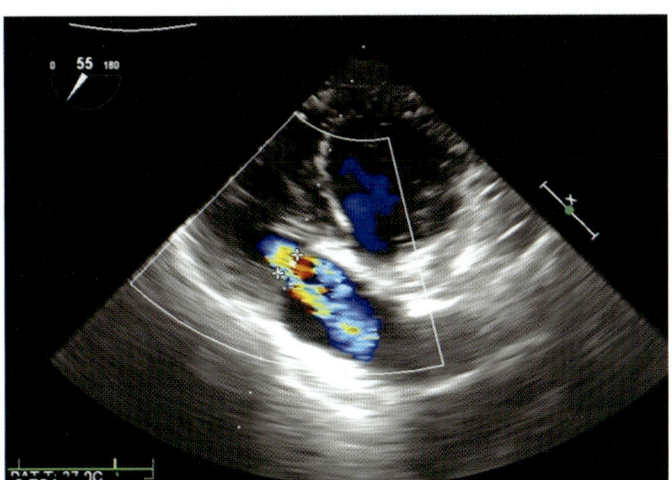

Figure 16 Color Doppler in right ventricle basal 60 degree view showing pulmonary stenosis; the gradient across PS may be measured here as Doppler alignment is good

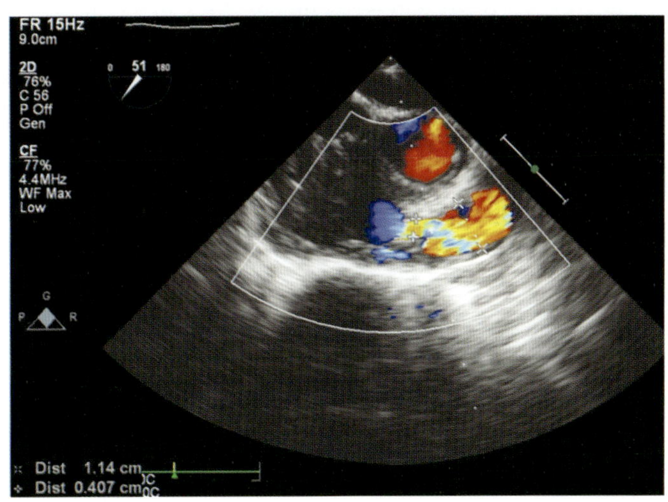

Figure 17 Color Doppler in RV inflow-outflow view showing pulmonary stenosis

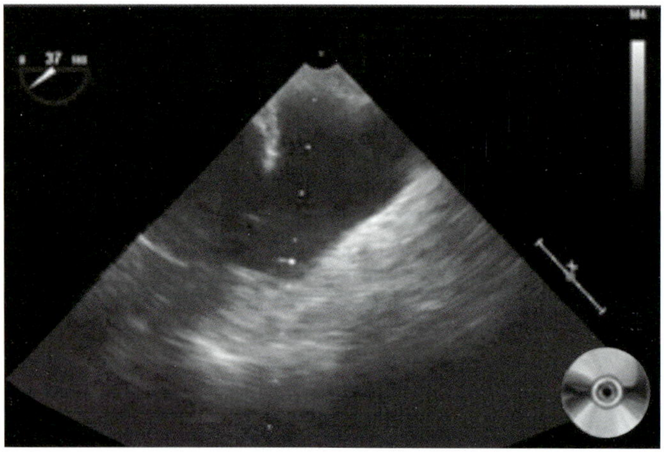

Figure 18 (Video 4) Transesophageal echocardiography of pulmonary stenosis

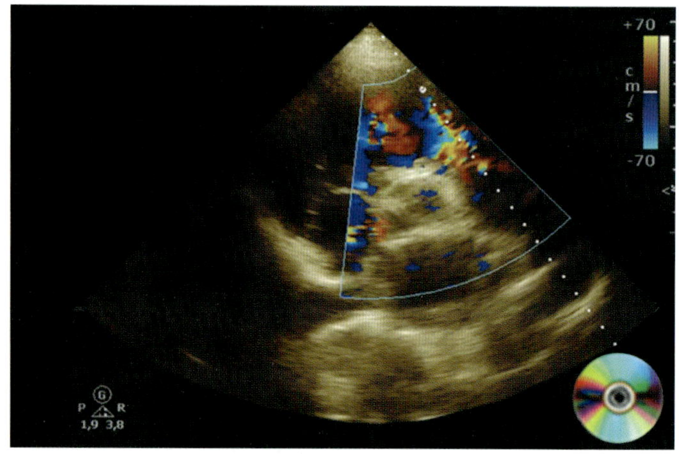

Figure 19 (Video 5) Atrial septal defects in pulmonary stenosis

- Residual RVOT obstruction
- *TR severity valve:* Thickened, calcified, immobile, systolic doming RVOT narrow in infundibular PS
- Right ventricular hypertrophy (RVH) (pressure overload), right ventricular (RV) dilated
- Poststenotic PA dilatation (> 20 mm).

POSTOPERATIVE PULMONARY STENOSIS ASSESSMENT (SEE FIGS 15 TO 17)

- Residual PR
- Post-PV stent ablation any PR?
- Residual gradient
- Pulmonary regurgitation
- Residual shunting in case of ASD or VSD.

REFERENCES

1. Waller BF, Howard J, Fess S. Pathology of pulmonic valve stenosis and pure regurgitation. Clin Cardiol. 1995; 18:45-50.
2. Bandin MA, Vargas-Barron J, Keirns C, Romero-Cardenas A, Villegas M, Buendia A. Echocardiographic diagnosis of rheumatic cardiopathy affecting all four cardiac valves. Am Heart J. 1990;120:1004-7.
3. Fox R, Panidis IP, Kotler MN, et al. Detection by Doppler echocardiography of acquired pulmonic stenosis due to extrinsic tumor compression. Am J Cardiol. 1984;53:1475-6.
4. Van Camp G, De Mey J, Daenen W, et al. Pulmonary stenosis caused by extrinsic compression of an aortic pseudoaneurysm of a composite aortic graft. J Am Soc Echocardiogr. 1999;12:997-1000.
5. Cassling RS, Rogler WC, McManus BM. Isolated pulmonic valve infective endocarditis: a diagnostically elusive entity. Am Heart J. 1985;109:558-67.
6. Roberts WC, Buchbinder NA. Right-sided valvular infective endocarditis. A clinicopathologic study of twelve necropsy patients. Am J Med. 1972;53:7-19.
7. Ramadan FB, Beanlands DS, Burwash IG. Isolated pulmonic valve endocarditis in healthy hearts: a case report and review of the literature. Can J Cardiol. 2000;16:1282-8.
8. Habib, et al. Echocardiography has a known key role in the diagnosis of infective endocarditis, the diagnosis of complications, follow-up evaluation after therapy, and prognostic assessment. Eur J Echocardiogr. 2011;11:202-9.

Chapter 8

TEE for Double-Chambered Right Ventricle

Poonam Malhotra Kapoor, Sarvesh Pal Singh, Sanjay Kumar, Balaswaroop Sahu

Chapter Outline

- Natural History of DCRV
- Associated Anomalies
- Transesophageal Echocardiography Views of DCRV
- Role of Echocardiography in Diagnosing Double-chambered Right Ventricle in Adults
- Preoperative TEE Assessment
- Electrocardiogram of DCRV
- Postoperative TEE Assessment

INTRODUCTION

Double-chambered right ventricle (DCRV) (Video hyperlinked) is a rare defect characterized by a septated right ventricle (RV) caused by the presence of abnormally located or hypertrophied muscular bands.[1] The right ventricle is divided into a proximal high-pressure and distal low pressure chamber, the obstruction being caused by an anomalous muscle bundle extending from the interventricular septum (beneath the level of the septal leaflet of the tricuspid valve) to the right ventricular free wall which is often associated with a malaligned VSD. It can be caused by the presence of anomalous muscle tissue, hypertrophy of the endogenous trabecular bands, or an aberrant moderator band; all of which will typically result in progressive obstruction of the right ventricular outflow tract.

NATURAL HISTORY OF DCRV

Double-chambered right ventricle occurs with an incidence of 0.5–2% of all congenital heart diseases and occurs in as many as 10% of patients with VSD. Although sporadic cases have been associated with Noonan's syndrome and Down syndrome, it has not been associated with any particular genetic abnormality.

The DCRV typically presents in childhood or adolescence. Most patients with (DCRV) initially present with no symptoms with the most common reason for referral being the detection of a murmur. Symptoms may include cyanosis, dyspnea, failure to thrive, excessive sweating, and congestive heart failure and are dependent on any associated VSD (presence, location, and size), degree of RVOT obstruction, and other associated cardiac anomalies.

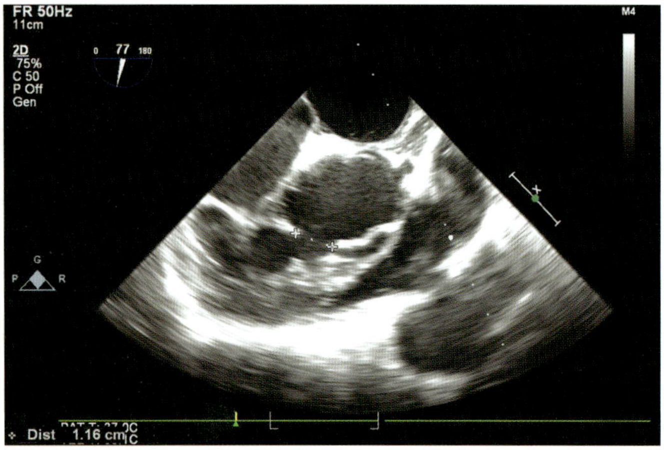

Figure 1 Patient who underwent a DCRV repair with a diverge repair for the tricuspid valve

ASSOCIATED ANOMALIES

Some of the associated cardiac anomalies, in a series of DCRV patients are:

TOF
Associated CHD
VSD
Subaortic ridge
Infundibular aneurysm
RCC prolapsed
Tricuspid insufficiency **(Fig. 1)**
Patent foramen ovale
Mitral valve prolapsed
Rheumatic aortic stenosis
Pulmonary valve stenosis
Pulmonary atresia

ECG in DCRV tall upright T waves in right precordial leads with RAD and RVH **(Fig. 2)**.

Echocardiography and cardiac magnetic resonance (CMR) imaging have increasingly become the modalities of choice for the noninvasive characterization of complex congenital heart lesions.

TRANSESOPHAGEAL ECHOCARDIOGRAPHY VIEWS OF DCRV

Echocardiography currently enables diagnosis on a 2-dimensional Doppler echocardiogram; before its advent, diagnosis of double-chambered right ventricle (DCRV) could not be made noninvasively.

TEE Views for DCRV

- *In infancy:*
  - Midesophageal (ME) 4 chamber view is optimal.
  - RV inflow-outflow and bicaval view may be more useful in older patients **(Fig. 3)**.
- The cardinal feature is demonstration of muscle bundles that traverse the RV cavity, with an accompanying gradient starting proximal to the infundibulum.
- Deep transgastric imaging is always required for Monoplane examination as the right ventricular outflow tract is poorly visualized from within the esophagus, in contrast to the omniplane approach.

ROLE OF ECHOCARDIOGRAPHY IN DIAGNOSING DOUBLE-CHAMBERED RIGHT VENTRICLE IN ADULTS

A recent case series showed that the discrete form of the obstruction was more common than the diffuse (20 v 6 patients), while low localization was more common than high (23 v 3 patients). The maximum systolic pressure gradient between the inflow and outflow chamber ranged between 20–135 mm Hg and exceeded 50 mm Hg in 19 cases (59.4%) **(Figs 4A to E)**. The authors found a perimembranous VSD to being the most common associated cardiac anomaly. Both TTE and TOE (particularly with the use of transgastric planes) were helpful in measuring pressure gradients.[2]

In the largest series of DCRV diagnosed echocardiographically in adults was recently published by Lascano and colleagues.[3] In their experience also, TOE was an excellent technique for demonstrating the lesion. TTE was of limited value but worked better in the context of a congenital echocardiography laboratory. Interestingly, cardiac catheterization failed in three patients. The authors emphasized that both echocardiography and right sided cardiac catheterisation should be interpreted by personnel with experience in congenital heart disease, to increase the likelihood of a correct diagnosis.

PREOPERATIVE TEE ASSESSMENT

- *2D echo:*
  - Anomalous muscle bundle with its insertion
  - Site of obstruction—mid RV cavity, RVOT
  - VSD—site, size

ELECTROCARDIOGRAM OF DCRV

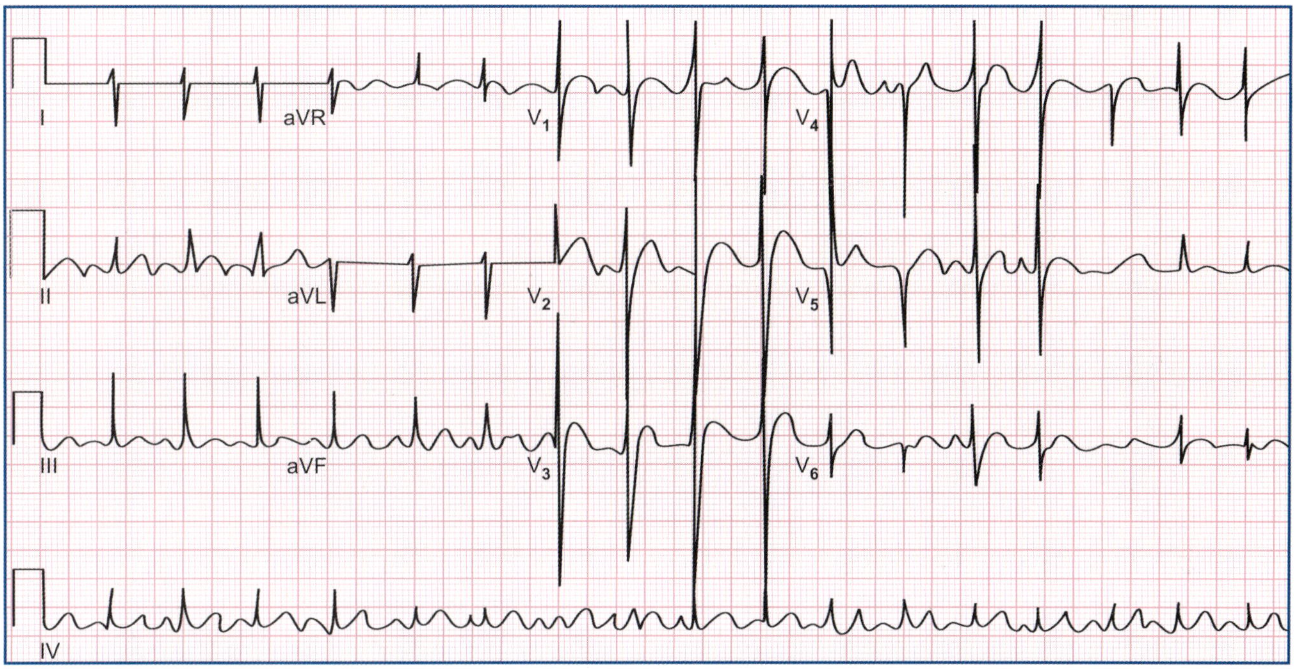

Figure 2 Electrocardiogram of an 18-month-old boy with double-chambered right ventricle. Note the upright T waves in the right precordial leads

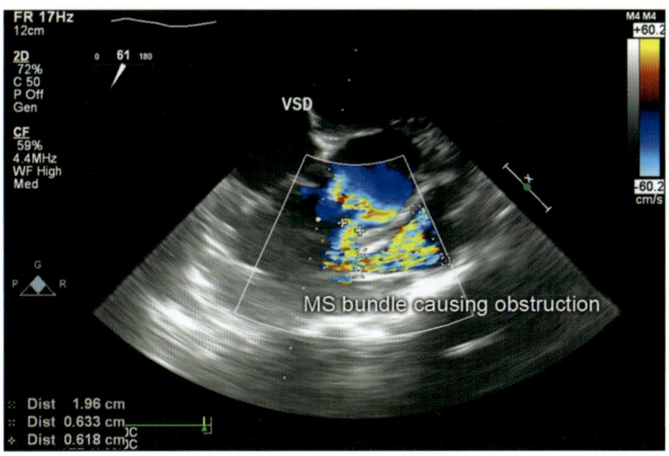

Figure 3 Color Doppler in ME RV inflow-outflow view showing right ventricular outflow tract obstruction, VSD and normal pulmonary valve

- *Color flow Doppler:*
  - RV obstruction was suggested by a turbulence
  - VSD shunting
- *Continuous wave Doppler:*
  - Gradient across obstruction
  - Gradient across the tricuspid valve: may be caused by a double-chambered right ventricle and not by pulmonary hypertension
- Assessment of pulmonary valve—annulus size and stenosis
- *Assessment of pulmonary arteries:*
  - Diameter—RVOT, MPA, RPA, LPA
  - Ostial stenosis of LPA/RPA
- Double-chambered right ventricle should be differentiated from tetralogy of Fallot by the absence of infundibular hypoplasia and pulmonary artery anomalies in double-chambered right ventricle.
- *Displacement index*[4]*:*
  - Dividing the distance from the pulmonary annulus to the septal insertion of the moderator band by the tricuspid annulus diameter, the displacement index is achieved.
  - An index less than 1 may predict that infants with ventricular septal defect (VSD) are at risk of developing an obstruction from a displaced moderator band.

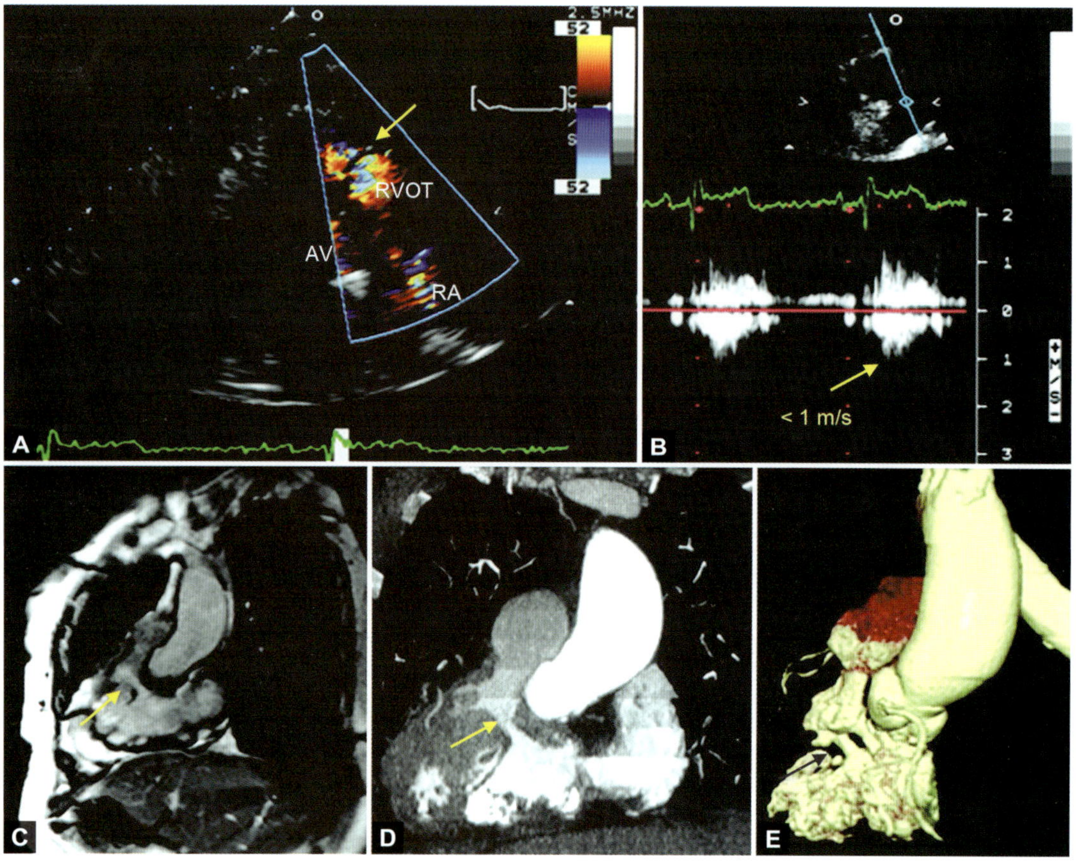

Figures 4A to E Anatomic assessment of the double-chambered right ventricle with infundibular stenosis. (A) In the RV inflow-outflow view, the RA and RVOT are located to the right of the aortic valve (AV) and the aorta is seen with color flow acceleration across the infundibular stenosis; (B) CWD across the pulmonary valve, demonstrates lack of a significance gradient (<1 m/s) and there is no evidence of pulmonary stenosis in these patients generally; (C) Cardiac MRI with balanced steady-state free precession sequence, also demonstrates infundibular stenosis (arrow). Maximum-intensity projection image in the coronal view; (D) and volume-rendered 3-dimensional image; and (E) obtained from contrast-enhanced cardiac computed tomography, showing infundibular stenosis (arrow)

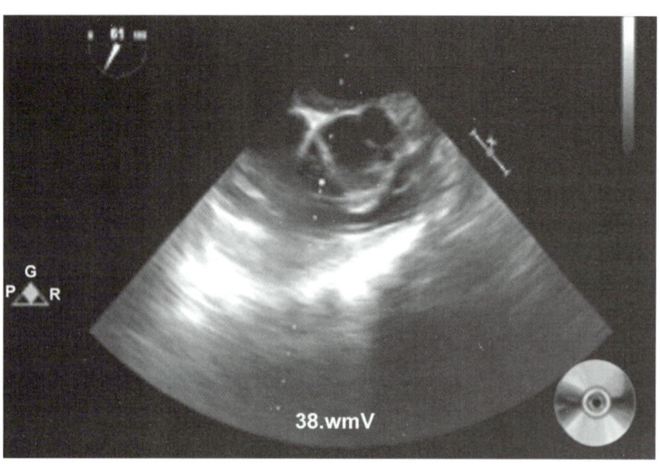

Figure 5 (Video 1) 2D echo in midesophageal right ventricle inflow-ouflow view showing a perimembranous ventricular septal defect and a muscle bundle obstructing the flow in right ventricular outflow tract in a patient with double chambered right ventricle

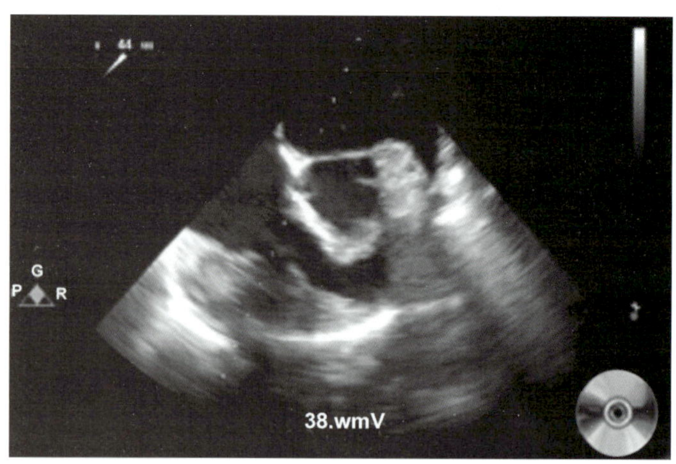

Figure 6 (Video 2) 2D echo in midesophageal right ventricle inflow-ouflow view showing the repair of ventricular septal defect with a Dacron patch and resection of the muscle bundle leading to a patent right ventricular outflow tract

POSTOPERATIVE TEE ASSESSMENT (FIGS 5 AND 6)

- Residual gradient
- Residual shunt
- Preload of right ventricle
- Aortic valve.

CONCLUSION

Double-chambered right ventricle is a rare congenital cardiac anomaly in adults. Echocardiography is very useful in diagnosing the anomaly in adult patients. TOE, however, is much more capable than TTE of defining the full details of the pathology, including estimation of the pressure gradient. High localization of the abnormal bundle is invariably associated with discrete morphology, whereas a low obstruction may be either discrete or diffuse, the latter being less common. DCRV is usually associated with a VSD or, less often, with membranous subaortic obstruction. Surgical treatment carries a low risk and provides excellent immediate results in these patients.

REFERENCES

1. Oliver JM, Garrido A, Gonzalez A, Benito F, Mateos M, Aroca A, et al. Rapid progression of mid ventricular obstruction in adults with double chambered right ventricle. J Thorac Cardiovasc Surg. 2003;126:711-7.
2. Hoffman P, Wojcik AW, Rozanski J, Siudalska H, Jakubowska E, Włodarska EK, et al. The role of echocardiography in diagnosing double chambered right ventricle in adults. Heart. 2004;90:789-93.
3. Lascano ME, Schaad MS, Moodie DS, et al. Difficulty in diagnosing double chambered right ventricle in adults. Am J Cardiol. 2001;88:816-7.
4. Wong PC, Sanders SP, Jonas RA, et al. Pulmonary valve-moderator band distance and association with development of double-chambered right ventricle. Am J Cardiol. 1991;68(17):1681-6.

CHAPTER 8

Chapter 9

TEE for Patent Ductus Arteriosus

Poonam Malhotra Kapoor, SN Das, Sarvesh Pal Singh, RS Rajput

Chapter Outline

INTRODUCTION

Patent ductus arteriosus (PDA) is also sometimes referred to as persistent ductus arteriosus. In the fetus, the ductus arteriosus acts as a shunt connecting the pulmonary artery (at the junction of the main and left pulmonary arteries) to the aortic arch (just after the origin of the left subclavian artery). This allows most (90%) of the blood pumped by the RV to reach the systemic circulation directly, bypassing the lungs. The ductus arteriosus normally starts to close immediately after birth, and is normally fully closed within a few days, leaving behind just a cord-like remnant (the ligamentum arteriosum). Failure of the ductus arteriosus to close means that a left-to-right shunt persists between the aortic arch and the pulmonary artery, with blood flow from the high-pressure aorta to the lower-pressure pulmonary artery. This leads to excessive blood flow through the pulmonary circulation and, in the longer term, can cause pulmonary hypertension.[1]

CLINICAL FEATURES OF PATENT DUCTUS ARTERIOSUS

Neonates with PDA are usually asymptomatic, but may sometimes have difficulty feeding or failure to thrive. The clinical features of PDA may include tachycardia, a wide pulse pressure and bounding pulse, a continuous systolic—diastolic 'machinery murmur', clubbing, and cyanosis.[2]

X-RAY

Findings on chest radiographs range from normal to those consistent for congestive heart failure (CHF). Cardiomegaly may be present with or without CHF.

If significant left-to-right shunt through the patent ductus arteriosus (PDA) is present, the pulmonary arteries, pulmonary veins, left atrium, and left ventricle are enlarged on chest films. Also, the ascending aorta may be prominent **(Fig. 1)**.

Usually, chest radiographic findings are normal until the magnitude of the ratio of pulmonary to systemic circulation (QP/QS) exceeds 2:1. Prominence of the main pulmonary artery segment is an early sign of increased pulmonary artery pressure and flow. With marked pulmonary overcirculation, pulmonary edema may occur. Accentuated peripheral pulmonary vascular markings and increased pulmonary venous markings may be noted. In elderly individuals, the patent ductus arteriosus (PDA) may calcify and may be visible on a standard radiograph.

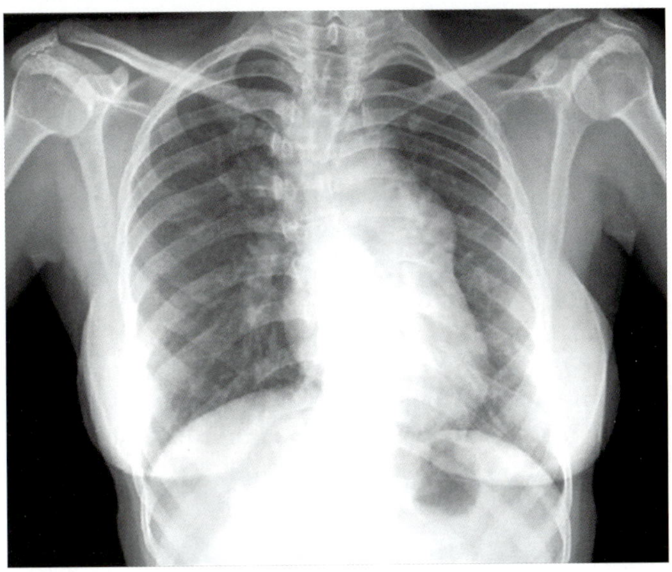

Figure 1 X-ray chest from a 22-year-old lady with large patent ductus arteriosus and severe pulmonary hypertension. Normal heart size, dilated pulmonary artery segment

TABLE 1 Chest X-ray findings in PDA

1. LA dilatation
2. RA dilatation
3. Large pulmonary artery
4. Dilated UL and LL veins
5. Small aortic arch < PA diameter
6. Large aorta
7. RV dilation

Studies have shown that chest radiographs have limited predictive value in determining which infants will benefit from ligation **(Table 1)**.

ECG

With a small patent ductus arteriosus (PDA), the electrocardiographic (ECG) findings are typically normal. Left ventricular hypertrophy may be present with a larger PDA. Left atrial enlargement may also be present with large shunts. In the presence of significant pulmonary hypertension, there may be evidence of right ventricular hypertrophy **(Fig. 2)**.

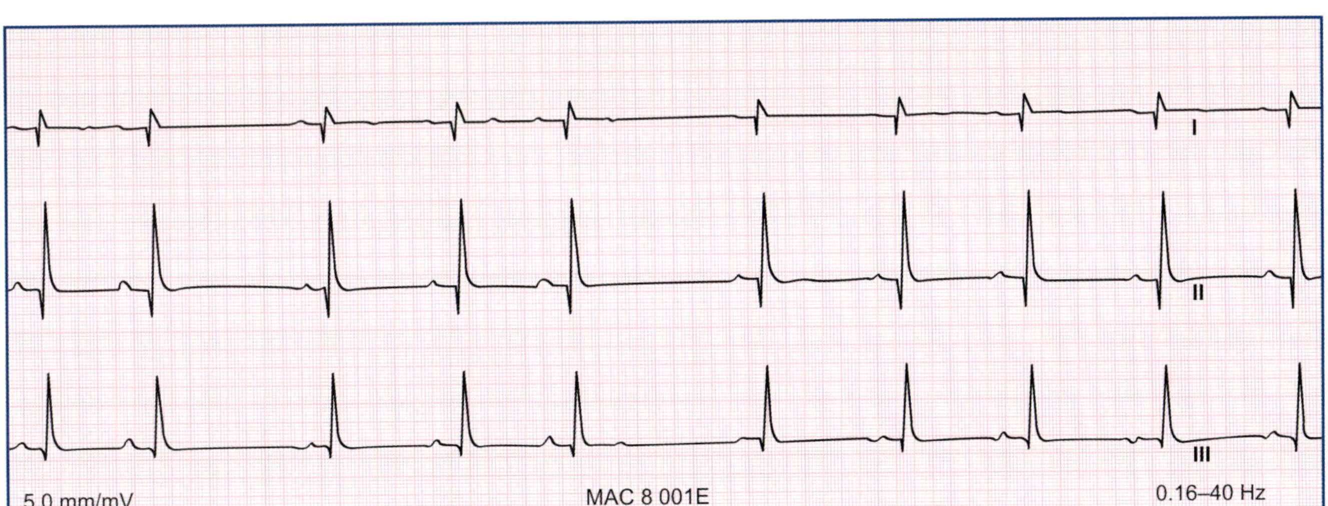

Figure 2 Patient who diagnosed patent ductus arteriosus

In the neonate, especially the premature neonate with a large patent ductus arteriosus (PDA), T-wave inversion and ST segment depression may be present, suggesting ischemia or a supply-demand mismatch. This is thought to be related to increased myocardial work due to the left-to-right shunt and pulmonary overcirculation in the face of low aortic and coronary diastolic blood pressure due to the run-off of blood from the aorta into the pulmonary arteries.

ROLE OF TEE IN PDA

Transesophageal echocardiography for isolated PDA ligation is not practically convincing. Being a short procedure in lateral decubitus position and the limitations of TEE in imaging the left pulmonary artery preclude the use of TEE in such children. However, every child undergoing intracardiac repair should be evaluated for PDA and these are the children from which most of our images for TEE are recorded.

- True communication is usually not seen.
- A flow on color Doppler emerging from aorta to left pulmonary artery (LPA) is usually understood as PDA until proved otherwise. This is seen on TEE as mosaic area of increased flow.

TEE VIEWS FOR PATENT DUCTUS ARTERIOSUS: FOR SIMULTANEOUS COARCTATION OF AORTA TO BE RULED OUT

- Upper esophageal DTA long axis view
- Upper esophageal DTA short axis view
- Upper esophageal aortic arch short axis view
  - Detect size
  - Gradient across PDA
- ME ascending aortic short axis view
  - Ductal flow detected
  - Abnormal continuous high velocity aliased flow
- ME AS AO SAX view
  - Size of left-sided heart chambers
  - Left ventricular volume overload
  - Valvular regurgitation
  - Pulmonary artery hypertension

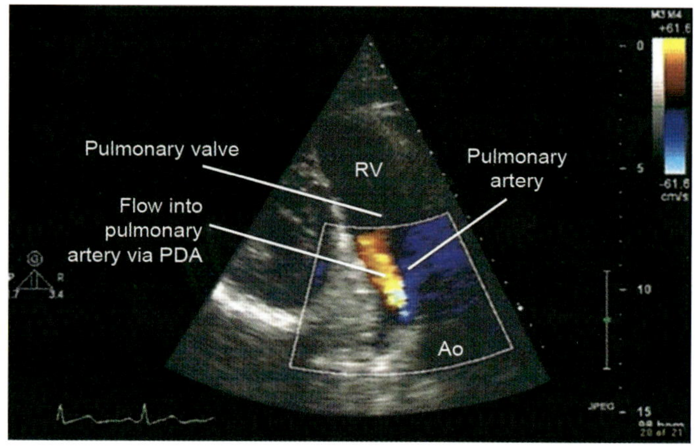

Figure 3 TEE view of transgastric right ventricular outflow with CFD showing flow into pulmonary artery via PDA

  - Infective endocarditis of pulmonary artery: size, shape and mobility of vegetations
  - Associated cardiac conditions: ASD/VSD
- Right ventricular outflow view **(Fig. 3)**

In either of these views, use color Doppler to assess flow in the pulmonary artery, looking in particular for evidence of blood flow into the pulmonary artery via a PDA.

Look carefully for any knock-on effects of the shunt on the rest of the heart, such as the development of pulmonary hypertension and right heart dilatation.

PREOPERATIVE TEE ASSESSMENT

- May be seen when pulmonary artery and its bifurcation is imaged in the long axis and probe is rotated slightly to the left to image LPA and the DTA.
- The communication is difficult to measure but may be done in rotated hearts
- Left ventricular volume overload
- Coarctation of aorta—UE DTA LAX and SAX view
- ASD/VSD to be ruled out
- Difficult to visualize the ductus directly
- Views of the descending aorta limited
- Suspected when there is retrograde systolic and diastolic flow in the pulmonary artery
- Continuous flow throughout systole and diastole in pulmonary artery through PDA

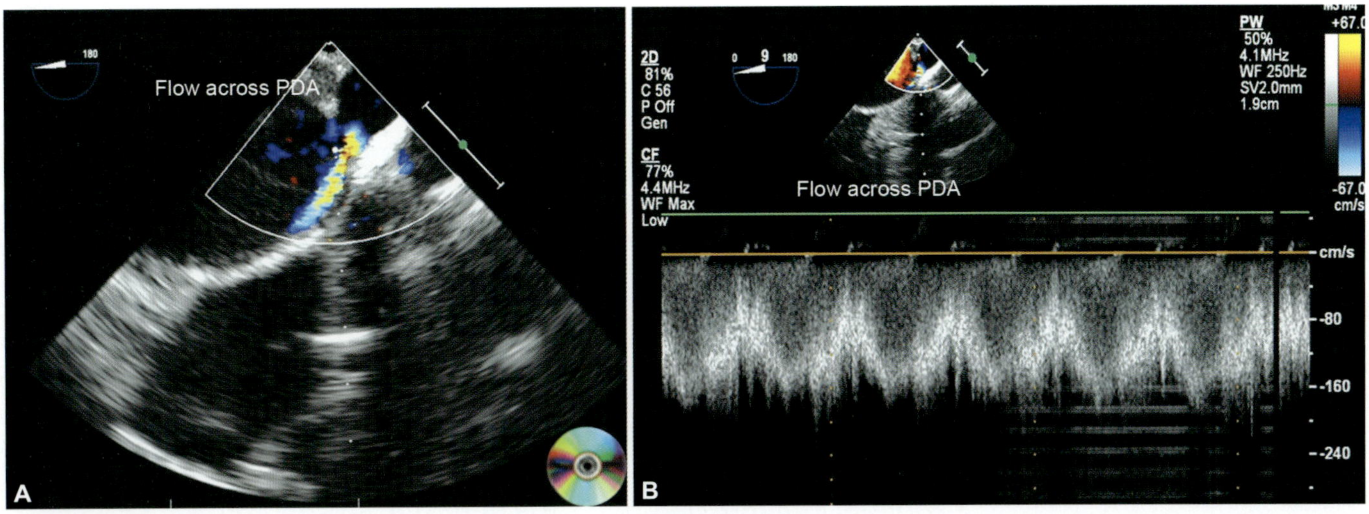

Figures 4A (Video 1) and B (A) Color flow Doppler in modified ME descending thoracic aorta short axis view (Probe rotated to right to visualize left pulmonary artery) showing patent ductus arteriosus; (B) Continuous wave Doppler showing continuous flow across PDA

- *Restrictive PDA:* Pressure in aorta exceeds pressure in pulmonary artery throughout the cardiac cycle leading to high velocity continuous flow in the PDA.

POSTOPERATIVE TEE ASSESSMENT

- Residual shunting or gradient
- Evaluation of effectiveness of ductal ligation
- Residual shunt detected with color flow Doppler
- Biventricular function assessment
- Valvular regurgitation
  - Color flow Doppler in modified ME descending thoracic aorta short axis view (probe rotated to right to visualize left pulmonary artery) showing patent ductus arteriosus **(Figs 4A and B)**
  - Continuous wave Doppler showing continuous flow across PDA.

ROLE OF TEE IN PERCUTANEOUS DEVICE CLOSURE OF PDA

- Double umbrella device used
- TEE for exact location of the device
- Adequacy of occlusion and any residual shunt assessed by color flow Doppler.

ECHO ASSESSMENT FOLLOWING REPAIR USING THE SAME VIEWS AS FOR UNREPAIRED ASD

- Comment on the presence of a septal occluder device or patch
- Check for any residual shunt
- Assess right heart size and function
- Assess pulmonary artery pressure.

CONCLUSION AND FUTURE DIRECTIONS

Echo is an imperative diagnostic tool in left-to-right shunts like PDA. Sizing and availability of the TEE probe will make this surgery have better outcomes.

REFERENCES

1. Sinha B. Controversies in Management of Patent Ductus Arteriosus in the Preterm Infant. J Pulmon Resp Med. 2013;S13:007.
2. Hermes-DeSantis ER, Clyman RI. Patent ductus arteriosus: pathophysiology and management. J Perinatol. 2006;26: S14-8.

Chapter 10

TEE for Aortic Coarctation

Poonam Malhotra Kapoor, Suruchi Hasija, Pawan Jain

Chapter Outline

- Clinical Features of Aortic Coarctation
- Physiology
- Transesophageal Echocardiographic Evaluation
- Transesophageal Echocardiography Assessment of Aortic Coarctation
- Management of Aortic Coarctation
- Transesophageal Echocardiography Assessment Following Coarctation Repair

INTRODUCTION

Aortic coarctation is a narrowing of the aorta that most commonly occurs just distal to the origin of the left subclavian artery. It accounts for 5–8% of congenital heart disease, occurring in 1 in 3000 live births (more commonly in males). There is more to aortic coarctation than just a narrowing of the aorta, however, and the condition should be considered to be part of a more generalized arteriopathy **(Fig. 1)**.

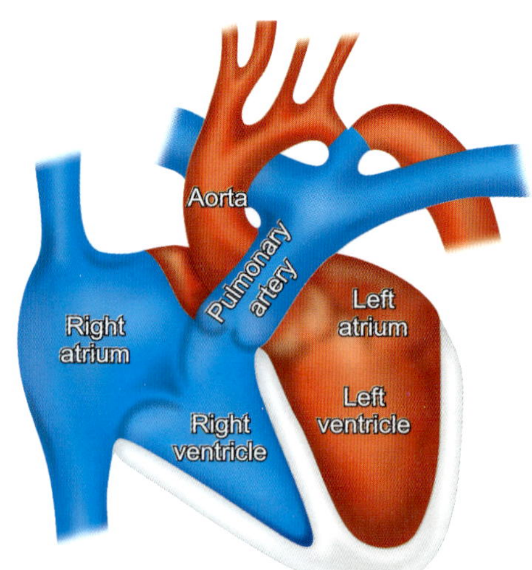

Figure 1 Coarctation of aorta: Outline diagram

CLINICAL FEATURES OF AORTIC COARCTATION

Children with aortic coarctation may present with heart failure and problems resulting from reduced arterial perfusion to the lower half of the body. Adults

TABLE 1 Clinical features of aortic coarctation

Symptoms	*Signs*
Often asymptomatic	Hypertension
	Systolic murmur
	Weak femoral pulse
	Radiofemoral delay (femoral pulse occurs after radial)

with aortic coarctation are often asymptomatic and the diagnosis is made during assessment of hypertension or as an incidental finding **(Table 1)**. Patients may have the clinical features of an associated condition such as bicuspid aortic valve or Turner syndrome. It is also associated with subvalvular, valvular and supravalvar aortic stenosis and with parachute mitral valve.[1]

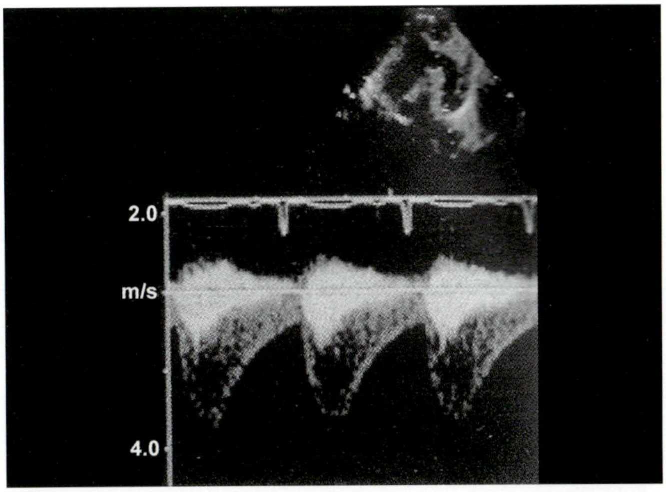

Figure 2 Coarctation of the aorta. Typical spectral Doppler flow pattern across the coarctation site. The lighter and darker velocities correspond to the dual population of blood elements across the region. The peak Doppler velocity allows the degree obstruction to be quantified

PHYSIOLOGY

The main physiologic consequence of coarctation of the aorta (CoA) is increased LV afterload. The systolic arterial blood pressure is increased proximal to the coarctation site and decreased distal to it, and systemic hypertension develops subsequently.[2] Most adults with coarctation of the aorta (CoA) are asymptomatic, although recurrent epistaxis, headache, claudication, dizziness, and palpitations may occur. Major complications include aortic dissection, rupture, or endarteritis of the aorta, cerebral hemorrhage, infective endocarditis, and LV failure.

TRANSESOPHAGEAL ECHOCARDIOGRAPHIC EVALUATION

The anterior position of the air-filled trachea relative to the esophagus limits the TEE examination of the distal ascending aorta and proximal aortic arch, thereby making this a difficult lesion to examine by TEE.[3] Images are obtained most reliably by transthoracic echocardiography **(Fig. 2)**. Suggested cross-sections for focused TEE examination: upper esophageal (UE) Ao Arch SAX and LAX, ME 4-CH, AV LAX, and TG SAX.

Goals of the two-dimensional examination are:

- Identification of associated lesions and limited evaluation of the aortic arch.
- Monitoring of LV function during aortic-clamp application.

Goals of Doppler examination are:

- Detection of turbulent, eccentric jets or flow acceleration in the descending aorta by color-flow Doppler.
- Determination of flow velocities across the area of narrowing by spectral Doppler; this examination is complicated by the limited ability to align the Doppler beam to the direction of flow.

Goals of the examination after surgical repair or during/after catheter intervention are:

- Detection of residual obstruction.

TRANSESOPHAGEAL ECHOCARDIOGRAPHY ASSESSMENT OF AORTIC COARCTATION

With the echo probe in the upper esophageal aortic arch, obtain an aorta view to visualize the aortic arch:

- Use 2D echo to assess the appearances and dimensions of the aortic arch. Aortic coarctation is seen most commonly just distal to the origin of the left subclavian artery. There may be dilatation of the aorta on either side of the coarctation.

- Use color Doppler to assess flow in the aorta, looking in particular for evidence of high-velocity or turbulent flow in the region of a suspected coarctation.
- Use continuous wave (CW) Doppler to assess flow in the descending aorta with the TEE probe in the descending aorta SAX view position, looking for evidence of increased flow velocity through the coarctation. However, be aware that high flow velocities measured with CW Doppler are not a reliable guide to coarctation severity. A better guide is the presence of "sustained anterograde diastolic flow" in the aorta (diastolic 'tail' or 'run-off'), the presence of which suggests a significant coarctation **(Fig. 3)**.

Perform a complete echo study to look carefully for any other abnormalities that can be associated with, or result from, aortic coarctation, including:

- Bicuspid aortic valve (present in at least 50% of cases)
- Subvalvar or supravalvar aortic stenosis
- VSD
- LV hypertrophy (LVH) or dysfunction (as a consequence of hypertension).

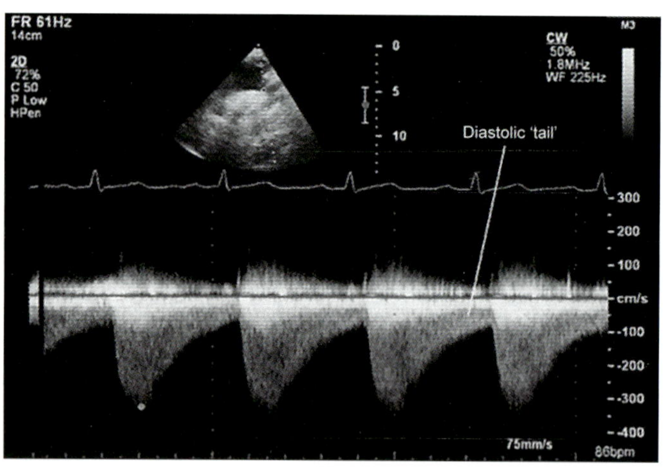

Figure 3 Aortic coarctation—continuous wave Doppler study from suprasternal window showing diastolic 'tail' and a peak velocity of 3.5 m/s in the descending thoracic aorta

MANAGEMENT OF AORTIC COARCTATION

- Aortic coarctaion can be managed by surgical excision of the area of coarctation (followed either by end-to-end anastomosis of the aorta, or with the use of a graft to bridge the resulting gap).
- It can also be managed percutaneously by angioplasty and/or stenting of the coarctation.

TRANSESOPHAGEAL ECHOCARDIOGRAPHY ASSESSMENT FOLLOWING COARCTATION REPAIR

Following correction, patients with aortic coarctation require lifelong follow up with annual echo studies. Using the same views as for unrepaired coarctation:

- Measure any residual gradient
- Check for the development of any dilatation of the aorta.

In addition:

- Assess any LVH (patients may remain hypertensive)
- Assess any associated abnormalities such as bicuspid aortic valve.

Recoarctation is more common in those who underwent repair as a neonate (recoarctation incidence 2.4–5.5%) than later in life (incidence <1%). It can be challenging to assess recoarctation (and residual coarctation) using echo, as the repaired area can be difficult to visualize and Doppler gradients tend to be overestimated.

REFERENCES

1. Hernández-González M, Solorio S, Conde-Carmona I, Rangel-Abundis A, Ledesma M, et al. Intraluminal aortoplasty vs. surgical aortic resection in congenital aortic coarctation. A clinical random study in pediatric patients. Arch Med Res. 2003;34:305-10.
2. Rao PS. Diagnosis and management of cyanotic congenital heart disease: part I. Indian J Pediatr. 2009; 76:57.
3. Chandar JS, Wolfe SB, Rao PS. Role of stents in the management of congenital heart defects. J Invasive Cardiol. 1996;8:314-25.

Look for sustained anterograde diastolic flow in the aorta as an indicator of a significant recoarctation.

Chapter 11

TEE for Tetralogy of Fallot

Poonam Malhotra Kapoor, Milind Hote, Sameer Taneja, Dinesh Chandra

Chapter Outline

DEFINITION

Cyanotic congenital heart disease characterized by the cephaloanterior displacement of the conotruncal septum manifesting as ventricular septal defect, aortic override, right ventricular outflow tract obstruction and hypertrophy.

ETIOLOGY

Most common congenital heart disease above 2 years of age (25% of cyanotics):

- 80–100 for 10,000 population, i.e. 8–10/1,000 population.

COMPONENTS OF TOF (FIG. 1)

- Infundibular stenosis of pulmonary artery (PA) (RV outflow obstruction)
- Large nonrestrictive type of ventricular septal defect (VSD)
- Right ventricular hypertrophy
- Overriding aorta (biventricular origin of aorta)

Right outflow through ventricle, i.e. pulmonary artery; may be:

- Infundibular stenosis (80%)
- Valvular (20%).

EMBRYOLOGY

Truncus arteriosus gives two parts: (i) aorta and (ii) pulmonary artery.

The truncus arteriosus has a septum to divide the aorta/PA—conotruncal/infundibular septum → spiral septum which divides the pulmonary artery and aorta.

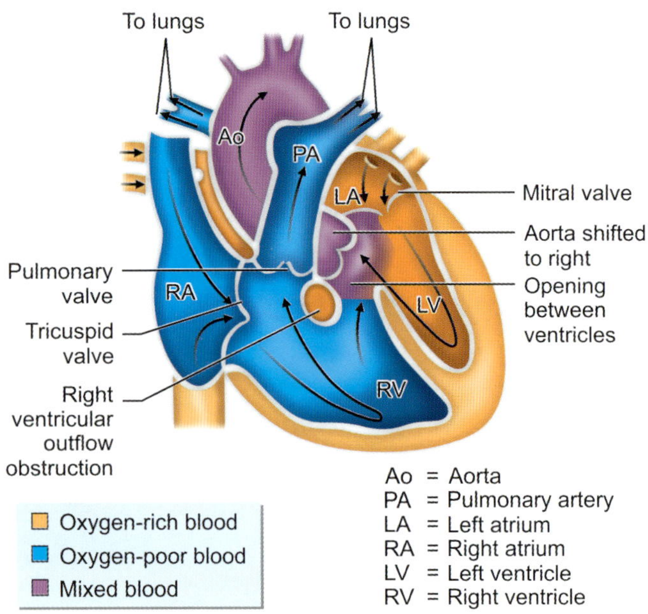

Figure 1 Components of TOF

In tetralogy of Fallot (TOF), spiral septum is displaced anterior and cephalad direction with a small pulmonary artery, overriding aorta.

ASSOCIATED ANOMALIES IN TOF

- Right side aortic arch (25%)
- Left side superior vena cava
- Mirror image type
- *Associated:* Atrial septal defect (ASD), patent ductus arteriosus (PDA), coarctation of aorta
- Anomalous origin of left coronary artery
- Dextrocardia
- Berry aneurysm
- Anomalies of coronary arteries
- Aberrant left anterior descending coronary artery arising from right coronary artery
- Abnormalities of the pulmonary artery and its branches
- Peripheral PA coarctations, unilateral
- Absence or hypoplasia of pulmonary artery
- Absence of pulmonic valve
- Bicuspid pulmonic valve.

SYNDROMES ASSOCIATED WITH TOF

- *Poland's syndrome:* TOF + absent pectoral mayor (left)
- *Goldenhar syndrome:* TOF + oculoauriculovertebral dysplasia
- *Digeorge syndrome:* TOF + immunodeficiency
- *Klippel-Feil syndrome:* TOF + fused cervical vertebra
- *Laurence-Moon-Biedl:* TOF + hypogonadism + retinitis pigmentosa + polydactyly + obesity
- Fetal alcohol syndrome
- *CHARGE association:*
  - C: Coloboma
  - H: Heart anomaly (TOF/VSD)
  - A: Choanal atresia
  - R: Renal anomaly
  - G: Growth retardation
  - E: Ear anomaly
- *TAR syndrome:* Thrombocytopenia + Absent/hypoplastic radius + TOF/VSD
- *Down's syndrome:* TOF + VSD + ASD.

CYANOTIC SPELLS IN TOF (FLOW CHART 1)

Why in TOF cyanosis occurs after 6 months of Life? Remember adult hemoglobin is responsible for cyanosis Increased O_2 binding capacity of fetal Hb.

- Hb fetal type is present up to 6 months
- Reduced pulmonary vascular resistance in neonate and more shunt left to right
- O_2 requirement (demand) is less in infants
- Neonatal baby dose not cry more and lies silent whereas infants cry more resulting in cyanosis
- Sensitivity of infundibular receptors for catecholamines not well-developed.

Cyanotic (Hypoxic) Spells

It is vicious cycle with paroxysmal spell occurs when the baby cries in early morning hours associated with:

- Deepening of cyanosis
- Decreasing intensity of ejection systolic murmur
- Hyper (tachypnea)
- May develop fits at times.

Treatment of Cyanotic Spells

- Knee chest position
- *Humidified O_2 therapy:* $\downarrow O_2$ content
- *Acidosis:* To prevent stimulation of respiratory center Na bicarbonate: 2–3 meq/kg added to drip
- *Morphine:* Depresses respiratory center 0.1 mg/kg SC

CHAPTER 11

Flow chart 1 Pathophysiology of TOF

Pulmonic stenosis
↓
Concentric right ventricular hypertrophy (RVH) without cardiac enlargement
↓
Increased right ventricular pressure than left
↓
Right to left shunt appears to decompress RV
↓
As the systolic pressures between the two ventricles are identical, there is little or no left to right shunt
↓
VSD is silent
↓
Flow across pulmonary valve produces ejection systolic murmur (ESM)
↓
More severe PS
↓
Less blood flows through pulmonary valve
↓
Shorter the ESM + cyanosis

- Propranolol ↓infundibular spasm 0.1 mg/kg slow IV
- *Phenylephrine injection:* To systemic vascular resistance
- Beta blockers
- *Vasopressors:* Phenylephrine
- Correction of anaemia, dehydration
- Indication for surgical correction.

SQUATTING EPISODE

Mechanism

- Reset decreases O_2 demand
- Compression of femoral artery:
  - Increased LV pressure (as there is increased systemic resistance)
  - Decrease of R → L shunt
- Compression of femoral vein:
  - Decreased venous return
  - Decreased R → L shunt
  - Decreased cyanosis.

Equivalents for Squatting

- Squatting
- Knee chest position
- Knee abdomen position
- Scissoring the lower limb
- Sitting with arms drawn underneath
- Standing on one leg
- Mother holding infant with thighs flexed
- Lying supine
- *In infants:* Put the child over the mother's shoulder.

CLINICAL FEATURES IN TOF

General Examination

- Cyanosis
- Tachypnea
- Clubbing
- *Jugular venous pulse (JVP):* 'a' wave prominent
- Polycythemia (conjunctival suffusion)
- Growth retardation
- Failure to thrive.

Fallot's trilogy: ASD + PS + Right ventricular hypertrophy (no VSD) Fallot's pentalogy—ASD + TOF.

Congestive cardiac failure (CCF) will never occur in TOF
↓
As there is nonrestrictive VSD ← no volume overload, all blood is diverted to aorta
If congestive heart failure (CHF) seen in TOF patients, there are high risk. Important then to rule out in this patient population, the following:
- Anemia
- Hypertension
- Infective endocarditis
- Myocarditis
- Other valve anomalies.

Palpation: Systolic thrill in pulmonary area (<30%)

Auscultation in the TOF Patient

- S1 normal
- S2 single loud A2
- ESM in pulmonary area
- *Constant ejection click:* Large aorta
- *Inconstant ejection click:* Valvular pulmonary stenosis (PS)
- Bilateral symmetrical systolic murmur in infra-clavicular/clavicular/supraclavicular.
  - Bronchopulmonary collaterals.

Investigations

- Blood: ***TCIDC***
  - *Hb% in TOF:* Because of polycythemia we, cannot detect anemia
  - *PCV:* Most reliable to find anemia
    - Keep PCV <60%
    - If PCV >65%—start treatment
- X-ray chest in TOF **(Figs 2A and B)**
  - Heart size normal, rarely enlarged
  - Cardiac apex displaced upward "coeur en sabot" (Apex of the heart raised above the hemidiaphragm)
  - PA segment concave
  - Pulmonary oligemia
  - Dilated aorta
  - Pulmonary arteries small
- Decreased vasculature R aortic arch in 25%.[1]
- *ECG in TOF:* RAD (+120 degrees to +150 degrees) in cyanotic form **(Fig. 3)**. Tall R wave in V_1 abruptly changes to an rS in V_2.

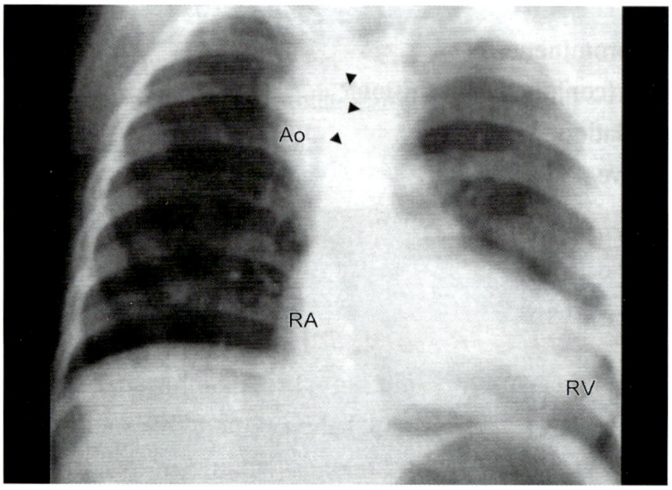

Figure 2A X-ray chest posteroanterior view (PAV) showing the typical boot

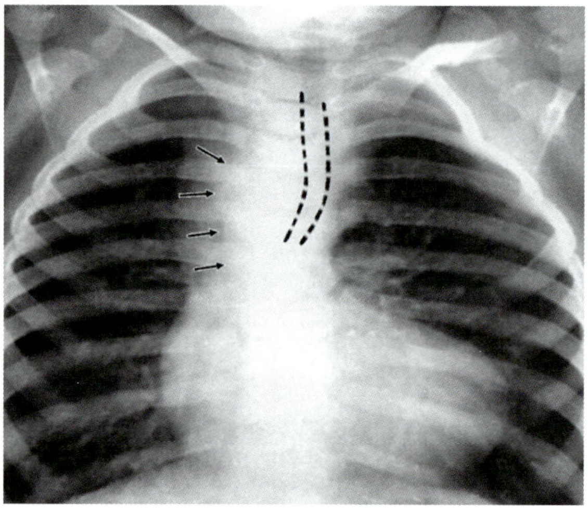

Figure 2B Shape heart with a displaced RV

Palliative Surgeries in TOF

- *Blalock-Taussig shunt:* (>3 months age) line, on the side opposite to aortic arch R/L subclavian artery with R/L pulmonary artery.
- *Modified Blalock-Taussig:* 'Goretex interposition shunt'. Placed between subclavian artery and ipsilateral artery.
- *Potts shunt:* Descending aorta to left pulmonary artery
- *Waterston shunt:* Ascending aorta to right pulmonary artery.
- *Davidsons operation:* Ascending aorta to pulmonary trunk anastomosis.
- *Glen's operation:* For tricuspid atresia—SVC with pulmonary artery anastomosis.

Definite Surgery

Ideal-age: 3–5 years—total correction

- Closing VSD
- Resecting infundibular obstruction.

COMPLICATIONS

- Right bundle branch block (RBBB) with or without left anterior hemiblock

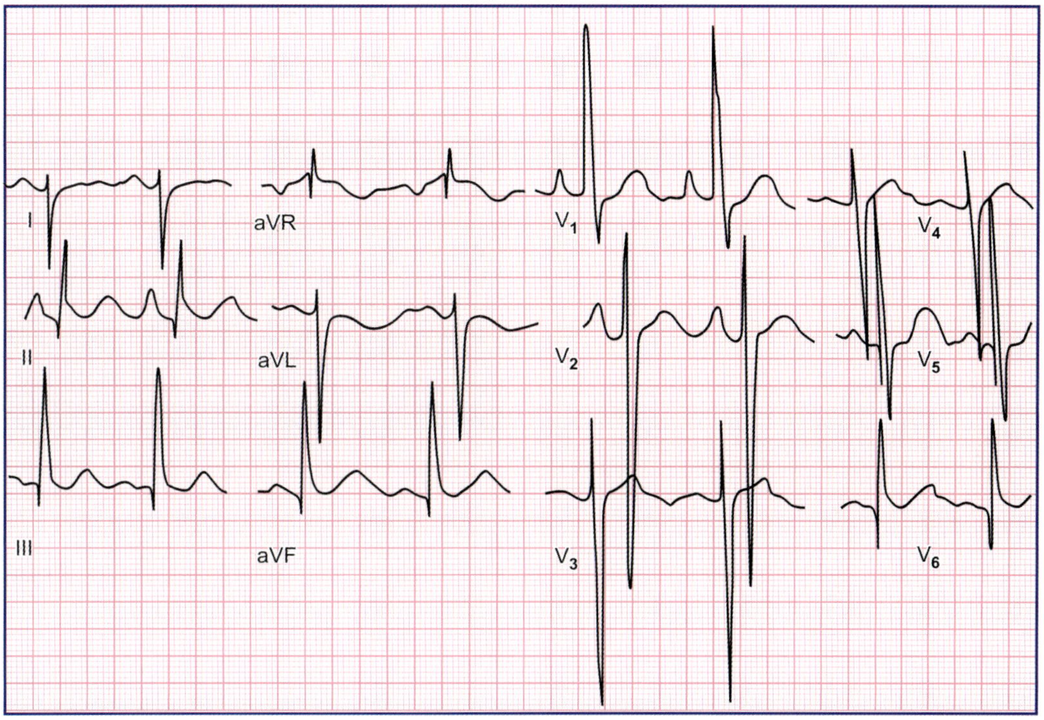

Figure 3 ECG of a patient with TOF shows right axis deviation (RAD) and right ventricular hypertrophy (RVH)

- Complete heart block
- Residual VSD/PS
- Pulmonary regurgitation.

Definite Procedure

Complete correction of TOF = Lilley's procedure.

Important Points to Remember in TOF

- No VSD murmur/on ESM at PS
- *Loud ESM:* Good prognosis
- *Importance of respiratory system examination:* Continuous murmur
  Central nervous system examination: Plantar extensor + (cerebral thrombus/abscess)
- If cyanotic occurs early neonatal:
  - Rule out (R/o) either cyanotic heart diseases
  - Tricuspid atresia ASD
  - The great arteries (TGA)
  - Total anomolous pulmonary venous connection (TAPVC)

  Most important differential diagnosis for TOF: Double outlet right ventricle with pulmonary stenosis with VSD.
- *TEE:* Demonstrate all defects posterior; great vessel being aorta.

ANESTHESIA CONSIDERATION IN TOF

Tetralogy of Fallot

- Preoperative preparation
  - Heavy premedication
- Consider IM ketamine or inhalation induction but get rapid control of airway
- Keep SVR up and PVR down, maintain heart rate
- Intraoperative TEE
- Perioperative concerns
  - Increase in PVR or decrease in SVR leading to right to left shunt
  - Tet Spells preinduction (crying/anxiety)
  - Polycythemia and bleeding
  - Air embolus
  - RV failure.

Palliative Shunts: Concerns

Reduce, but, not abolish the frequency of Tet Spells

Pulmonary blood flow depends on

Radius of shunt → PVR : SVR

Radius of shunt ↓

Too small → Hypoxia, cyanosis

Too large → Pulmonary edema
CHF

BP monitoring not accurate in upper extremity ipsilateral to shunt

Antibiotic prophylaxis required

Post-total Correction of TOF: Concerns

- Residual RVOT obstruction
- Residual VSD
- Pulmonary insufficiency
- Ventricular arrhythmias
- Risk of sudden death.

Utility of 2D TEE in TOF Intraoperatively

Tetralogy of Fallot (TOF) is the most common cyanotic congenital heart disease. Unrepaired, survival to adulthood is uncommon with only 3% reaching the age of 40. This patient was able to survival to adulthood is due to the mild degree of pulmonic obstruction which may be missed on 2D TEE as mild, because the latter is unable to determine the number of leaflets of the PV but gives a good evaluation of VSD.

3D TRANSESOPHAGEAL ECHOCARDIOGRAPHY IN TOF

3D TEE further delineates, intraoperatively:

- Location of the supravalvular stenosis and may reveal a bicuspid pulmonic valve.
- Show a subvalvular stenosis for a PV replacement is done with pulmonary arterioplasty with good prognosis. Thus 3D TEE scores over 2D TEE wherein, the pulmonic valve is usually not well visualized **(Fig. 4)**.
- The surgeon performed infundibular muscle resection, pulmonic valve replacement, pulmonary arterioplasty.

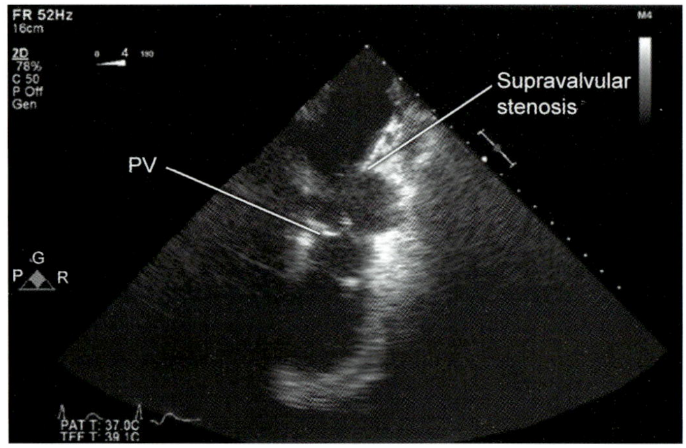

Figure 4 Supravalvular stenosis for a PV replacement is done with pulmonary arterioplasty with good prognosis

- Although the 3D TEE findings did not necessarily alter the surgical management but illustrates another advantage of 3D over 2D TEE is that the pulmonic valve is usually not well visualized by 2D TEE imaging but all three leaflets of PV well seen on 3D TEE.

PREOPERATIVE TEE ASSESSMENT (FIGS 5A TO C)

- VSD—size, site, shunting (pink TOF), gradient (restrictive or unrestrictive), extension to inlet or muscular septum, prolapse of septal tricuspid leaflet (STL) of tricuspid valve (TV) or right coronary cusp (RCC) (TR or AR)
- Additional VSDs, muscular
- Aortic override (percentage)
- Right ventricular hypertrophy
- *Right ventricular outflow tract obstruction:* Site (infundibular and/or valvular), type (uniform narrowing or muscle bundle); gradient
- Pulmonary valve—morphology, bicuspid or tricuspid, annulus size, absence of PV (PAH)
- Size and anatomy of main pulmonary and branch pulmonary arteries, osteal stenosis of LPA is common due to presence of ductal tissue.

MaGoon ratio: This is sum of diameters of immediately prebranching left and right pulmonary arteries to descending aorta just above level of diaphragm. Normal value more than 2–2.5. TOF survivor with pulmonary artesia have MaGoon ratio more than 1.

Nakata index: Nakata index is cross sectional area of left and right pulmonary artery in mm^2 divided by total

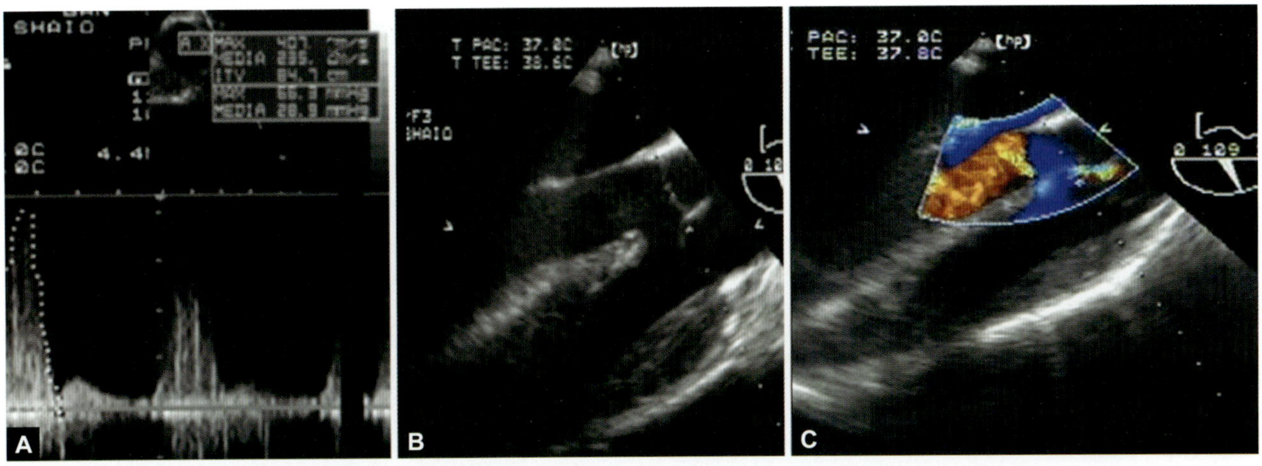

Figures 5A to C Precorrection. (A) Continuous Doppler of the RVOT with peak and mean gradient of 66 mm Hg and 29 mm Hg, respectively, in a deep transgastric of the right ventricle (Deep TG RV). The arrow indicated the peak gradient; (B) Long axis of the aortic valve in the mid-esophagus (ME AV LAX) showing the classical characteristics of the TOF; overriding aorta and broad VSD. The arrow points the VSD; (C) Color Doppler interrogation of the previous view, showing right to left shunting through the VSD, the arrow points the flow

body surface area (BSA). Normal Nakata value is 330 ± 30 mm^2/BSA. TOF with PS should have value more than 100 mm^2/BSA for survival.

Atrial septal defect, patent ductus arteriosus, coarctation of aorta, left superior vena cava to be ruled out.

- *LV and MV size:* If left ventricular end-diastolic volume (LVEDV) <30 mL/m^2; left ventricular end-diastolic diameter (LVEDD) <60% of normal for that weight or MV area is <2 Z value—contraindication for intracardiac repair.
- Proximal coronary arteries, branching of left main coronary artery (LMCA)
- *The classical findings of a TOF:* Extensive ventricular septal communication with right to left shunt, severe hypertrophy of the right ventricle with mild RVEF depression calculated at 35%, RV outlet tract obstruction with peak and mean gradients of 66 and 29 mm Hg, respectively (*see* **Fig. 1**).

POSTOPERATIVE TEE ASSESSMENT (FIGS 6 TO 13)

- Residual VSD—size, shunt, gradient
- Residual gradient across PV
- Pulmonary regurgitation—valvotomy or trans-annular patch
- Tricuspid regurgitation
- Position of interatrial septum (IAS) and interventricular septum (IVS)
- Aortic valve and its leaflets and opening
- Patent foramen ovale (surgically created), if so direction of shunting.

What is really important is the comparison between before and after the correction. The obstruction of the right ventricular outflow tract (RVOT) determines the severity of the symptoms in this particular heart disease and hence determining the RVOT gradient during the postrepair period is key to only to prevent a low cardiac output in the immediate postoperative, but during reoperations in the long-term.

The classical approach to estimate the RVOT gradient is to calculate the ratio between the right ventricle systolic pressure divided into the systemic systolic pressure; if the result is equal or less than 0.75, the correction is considered acceptable.[2]

The exact determination of the peak and mean RVOTF gradient using the continuous Doppler method according to Bernoulli's principle that establishes the relationship between flow acceleration and the increase in pressure through an orifice. In the case of correcting a TOF, a mean gradient above 54 mm Hg is an indication for revision of surgery.[3]

CONCLUSION

Although patients with TOF repaired within first 6 months of life had prolonged postoperative recovery and an increased chance of transannular patch usage, outcomes were comparable to those patients with TOF repaired later. Therefore, symptomatic infants can receive total repair of TOF early to avoid the need for use of a palliative shunt. However, when total repair is undertaken on an elective basis, the procedure may be delayed until the patient is older than 6 months of age.[4]

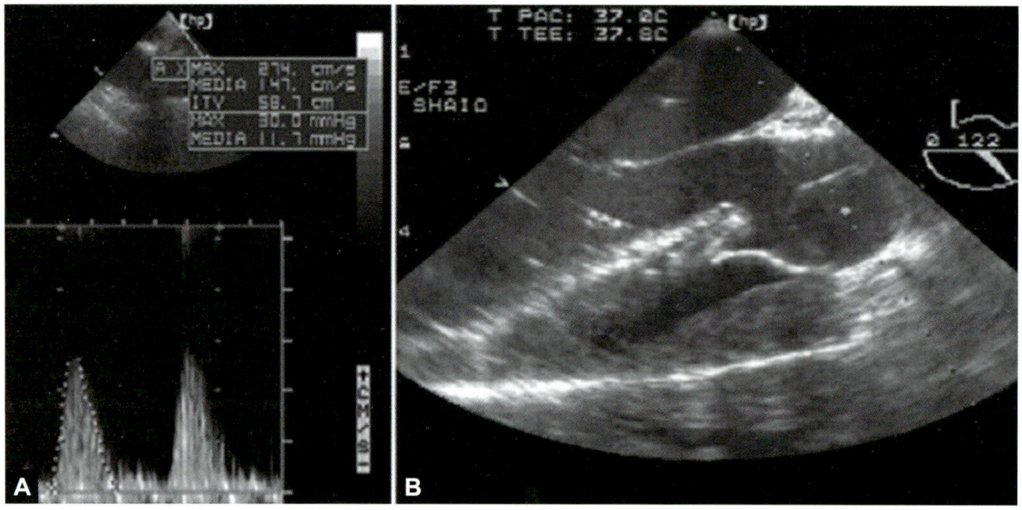

Figures 6A and B Corrected. (A) Continuous Doppler of the RVOT with peak and mean gradients of 30 and 11 mm Hg in a deep transgastric of the right ventricle (Deep TG RV). The arrow indicates the peak gradient; (B) Long axis of the aortic valve in the midesophagus (ME AV LAX) indicating the correction of the aorta aligned to the right with the patch. The arrow indicated the patch. *Abbreviations:* LA–left atrium; LV–left ventricle, RV–right ventricle, AO–aorta

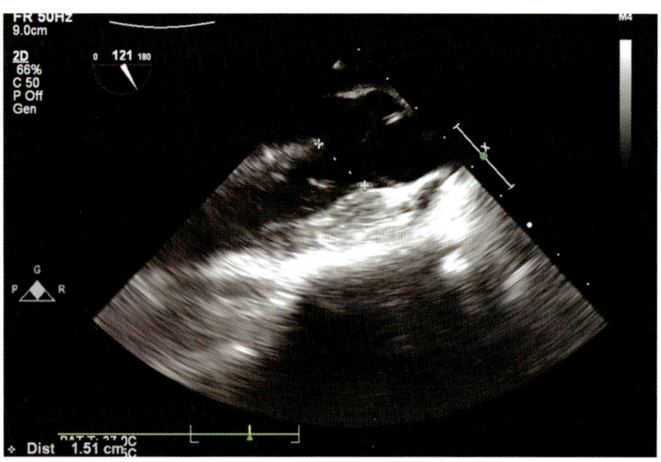

Figure 7 Midesophageal LAX view showing a subaortic VSD of 1.51 cm and override of aorta. In patients with tetralogy of Fallot the size of aortic root is enlarged because of the override. The ME long axis view the ideal view for interrogating flow across the subaortic VSD and to measure the gradient across it. Since in TOF, the VSD is usually large the gradient is essentially insignificant

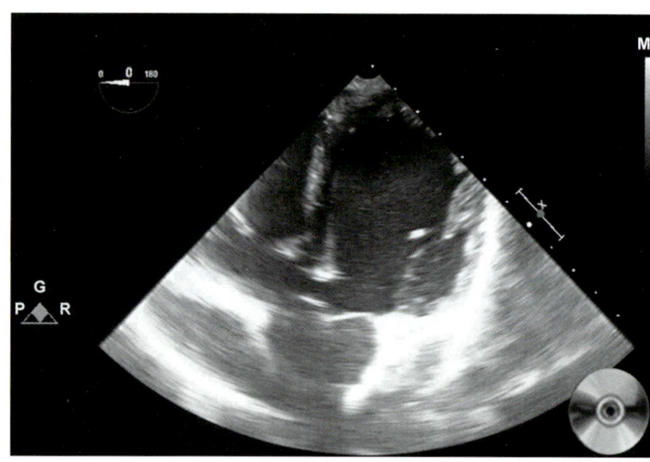

Figure 8 (Video 1) 2D echo deep transgastric view showing a subaortic ventricular septal defect and aortic over-ride in a patient with Tetralogy of Fallot. The aortic root is always enlarged because of the over-ride

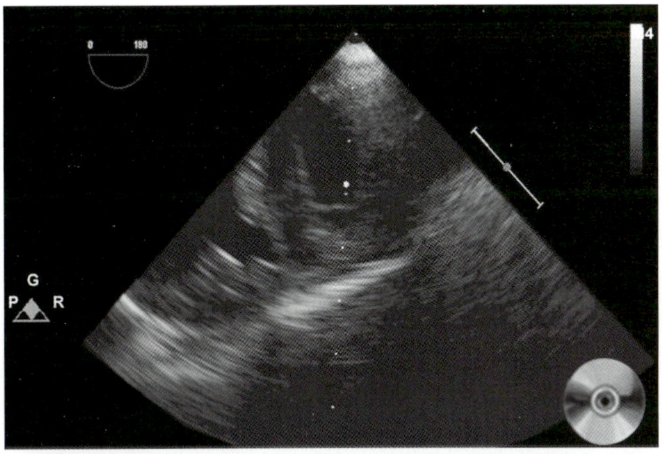

Figure 9 (Video 2) 2D echocardiography in mid papillary transgastric view showing normal left ventricular function

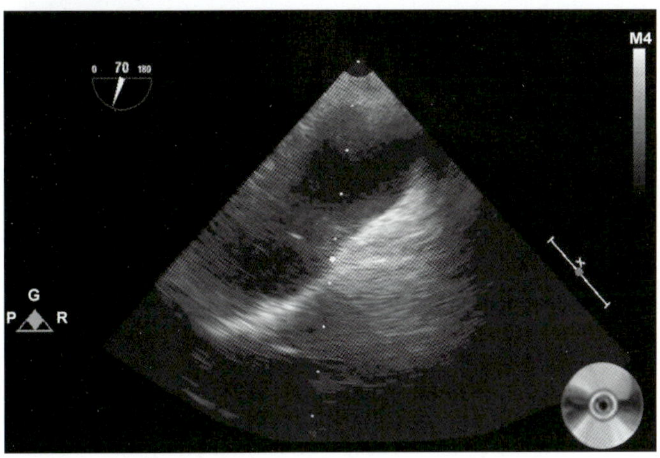

Figure 10 (Video 3) 2D echocardiography in upper esophageal ascending aortic short axis view showing pulmonic valve stenosis

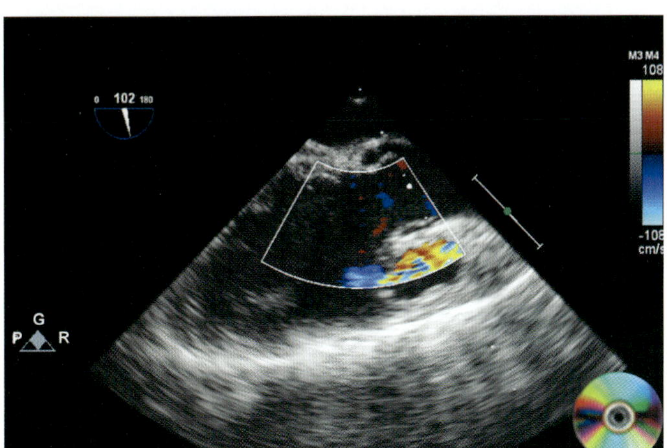

Figure 11 (Video 4) Color Doppler in midesophageal long axis view showing a subaortic ventricular septal defect shunting from left to right and infundibular pulmonary stenosis in a patient with Tetralogy of Fallot

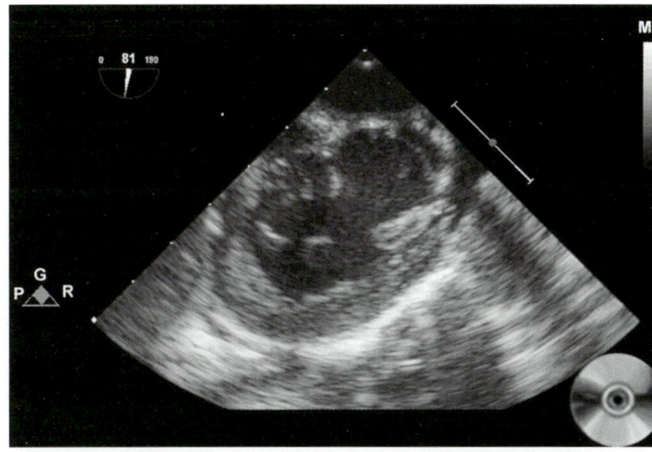

Figure 12 (Video 5) 2D echo in midesophageal right ventricle inflow-outflow view showing subaortic ventricular septal defect and infundibular pulmonary stenosis in a patient with Tetralogy of Fallot

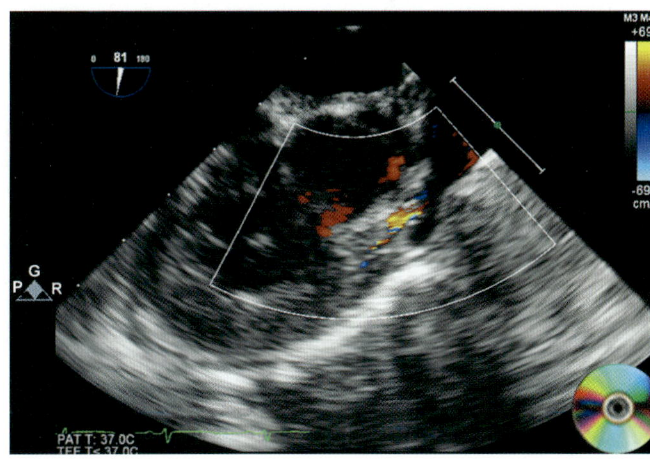

Figure 13 (Video 6) Color Doppler in midesophageal right ventricle inflow-outflow view showing subaortic ventricular septal defect and infundibular pulmonary stenosis in a patient with Tetralogy of Fallot

REFERENCES

1. William Herring. Cyanotic Heart Disease. Slide show mode, 2003.
2. Joyce J, Hwang E, Wiles H, et al. Reliability of intraoperative transesophageal echocardiography during tetralogy of Fallot repair. Echocardiography. 2000;17:319-27.
3. Kaushal S, Radhakrishanan S, Dagar K, Iyer P, Girotra S, Shrivastava S, et al. Significant intraoperative right ventricular outflow gradients after repair for tetralogy of Fallot: to revise or not to revise? Ann Thorac Surg. 1999;68:1705-13.
4. Shuenn-Nan Chiu, Jou-Kou Wang. Long-term outcomes of patients with tetralogy of Fallot repaired in young infants and toddlers. Acta Cardiol Sin. 2012;28:137-44.

Chapter 12

TEE for Double-Outlet Right Ventricle

Poonam Malhotra Kapoor, Sarvesh Pal Singh, Jitin Narula, Suruchi Ladha

Chapter Outline

- Various Criteria for Classification of DORV
- Other Anomalies with DORV
- Aortic Over-Ride
- Chest X-ray
- Electrocardiography
- Use of TEE in DORV
- Two-Dimensional TEE for DORV in TOF
- Ventricular Septal Defect
- Location of VSD in DORV
- Preoperative Assessment of DORV on TEE
- Assessment for Routability of VSD
- Anatomy and Suggested Two-Dimensional Views for Routability of Ventricular Septal Defect
- Postoperative Assessment of DORV on TEE

INTRODUCTION

Double-outlet right ventricle (DORV) is a "disease" that includes a family of anatomically related complex congenital heart lesions involving the right ventricular outflow tract. There are a number of variations within the diagnostic category of DORV that give rise to a wide spectrum of physiology ranging from that of tetralogy of Fallot to transposition of the great arteries (TGA) to true single ventricle physiology. It therefore encompasses virtually the entire spectrum of cardiac physiology.

Determining treatment requires an understanding of the specific relationship of the ventricular septal defect (VSD) to the great vessels, the size of the VSD, the size of the great vessels, the ventricular size, and the status of the atrioventricular (AV) valves. Understanding these components and their relationship allows one to predict the physiology and therefore consider appropriate treatment repair algorithms.[1]

DEFINITION

Double-outlet right ventricle refers to the ventriculoarterial connection where both great arteries are nearly or completely aligned with respect to the right ventricle. This is thought to be the result of abnormal conal development leading to pathologic great artery relationships. Various criteria have been proposed to characterize this pathology leading to significant controversy. These include the 50% rule, the absence of fibrous discontinuity between the aortic valve and adjacent atrioventricular valve, and the morphology of the conus septum. The anatomic and physiology diversity of DORV relates to the location of the ventricular septal defect and great artery relationships.

Normally, the aorta, which is the largest artery in the body, comes from the heart's left ventricle. But when DORV occurs, the aorta and the pulmonary artery are attached to the right ventricle.

Another heart defect called ventricular septal defect (VSD) usually occurs with DORV. DORV can be categorized into several types depending on the position of the VSD.

VARIOUS CRITERIA FOR CLASSIFICATION OF DORV

Various criteria have been used in the definition and classification of DORV.

- DORV morphology should be characterized by an exact description of the ventricular septal defect (VSD) in and its
  - Relationship to the semilunar valves
  - Relationship of the great arteries to each other
  - The presence of pulmonary outflow tract obstruction or aortic outfow tract obstruction
  - The tricuspid pulmonary annular distance
  - Finally the presence of other associated cardiac pathology.[1]

Types of DORV

- The relationship of VSD to the great arteries is the basis for the classification. The Association of European Pediatric Cardiology (AEPC) considers DORV is of four different types:
  - VSD type
  - Fallot-type
  - Transposition of great arteries type
  - Non-committed (remote) VSD type.
- Although ascent from the right ventricle of more than 50% of aorta may be accepted as a sufficient condition for DORV, demonstration of a total defect is liable to modify preoperative preparation. The diagnosis of DORV implies not only anatomical heterogeneity and difficulties with clinical classification, but also problems concerning surgical timing and the choice of appropriate technique.
- The characterization of malformations for a correct choice of diagnosis and treatment should include the:
  - Position of VSD
  - The relations between the great arteries
  - The presence or absence of pulmonary artery outlet obstruction
  - Pulmonary hypertension
  - Associated cardiac lesions.

Other anomalies seen are: Witham in 1957 first used the term double-outlet right ventricle to describe a partial transposition of the great arteries.[2] Several associated cardiac anomalies are associated with double-outlet right ventricle, and many of these affect the clinical presentations and limits of the repair.

OTHER ANOMALIES WITH DORV

Occurrence rates of associated cardiovascular anomalies include: pulmonary stenosis 21–47% (most commonly observed with subaortic type VSD), atrial septal defect 21–26%, patent ductus arteriosus 16%, atrioventricular canal 8%, subaortic stenosis 3–30%, coarctation/ hypoplastic arch/interrupted aortic arch 2–45%, mitral valve anomalies 30%.[3] Almost all our series had VSD, and some had ASD. The reason for VSD and ASD could be that their presence could help to reduce pulmonary resistance and, thus help to increase oxygen saturated blood to the system, thus averting cyanosis **(Fig. 1)**.

Along with these conditions, the pulmonary valve may be narrowed. DORV is thus a serious condition.[4]

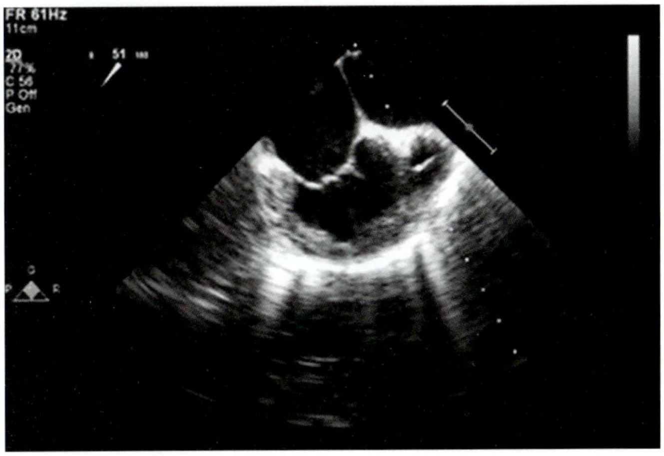

Figure 1 DORV with pulmonary stenosis and mitral stenosis in RV inflow-outflow view

AORTIC OVER-RIDE

In tetralogy of Fallot (TOF) the aortic root characteristically overrides the ventricular septum/defect. This is manifested as a biventricular connection of the leaflets of the aortic valve. In DORV the spatial relations of the arterial trunks ranges from normal to side-by-side to malposed, as in the case of the location of the VSD, are influencing the physiology and surgical approach.

Double-outlet right ventricle (DORV) lies in the middle of the spectrum between ToF and transposition of the great arteries (TGA). The right ventricle empties into both the pulmonary artery (PA) and aorta simultaneously. The relative fraction of CO being emptied in the individual arteries depends on whether the VSD is restrictive or unrestrictive. If unrestrictive the ratio will depend on the ratio of systemic vascular resistance (SVR) and pulmonary vascular resistance (PVR). Another issue unique to DORV is malaligned VSD and its routability. The VSD location may be such that it is difficult to route it and this is where TEE is very helpful, especially in adults with DORV.

CHEST X-RAY

Plain chest radiography shows cardiomegaly and pulmonary oligaemia.

Double-outlet right ventricle **(Figs 2A and B)**

1. Subaortic VSD, no pulmonary stenosis low pulmonary vascular resistance-resembles non-restrictive perimembranous VSD.
2. Subaortic VSD, no pulmonary stenosis high pulmonary vascular resistance resembles Eisenmenger's complex.
3. Subaortic VSD with pulmonary stenosis resembles tetralogy of Fallot (TOF).
4. Subpulmonic VSD, no pulmonic stenosis resembles complete transposition of great arteries with large VSD.
5. Complete transposition of great arteries.
6. Total anomalous pulmonary venous connection.

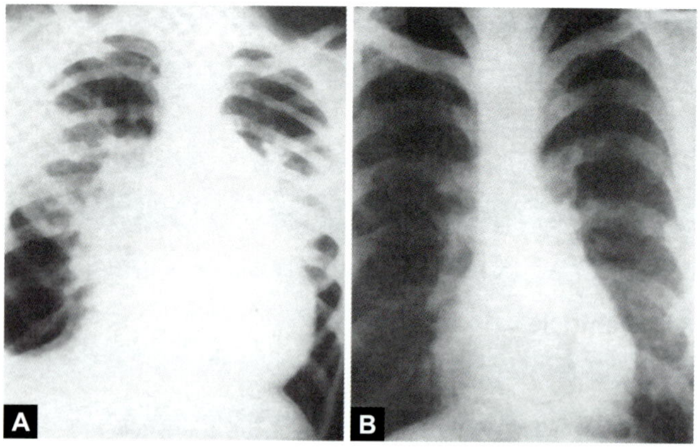

Figures 2A and B Chest films of two patients with double-outlet right ventricle. Figure (A) is that of a patient with ventricle septal defect with no pulmonary stenosis. X-ray resembles that of a nonrestrictive ventricular septal defect with pulmonary hypertension; Figure (B) is that of a patient with ventricular septal defect with pulmonary stenosis resembling tetralogy of Fallot

ELECTROCARDIOGRAPHY

Common electrocardiography (ECG) findings in a child with double-outlet right ventricle include right ventricular hypertrophy, right axis deviation, and occasionally, evidence of left ventricular hypertrophy. Prenatal diagnosis may be helpful in detecting this anomaly early and avert the morbidity and mortality that follow this disease. However, prenatal diagnosis is yet to gain grounds in the management of DORV in most countries and this service is not offered to patients in most setting.[5]

Angiography result showed a dilated branch of pulmonary artery and normal pulmonary venous drainage, and the 2-D echocardiography (ECG) result is attached **(Figs 3 and 4)**.

USE OF TEE IN DORV

The primary applications of transesophageal echocardiography (TEE) in patients with ToF or DORV include those related to the intraoperative setting, either during initial surgical correction or when reoperation is needed to address sequelae or less likely, residual or recurrent pathology. The main goals of the examination are the confirmation of the preoperative diagnoses, baseline assessment, and identification of hemodynamically significant defects immediately following the surgical intervention that may necessitate revision. Additional benefits of TEE include:

- Evaluation of associated defects
- Assessment of atrioventricular and semilunar valve competence
- Monitoring of ventricular preload and function
- Determining the adequacy of **cardiac dealring**
- Guidance of the surgical revision.

When TEE is contraindicated epicardial imaging may be considered. Imaging via the transesophageal

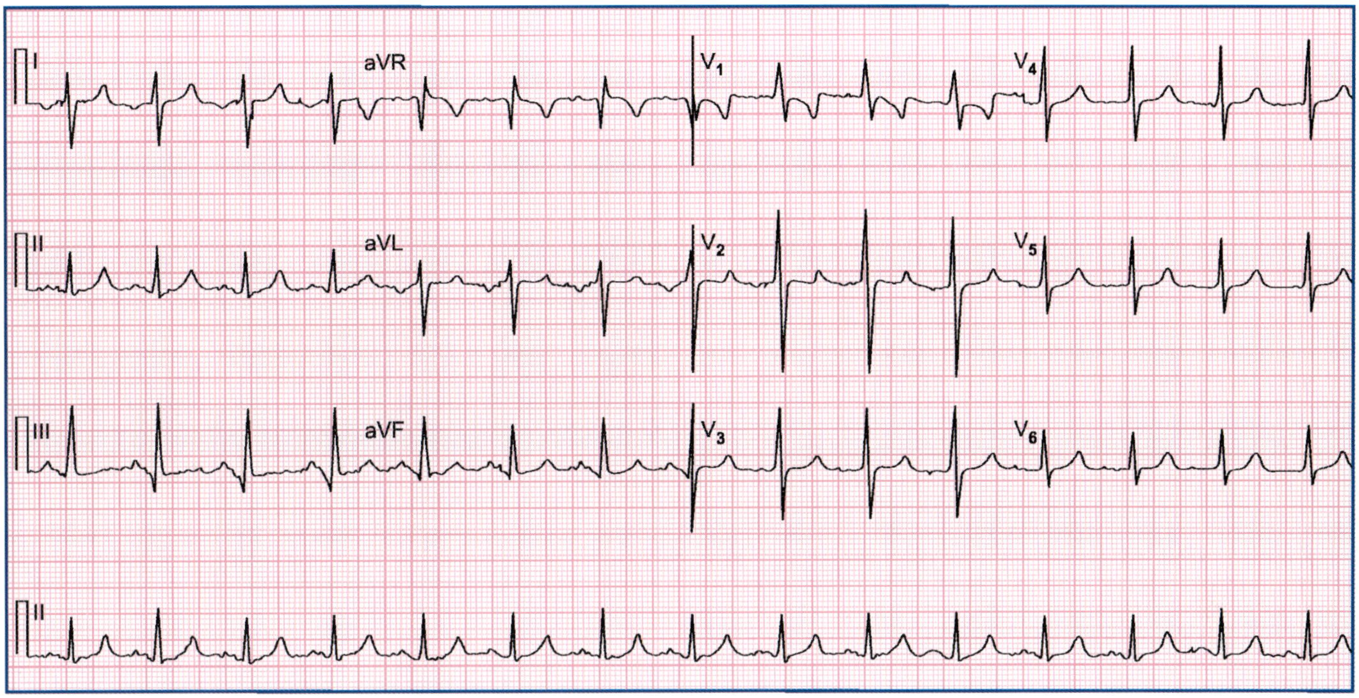

Figure 3 Complex congenitally corrected with double-outlet right ventricle, dextrocardia, subpulmonary stenosis

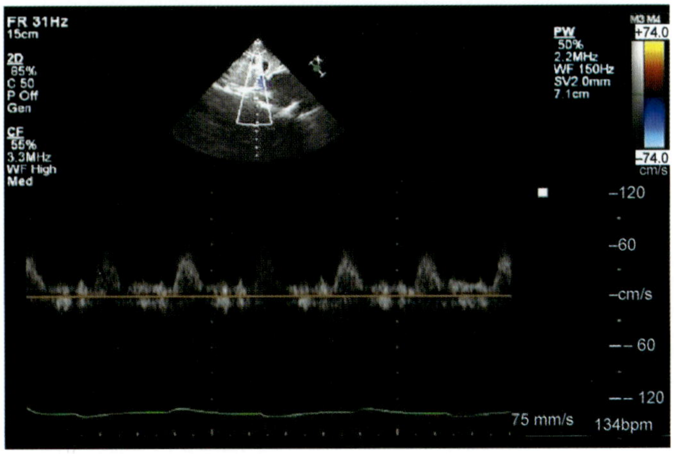

Figure 4 Echocardiogram (2-D)

approach in these patients may also be of benefit in the cardiac catheterization laboratory during catheter-based interventions for monitoring of the procedure, management of potential complications, minimizing the use of fluoroscopy as well as the need for angiography.

TWO-DIMENSIONAL TEE FOR DORV IN TOF (FIG. 5)

Anatomy and Suggested Two-Dimensional Views

Views for RVOT

- ME RV inflow-outflow
- ME Asc Ao SAX, Deep TG (RVOT)
- Additional RVOT/PA views.

Outflow tract obstruction occurs in the majority of patients with DORV (over 70%). This most commonly affects those with a subaortic VSD.

Color Doppler

- *Determine nature, location, and severity of the obstruction in the postoperative patient*: Assess for residual obstruction, degree of pulmonary/conduit regurgitation (patency of left ventricular outflow post DORV repair)
- Use spectral Doppler (obtained in views that allow for optimal alignment of the Doppler cursor to the direction of flow)

- *Evaluate severity of right ventricular outflow tract obstruction*: Estimation of gradient(s) derived from peak velocity.
- Assess direction of flow across VSD.
- Evaluate additional shunts (ventricular, atrial and great artery levels).
- Evaluate for residual ventricular level shunting.

  In some cases, closure of the large conoventricular defect in tetralogy of Fallot (TOF) may unmask smaller ventricular septal defects. This should be evaluated in the post bypass examination.
- *Spectral Doppler*: Determine peak velocity of VSD jet (usually low due to unrestrictive nature of defect).

  If residual defect, determine degree of restriction based on jet velocity.
- *Contrast echocardiography*: It may assist in the evaluation of residual intracardiac shunts.

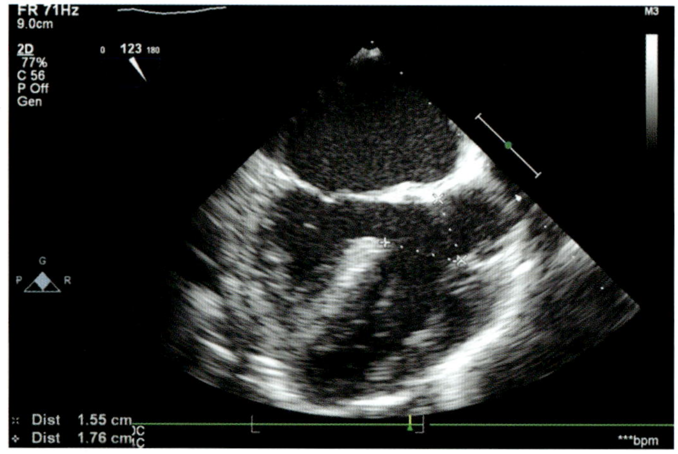

Figure 5 Midesophageal (ME) long axis view showing a subaortic ventricular septal defect and more than 50% override of aorta. The override is so much that the cardiac output of right ventricle ejects directly into the ascending aorta. Also seen in the left atrium and both the ventricles

VENTRICULAR SEPTAL DEFECT

The interventricular communication is generally unrestrictive in tetralogy of Fallot (TOF). The classic defect is an anterior malalignment-type outlet type (large conoventricular or subaortic defect). Other anatomic defects may be present in the ventricular septum are:

- Perimembranous
- Atrioventricular septal defect
- Inlet
- Muscular
- Doubly committed subarterial.

The direction of shunting across the defect is related to the right ventricular outflow obstruction. The shunt direction is left to right if minimal outflow obstruction is present and predominantly right to left during hypercyanotic episodes. In most cases the shunt is bidirectional and the ventricular pressures are equal.

LOCATION OF VSD IN DORV

The location of the VSD is variable in DORV accounting for the physiologic diversity of this defect.

- Subaortic location
- Subpulmonary location
- Doubly committed or noncommitted (remote) location.

PREOPERATIVE ASSESSMENT OF DORV ON TEE (FIG. 5)

- Ventricular septal defect (VSD)—size, site, shunting, gradient (restrictive or unrestrictive), extension to inlet or muscular septum, prolapse of septal tricuspid leaflet (STL) of tricuspid valve (TV) or RCC (TR or AR)
- Routability of VSD **(Fig. 6)**
- Additional VSDs, muscular
- *Aortic override*: Percentage
- Right ventricular hypertrophy
- *Right ventricular outflow tract obstruction*: Site (infundibular or valvular), type (uniform narrowing or muscle bundle); gradient
- Pulmonary stenosis or pulmonary artery hypertension
- Pulmonary valve—morphology, bicuspid or tricuspid, annulus size
- Size and anatomy of main pulmonary and branch pulmonary arteries
- LV size
- ASD, PDA, CoA, LSVC
- Mitral valve
- Proximal coronary arteries, branching of LMCA
- Juxtaposed appendages.

ASSESSMENT FOR ROUTABILITY OF VSD (FIG. 6)

- *Size of VSD in relation to aortic valve annulus*: The VSD should be atleast the size or more than the size of aortic annulus
- Aorto-mitral continuity should be uninterrupted
- Relation of Aorta and PA (Root) should be seen

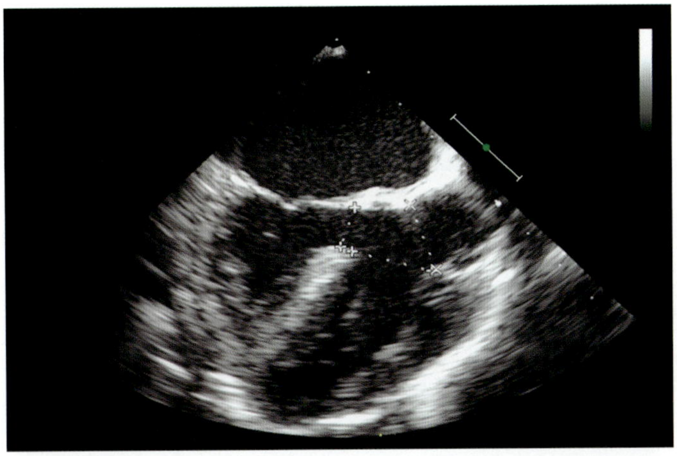

Figure 6 Midesophageal (ME) long axis view showing the VSD in a double-outlet right ventricle whose routability is in question. This image shows a large VSD (size larger than the aortic annulus), with aorto-mitral continuity present and a wide open left ventricular outflow, if the VSD is closed. Therefore this VSD is routable

- Taussig Bing physiology (DORV with doubly committed VSD, dextroposed aorta); RV output preferably goes to aorta and LV to PA. *Surgery*: Arterial Switch operation
- *Aortic valve*: In tetralogy of Fallot (TOF), the aortic root characteristically overrides the ventricular septum/defect. This is manifested as a biventricular connection of the leaflets of the aortic valve. In DORV the spatial relations of the arterial trunks ranges from normal to side-by-side to malposed, as in the case of the location of the VSD, influencing the physiology and surgical approach.

ANATOMY AND SUGGESTED TWO-DIMENSIONAL VIEWS FOR ROUTABILITY OF VENTRICULAR SEPTAL DEFECT

Aortic relationship to the ventricular septum: Deep TG (LVOT) LAX.

The degree of aortic override has been used as criteria for distinguishing between tetralogy of Fallot (TOF) and double-outlet right ventricle (less than and more than 50% override respectively). However, it is important to recognize that the degree of override may vary according to the angle of two-dimensional interrogation. Thus it is helpful to also consider additional criteria that would support one or the other diagnosis.

Aortic root dilation is a frequent finding, which may be associated with aortic regurgitation.

Suggested views for biventricular function and gradients LV/RV are:
- ME 4 Ch
- TG Mid SAX
- ME RV inflow-outflow
- TG RV inflow
- Deep TG LAX.

POSTOPERATIVE ASSESSMENT OF DORV ON TEE (FIGS 7 TO 9)

- *Residual VSD*: Size, shunt, gradient
- Residual gradient across PV
- Pulmonary regurgitation—valvotomy or trans-annular patch needed or not?
- Tricuspid regurgitation, PA pressures
- Position of IAS and IVS
- Aortic valve
- Patent foramen ovale (surgically created), if so direction of shunting.

CONCLUSION

Preoperatively, comprehensive multi-modal imaging that includes 3D Echo and 3D MRI is needed for evaluation of complex DORV. Joint surgical discussion should include manipulation of 3D images by echo-cardiographers and surgeon to assess different virtual options it should be possible to have planned the operation in the great majority of cases (rather than open up and look see!).

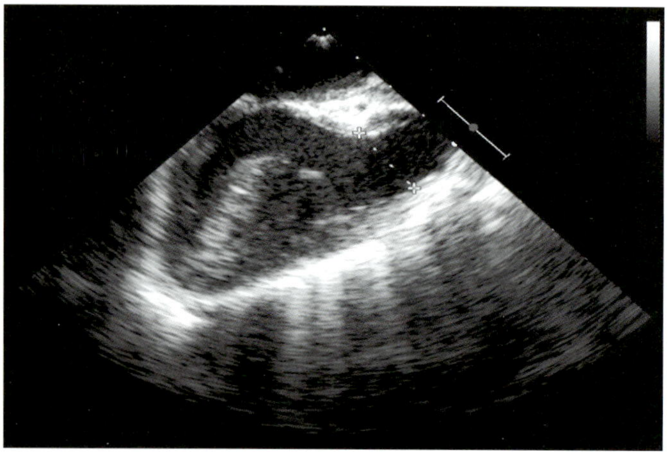

Figure 7 ME long axis view showing the VSD in a double-outlet right ventricle whose routability is in question. Although the VSD is large when compared with the aortic annulus but the aorta is dextroposed and thus the VSD, if routed may lead to a right ventricle outflow tract obstruction. In such cases, it is better to perform an arterial switch operation rather than an intracardiac repair

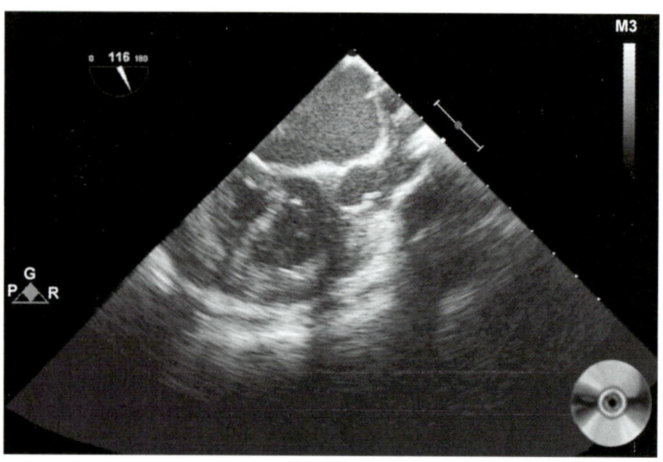

Figure 8 (Video 1) 2D echocardiography in midesophageal long axis view showing a subaortic ventricular septal defect with over-riding of aorta (>50% in this case) in a patient with double-outlet right ventricle

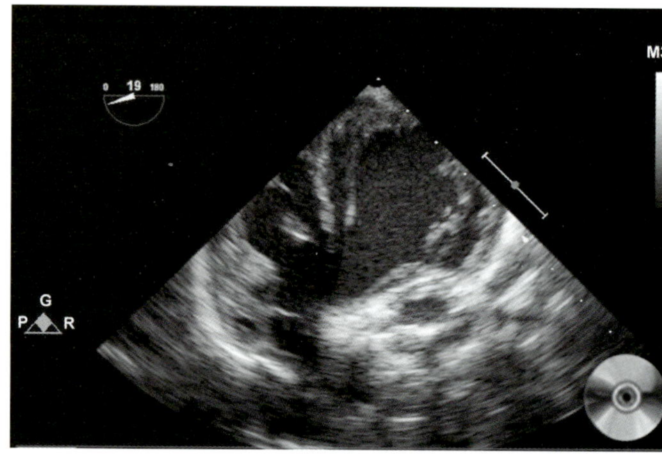

Figure 9 (Video 2) 2D echocardiography in deep transgastric long axis view showing a subaortic ventricular septal defect with over-riding of aorta (>50% in this case) in a patient with double-outlet right ventricle. Because of so much of over-ride the right ventricle ejects directly into the aorta. Note the mitral valve in its cross-section

REFERENCES

1. Walters HL 3rd, Mavroudis C, Tchervenkov CI, et al. Congenital heart surgery nomenclature and database project: double-outlet right ventricle. Ann Thorac Surg. 2000;69:249-63.
2. Belli E, Serraf A, Lacour-Gayet F. Double-outlet right ventricle with non-committed ventricular septal defect. Eur J Cardiothorac Surg. 1999;15:747-52.
3. Brown JW, Ruzmetov M, Okada Y. Surgical results in patients with double-outlet right ventricle: a 20-year experience. Ann Thorac Surg. 2001;72:1630-5.
4. Menahem S, Grimwade J. Pre-natal counseling—helping couples make decisions following the diagnosis of severe heart disease. Early Hum Dev. 2005;81:601-7.
5. Diagnosis and Management of Adult Congenital Heart Disease, 1st edition, Chapter 5, pp.242-4. Copyright © 2014 Elsevier Inc.

Chapter 13

TEE for Transposition of Great Arteries

Sarvesh Pal Singh, Jitin Narula, Poonam Malhotra Kapoor, Sachin Talwar

Chapter Outline

INTRODUCTION

Transposition of great arteries means the aorta arises from the right ventricle and pulmonary artery from the left ventricle. Therefore, the pulmonary and systemic circulations are in parallel rather in series. A communication between both the circulations is essential for the survival of the child.[1] This communication can be at atrial, ventricular or ductus arteriosus level **(Figs 1A and B)**.

Transposition of great arteries can be of two types: *d*-Transposition or *l*-Transposition.

1. *d-Loop*: The normal *rightward* (*dextro = d*) bend in the embryonic heart tube. The d-loop designation as applied to the developed heart indicates that the sinus or inflow portion of the morphologic right ventricle lies to the right of the morphologic left ventricle.
2. *l-Loop*: A *leftward (levo = l) bend* in the embryonic heart tube. The l-loop designation as applied to the developed heart indicates that the sinus or inflow portion of the morphologic right ventricle lies to the left of the morphologic left ventricle.

PREOPERATIVE TEE ASSESSMENT

Identify the valves and ventricles. Ventricles always go with the valves. Therefore, if mitral valve is identified then the corresponding ventricle is the morphologic left ventricle.

- Shape of ventricles (first two are consistent with ASO, third shows regressed LV) **(Table 1)**.
- Mass of left ventricle (preparedness of left ventricle)
- Identification of aorta and pulmonary artery: the great artery which arises and bifurcates is the

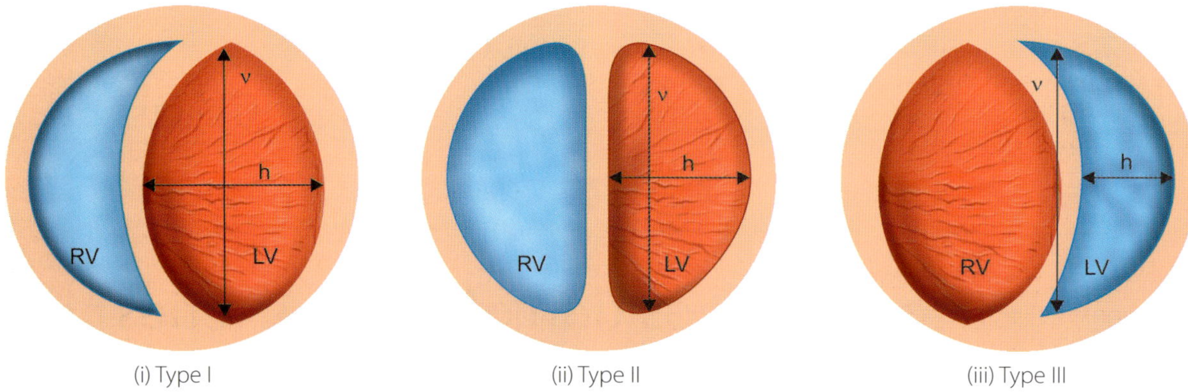

Figure 1A Schematic representation of the three patterns of LV geometry in patients with TGA: (i) "Favorable" (type I); (ii) "Acceptable" (type II); (iii) "Unfavorable" (type III). These three diagrams represent the end-systolic subcostal short-axis echocardiographic projections of the left and right ventricles at the level of the tips of the LV papillary muscles. The minor axis ratio is calculated as v/h. *Abbreviations:* RV = right ventricle; LV = left ventricle; v = superoinferior minor transverse axis; h = anteroposterior minor transverse axis

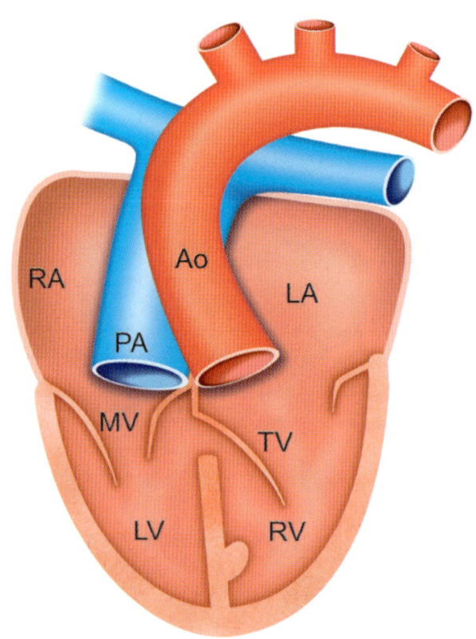

Figure 1B Anatomically corrected transposition of the great arteries. The atrioventricular and the ventriculo-arterial junctions are discordant. The anatomical left ventricle (LV), with the mitral valve (MV), is on the right side and connected to a pulmonary artery (PA). The anatomical right ventricle (RV), with the tricuspid valve (TV) and a septal papillary muscle, is on the left side and connected to the aorta (Ao)

TABLE 1 Ventricles: morphology—right, left and their differences

	RV	*LV*
Atrioventricular valve	Trileaflet	Bileaflet (unless AML cleft)
Leaflet attachment	Septum	No septal
Annulus location	More apical	More basal
Apex	Prominent	Less prominent trabeculations
Moderator band	Present	Absent
Infundibulum	Present	Absent

pulmonary artery whereas which continues as singular trunk is the aorta. Therefore, it is essential to trace the course of both the great vessels in case of TGA or CCTGA.

- Relation of aorta and main pulmonary artery
- IVS/VSD
- PS
- ASD.

Ventricular morphology is indeterminate if trabeculations are absent and there is a large VSD.

In univentricular physiology the morphology of the single ventricle is not stressed much because whatever morphology it is going to be the systemic ventricle after correction.

For Arterial Switch Operation

- Identify the ventricles and great arteries
- Relation of great arteries
- Evaluation of VSD and ASD (if present)
- Mitral and tricuspid annulus-size-development of both ventricles
- Mitral and tricuspid valve—regurgitation or tethering of TV
- Pulmonary artery size, branch PAs size
- Pulmonary valve—annulus, bicuspid or tricuspid (long term implications), regurgitation (future valve towards systemic circulation) or stenosis—mild (ASO) or severe (Rastelli)
- Left ventricular outflow tract—size, any accessory mitral tissue or membrane causing obstruction
- Left ventricle—any signs of regression—LV PWed, IVS ed and LV IDd
- LV mass = 0.8 $\{1.04\ (LVIDed + IVSed + LVPWed)^3 - (LVIDed)^3\} + 0.6$ g
- LVPWed < -2Z is suggestive of regressed left ventricle
- Pulmonary and systemic venous drainage.

Surgical Options Apart from ASO in Selected Patients (with Severe Pulmonary Stenosis)

Rastelli Procedure

- *Indications:*
  - Coronary artery crossing RVOT
  - Look for routability of VSD and relation of PA and RV
- *Disadvantage:* Conduit may get compressed with the sternum.

Nikaidoh Operation (Aortic Translocation)

- *Indications:*
  - Presence of an inlet or restrictive ventricular septal defect
  - A hypoplastic right ventricle
  - A straddling atrioventricular valve and/or
  - Anomalous coronary anatomy interfering with a distal right ventricular outflow tract incision.

Options for Regressed Left Ventricle

- *Two stage ASO:* PA band + MBTS followed by ASO
- *Senning's procedure* (Juxtaposed appendages are a contraindication for performing Senning procedure).

TRANSESOPHAGEAL ECHOCARDIOGRAPHY FOR SENNING PROCEDURE

The Senning operation for TGA was first reported by Senning in 1959 with later work by Quaegebeur in the late 1970s. It became the operation of choice for surgical repair of TGA during this time period.

- The Senning procedure uses a "baffle" between the atria resulting in the redirection of deoxygenated vena caval blood through the mitral valve to the morphological LV and pulmonary arteries and oxygenated pulmonary venous blood through the tricuspid valve into the morphological RV and aorta.
- The "baffle" created in the Senning procedure is derived from autologous atrial tissue that is cut and folded in a complex manner to allow for the redirection of blood flow.
- Because of the technical difficulty associated with the formation of the Senning "baffle," this procedure was not widely embraced.
- Mustard simplified the procedure by excising the atrial septum and placing a "single, synthetic pantaloon-shaped patch" between the atria to create the baffle, again redirecting the blood flow in the same manner as the Senning procedure.

- Owing to its simplified nature, the Mustard procedure quickly became the surgeon's operation of choice.
- Two main therapeutic approaches govern surgical treatment: redirecting the venous return at the atrial level (Mustard or Senning procedures), and switching the great arteries during the first 2–3 weeks of life. Examination of adult patients with previous arterial switch procedure should be close to normal. However, RVOT or LVOT obstruction, AV and semilunar valve regurgitation, possible residual shunt or left ventricular dysfunction may be found.[2]
- After Mustard or Senning operations, the echocardiographic images are more complex. The intra-atrial repair divides the biauricular cavity into an anterior and a posterior chamber, with a baffle redirecting the systemic venous return to the mitral valve (anterior chamber) and the pulmonary venous flow to the tricuspid valve (posterior chamber), wrapping in horseshoe fashion around the midatrial systemic venous channel where the flow should remain biphasic, mirroring the atrial pressure trace." A contrast study with saline injected into a systemic vein helps in the evaluation of cardiac anatomy. In the case of obstruction, the Doppler analysis reveals a loss of phasic pattern, an increased flow velocity (>1.5 m/s), and a turbulent flow on color mapping. Tricuspid regurgitation and progressive right ventricular dilation and dysfunction are frequently encountered in adulthood, as the right ventricle is small and squashed by the right ventricular because of septum encroachment on the left ventricular cavity. A dynamic LVOT obstruction, which is most frequently encountered by patients with intact septum, may occur progressively with advancing age because of the low resistance PA bed being connected to an anatomical left ventricular chamber. Left ventricular dilation and failure may supervene in case of increased pulmonary vascular resistance.

ASSESSMENT OF THE PULMONARY VENOUS PATHWAY

The pulmonary venous pathway is to be assessed for any obstruction. The pulmonary venous atrium (PVA) should be checked for any turbulence, the most common site being where it curves anteriorly towards the tricuspid valve (arrow in **Figure 2**). A continuous wave Doppler should be used to quantify the gradient. Individual pulmonary veins should be assessed for turbulence, the most common pulmonary vein to show turbulence is the right upper pulmonary vein (RUPV) **(Fig. 3)**. A pulsed wave Doppler should be used to quantify individual pulmonary veins especially RUPV. A gradient of more than 4–5 mm Hg in the pulmonary venous pathway or individual pulmonary veins is not acceptable.

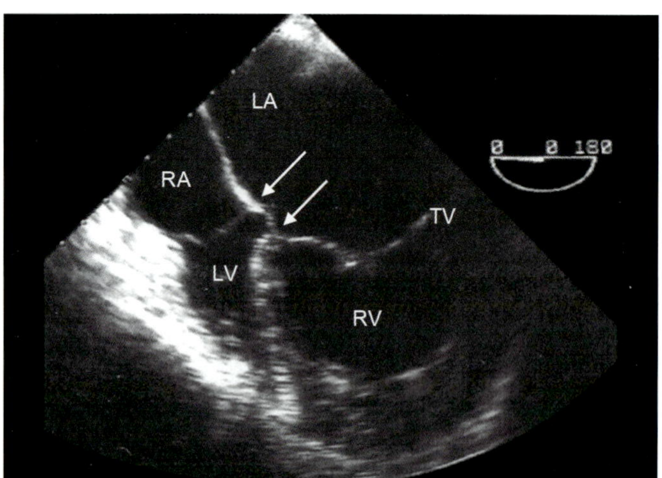

Figure 2 Anatomically corrected transposition of the great arteries four chamber view. The septal insertions of the MV and the TV (arrows) show that the MV is connected to the right atrium (RA) and the TV to the left atrium (LA). The enlarged anatomical RV is on the left side. The small triangular LV is on the right side

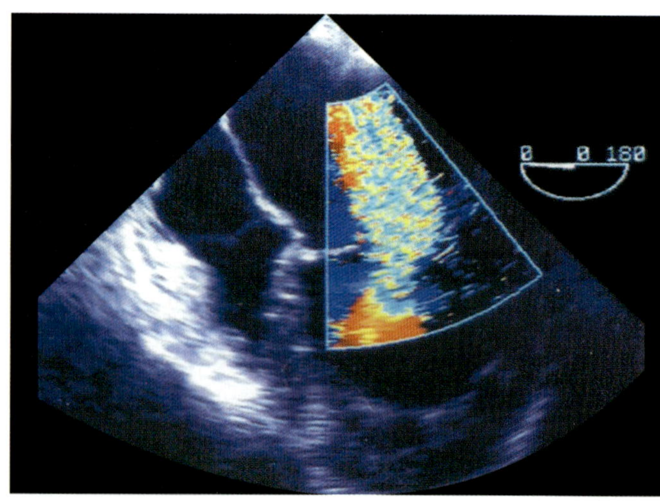

Figure 3 Anatomically corrected transposition of the great arteries. Severe tricuspid regurgitation of the dilated subaortic ventricle

ASSESSMENT OF SYSTEMIC VENOUS PATHWAY

The systemic venous atrium (SVA) should be assessed for any obstruction, the common site being an obstruction in the SVC. A continuous wave Doppler should be used to quantify the gradient, which will show the gradient to be either continuous or phasic. The gradient in SVC is significant if it is more than 6 mm Hg and it is continuous. A phasic gradient up to 6 mm Hg is acceptable **(Fig. 4)**.

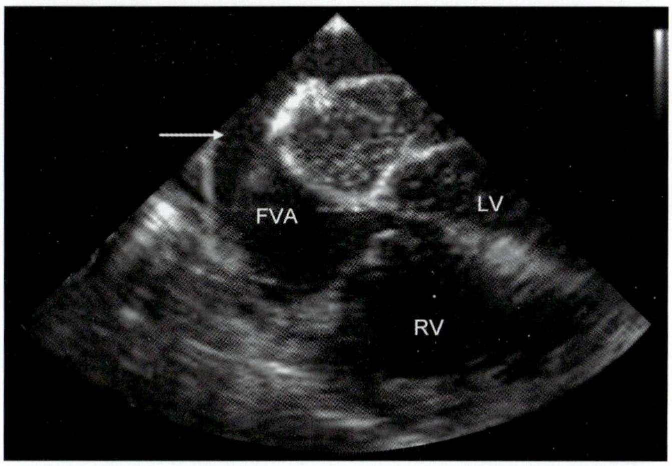

Figure 4 Midesophageal 4-chamber view of postoperative Senning showing contrast in the SVA to check baffle leak

ASSESSMENT OF BAFFLE

The baffle used to make the systemic venous pathway should be assessed for any leak that may lead to desaturation. The leak is checked by injecting a contrast through the cannula in the internal jugular vein and simultaneously examining the TEE and ensuring that it is not leaking into the pulmonary venous pathway. The baffle should also be examined for any redundant tissue that can project into the pulmonary venous pathway and it should not be too short that it causes high venous pressures **(Fig. 5)**.

PERIOPERATIVE CARE, POST-SENNING OPERATION

As noted above, patients may develop several late complications from the Senning and Mustard procedures. With current cardiology care, many of these patients are living into the 2nd and 3rd decades of life. As such, there are an increasing number of patients who may require anesthetic care during various types of surgical procedures. Given the complex nature of these patients and the potential for co-morbidities related to the primary defect or acquired during life, a thorough preoperative evaluation is necessary to ensure the safe perioperative care of such patients. The 3 major issues related to the

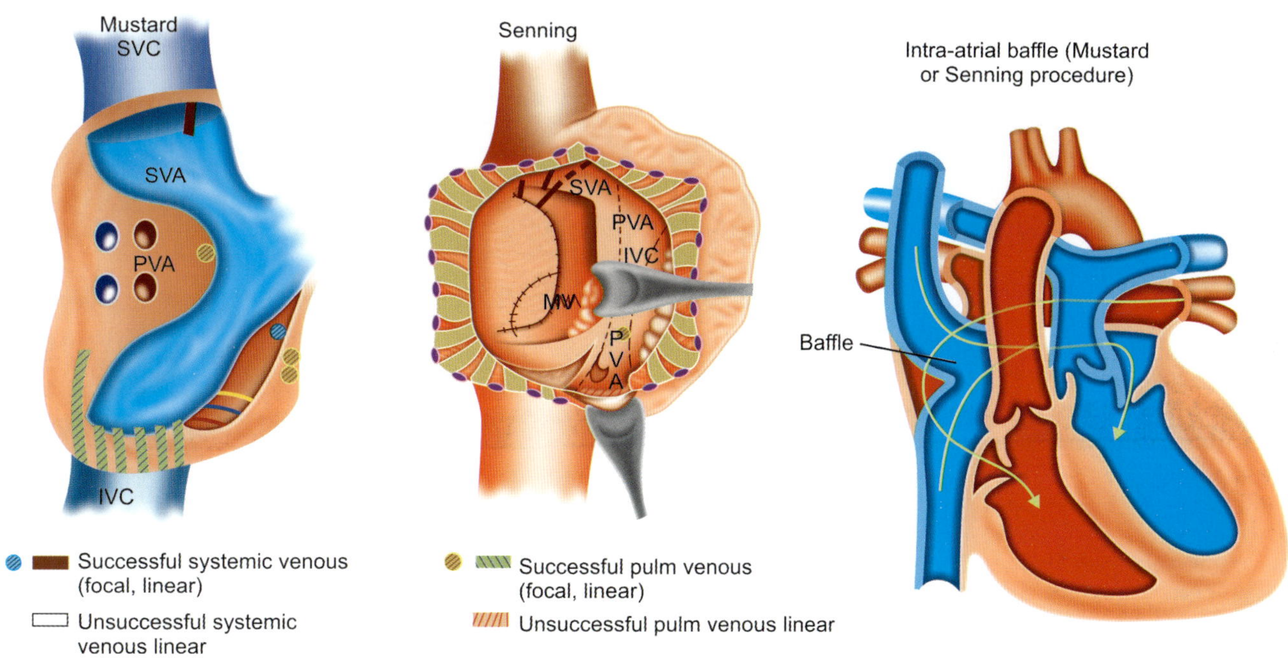

Figure 5 Baffle in Mustard and Senning procedure

anatomy of the Mustard or Senning procedure which should be addressed preoperatively include:[1]

1. An evaluation of myocardial function given that the systemic ventricle is the right ventricle
2. An evaluation for the presence of pulmonary hypertension
3. An evaluation of the baffle for obstruction or leaks.

Patients who have undergone a Senning or Mustard repair frequently have abnormal electrocardiograms (ECG). Common postatrial repair ECG findings include:

- Sinus bradycardia or a junctional rhythm
- Evidence of single or dual-chamber pacing
- Signs of right ventricular hypertrophy.

RVH can be identified on ECG by the presence of right-axis deviation large R-waves in leads V_1 and AVR, and evidence of right atrial enlargement. ST-segment depression and T-wave inversion in the right precordial leads may be indicative of severe RVH. Prior Holter monitor recordings should be evaluated for paroxysmal atrial fibrillation/flutter, frequent supraventricular extrasystoles, junctional escape rhythm at rest, or episodes of nonsustained ventricular tachycardia.

POSTOPERATIVE TEE ASSESSMENT (FIGS 6 TO 24)

- Biventricular function
- Position of IVS and IAS
- Residual shunt across VSD
- *Gradient across LVOT:* If resection done
- *Aortic regurgitation:* In case of bicuspid pulmonary valve, the valve may exhibit some regurgitation when exposed to systemic pressures postoperatively (as against pulmonary pressures preoperatively).

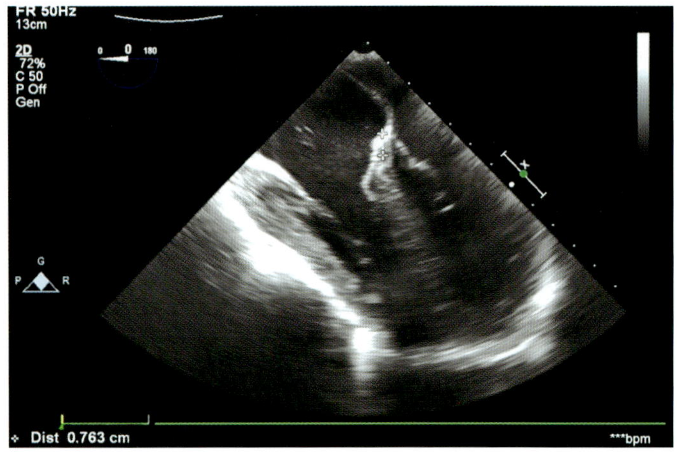

Figure 7 ME 4C view showing that the right atrioventriclar valve is more apical (by 7 mm) in comparison with the left atrioventricular valve and, therefore, should be the tricuspid valve. Thus the right chamber is the right ventricle

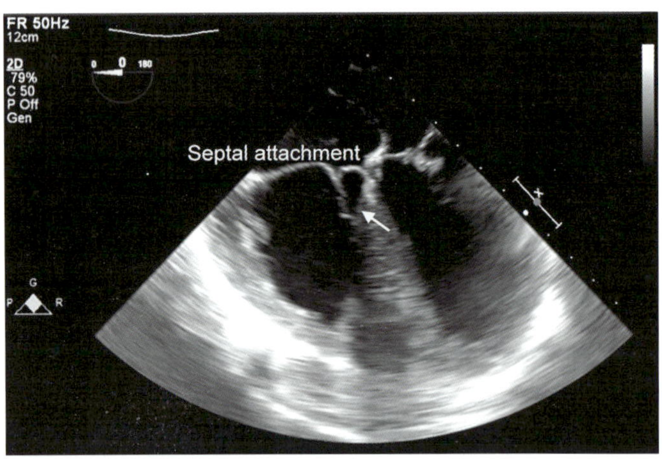

Figure 6 ME 4C view showing the septal attachment of the right atrioventricular valve implying that it is the tricuspid valve and the adjoining ventricle is right ventricle. Also seen is the moderator band in the right ventricle near the apex. On gross comparison, both the ventricles appear to be of the same size and well developed

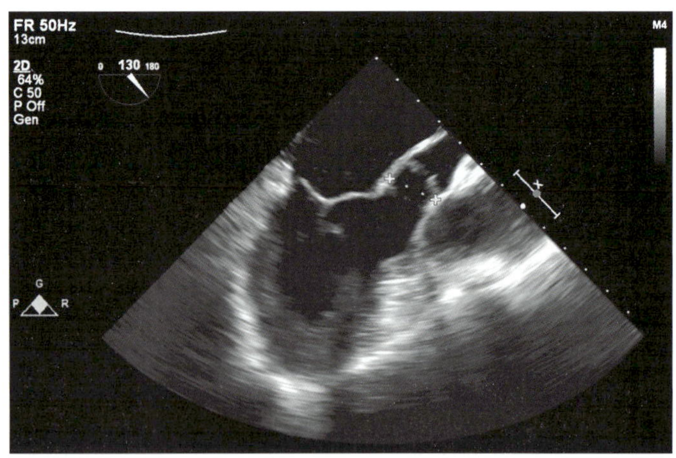

Figure 8 ME long axis view showing the relation of aorta and the pulmonary artery. Normally in the long axis view, the pulmonary artery is anterior and the aorta is posterior. In transposition of great arteries, the aorta is anterior (as seen here) and pulmonary artery posterior. To ensure whether the vessel is pulmonary artery or aorta, one should trace the course of the said vessel, if it bifurcates, then it is the pulmonary artery, otherwise it is the aorta

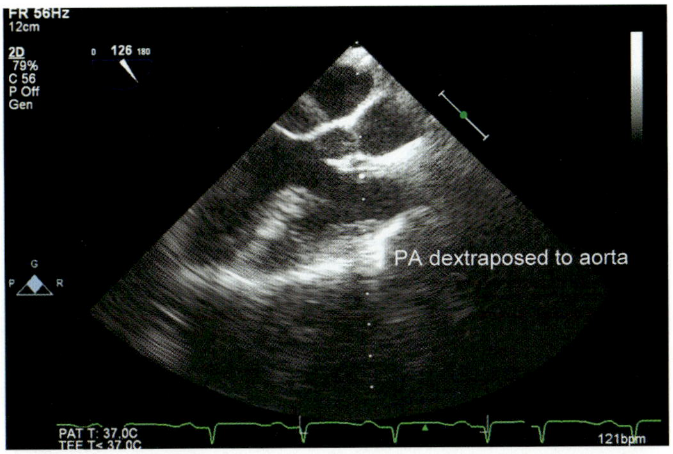

Figure 9 ME long axis view showing the relationship between aorta (anterior) and the pulmonary artery (posterior) in transposition of great arteries. Unlike the previous image in which both the great arteries are running parallel to each other, and so can be imaged in the same TEE view, in the image above only one vessel can be focussed at one time. This is because the pulmonary artery is dextroposed to the aorta and is not parallel to it. Therefore aortic valve and ascending aorta are not clearly seen together with the pulmonary artey. In such scenarios, arterial switch operation is not possible because the pulmonary artery is at a distance from aorta. Also since the pulmonary artery is dextroposed, there is the possibility of a conduit being compressed by the sternum and Rastelli operation may not be a choice as well. Patients with such an anatomy are destined for single ventricle repair

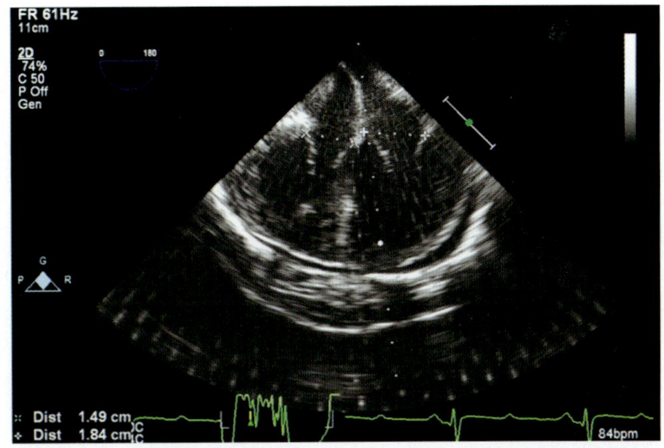

Figure 11 ME 4C view showing the dimensions of the tricuspid and mitral annuli. The tricuspid valve is identified by septal attachment and apical location. The measured annuli are compared with the dimensions normalized for body surface area. If it is < –2 Z value, then the said valve and possibly the corresponding chamber is underdeveloped. The dimensions of the corresponding ventricle should be measured and evaluated for underdevelopment by comparing with the normal values adjusted for body surface area

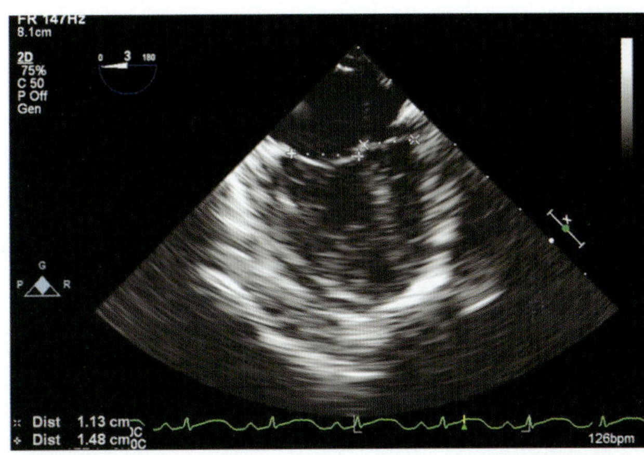

Figure 12 ME 4C view showing the comparative sizes of right and left ventricle. On gross inspection, it appears the left ventricle is small. The reason for a small ventricle may be underdevelopment or "regression". Regression is a phenomenon unique to patients with transposition of great arteries. In transposition of great arteries, the left ventricle ejects blood into pulmonary circulation. In the postnatal period because of high pulmonary vascular resistance the left ventricle has to empty against high afterload and therefore maintains its myocardial mass and thickness. As a child grows the pulmonary vascular resistance begins to decrease and thus the afterload to the left ventricle decreases progressively. The myocardial mass and thickness, thus, begin to decrease and after some time the left ventricle is no longer capable of tolerating the afterload of the systemic circulation. On transesophageal echocardiography, the measurement of mitral valve annulus helps differentiate between hypoplastic left ventricle or regressed left ventricle. If the left ventricle is small and mitral valve annulus is normal when adjusted for body surface area, then the ventricle has regressed. If the mitral valve is hypoplastic and left ventricle is small, then the left heart is underdeveloped

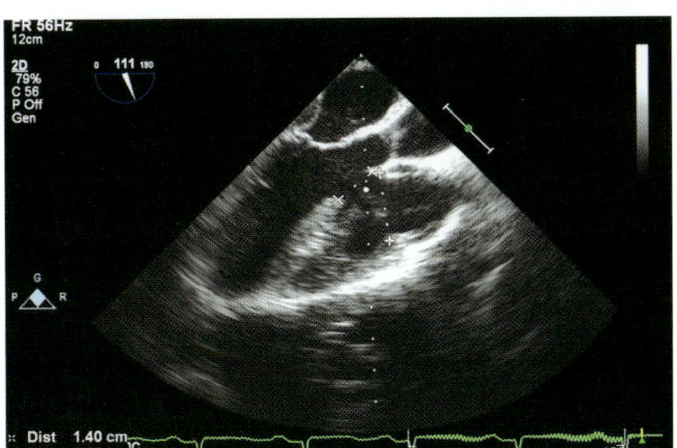

Figure 10 ME long axis view showing the dimensions of a ventricular septal defect and aortic annulus in a patient with *d*-transposition of great arteries

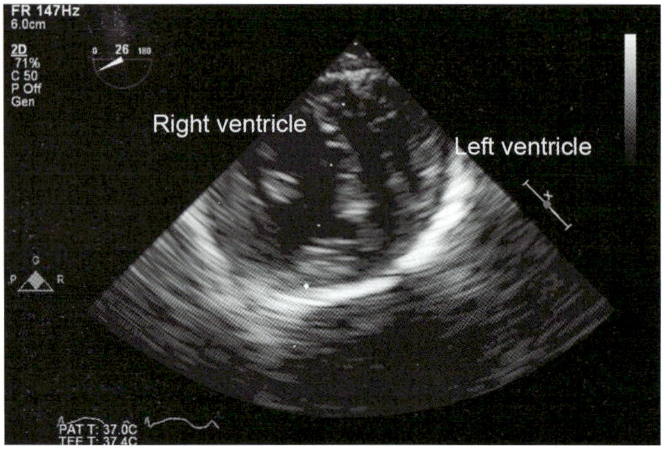

Figure 13 2D echo for evaluation of regressed left ventricle in transposition of great arteries. Transgastric mid papillary short axis view showing the comparative shape and size of both the right and left ventricles. Note the banana-shaped left ventricle and well developed right ventricle. The interventricular septum is convex towards left ventricle and moves with the right ventricle. Not shown here is the measurement of the thickness of the interventricular septum, posterior wall of left ventricle and internal diameter of left ventricle on basis of which left ventricular mass may be calculated. This subset of patients are at high-risk of left ventricular failure after arterial switch operations. If an arterial switch operation is to be done, then the possibility of patient requiring extracorporeal membrane oxygenation in the postoperative period should be kept in mind

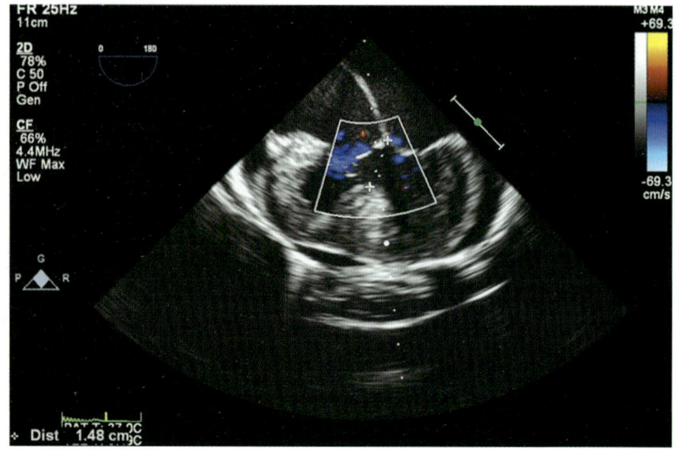

Figure 15 2D echo for assessment of ventricular septal defect in transposition of great arteries. The image shows a 1.48 cm inlet ventricular septal defect in a child with transposition of great arteries. Inlet ventricular septal defect with severe pulmonary stenosis is one of the indications for performing a Nikaidoh procedure (aortic translocation)

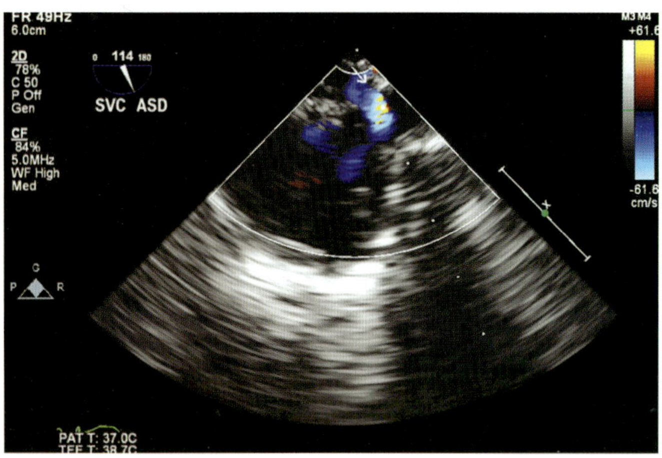

Figure 14 2D echo for assessment of sinus venosus atrial septal defect in transposition of great arteries. The arrow shows a superior vena cava type sinus venosus atrial septal defect, shunting form left to right, in a child with transposition of great arteries. Ostium secundum atrial septal defect is commonly found in transposition of great arteries but sinus venosus atrial septal defect is uncommon

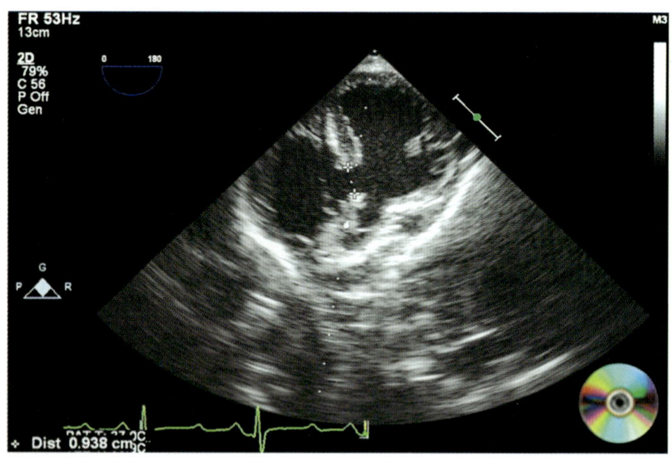

Figure 16 (Video 1) 2D echo for assessment of ventricular septal defect in transposition of great arteries. The echocardiogram shows an anterior muscular ventricular septal defect with a subpulmonic extension. In transposition of great arteries, the pulmonary artery is arising from left ventricle, hence the extension towards systemic outflow is no more subaortic but subpulmonic

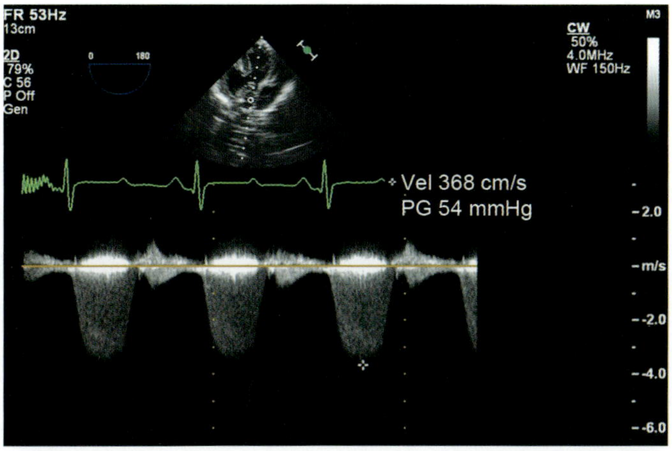

Figure 17 Continuous wave Doppler for assessment of left ventricular outflow tract. Although uncommon but in some patients with transposition of great arteries, there may be an accessory mitral tissue present in the left ventricular outflow tract. This accessory tissue may cause obstruction presenting as gradient across left ventricular outflow on echocardiography. It is important to measure the dimensions of left ventricular outflow in such children to confirm adequate development and predict postexcision patency of the outflow

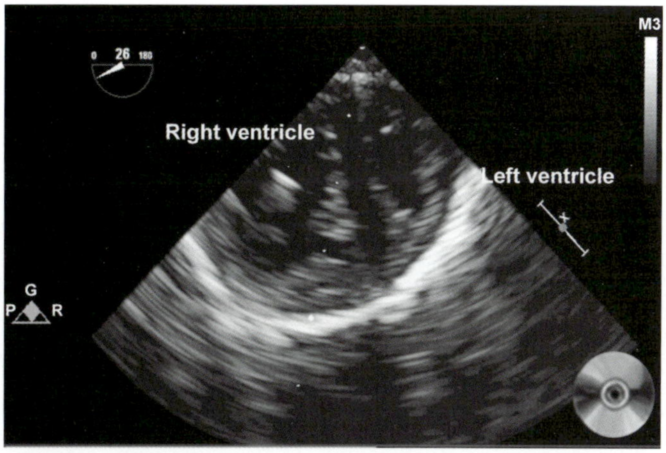

Figure 19 (Video 3) 2D echo for evaluation of regressed left ventricle in transposition of great arteries. Transgastric midpapillary short axis view showing the comparative shape and size of both the right and left ventricles. Note the banana shaped left ventricle and well developed right ventricle

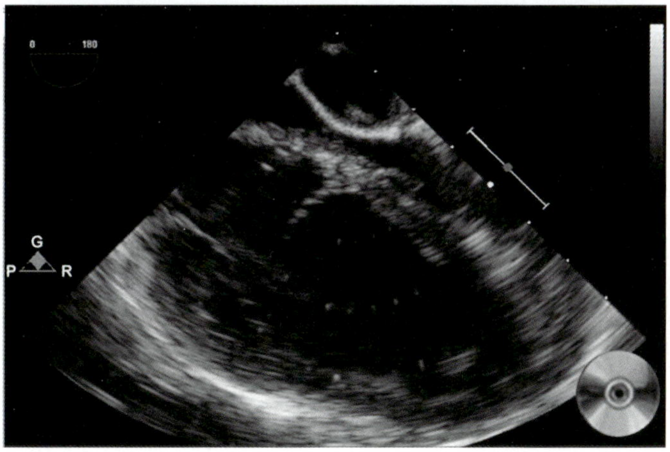

Figure 18 (Video 2) 2D echo showing the atrial baffle post-double switch operation. Left atrium (constructed by pericardium posteriorly is now directed to the left ventricle and the left ventricle now ejects into the aorta (arterial switch done)

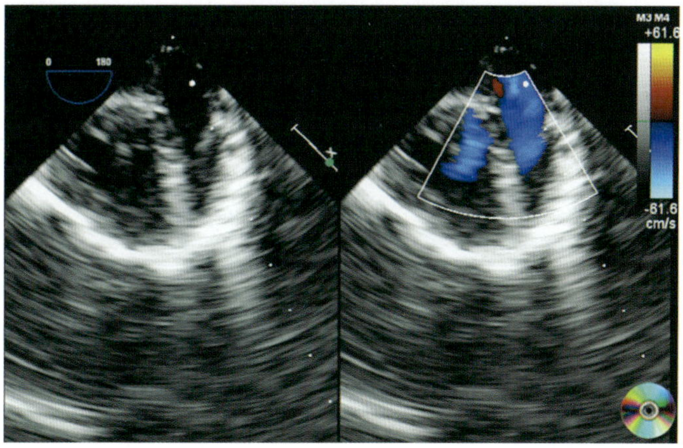

Figure 20 (Video 4) 2D echo for evaluation of regressed left ventricle in transposition of great arteries. Midesophageal 4 chamber view showing a restrictive upper muscular ventricular septal defect in a patient with transposition of great arteries

CHAPTER 13

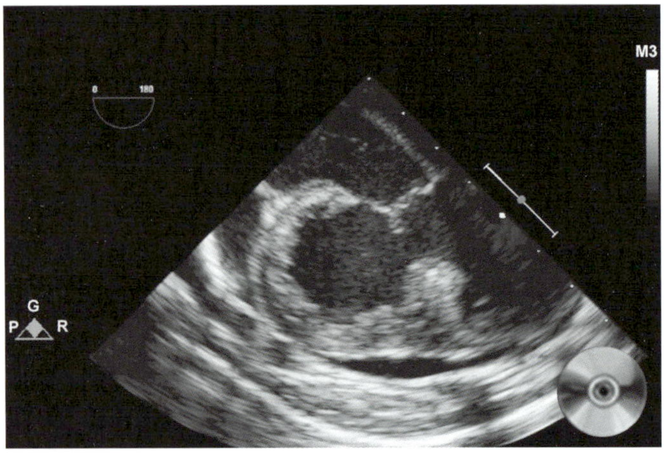

Figure 21 (Video 5) 2D echo for assessment of ventricular septal defect in transposition of great arteries. The midesophageal 4 chamber view shows a large inlet ventricular septal defect with both the ventricles lying side by side

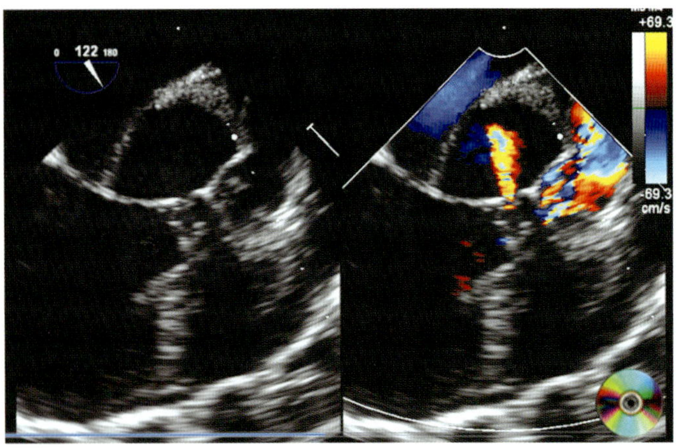

Figure 22 (Video 6) 2D echo and color Doppler assessment of transposition of great arteries. The midesophageal long axis view shows accessory mitral tissue in the left ventricular tract causing obstruction and gradient across left ventricular outflow tract

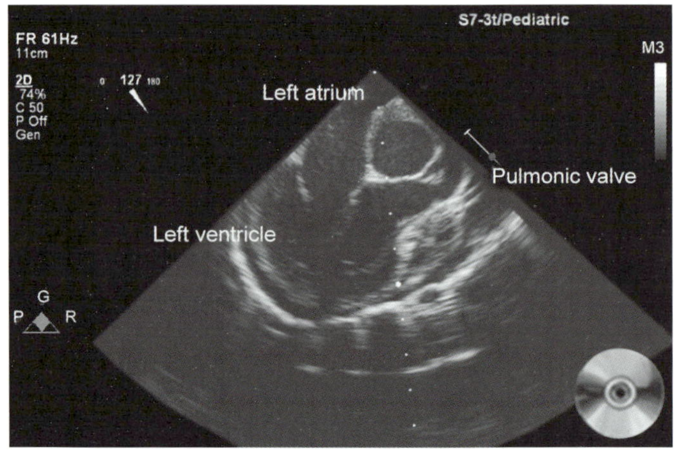

Figure 23 (Video 7) 2D echo for assessment of transposition of great arteries. The midesophageal long axis view showing the connection from left atrium to left ventricle to pulmonary artery

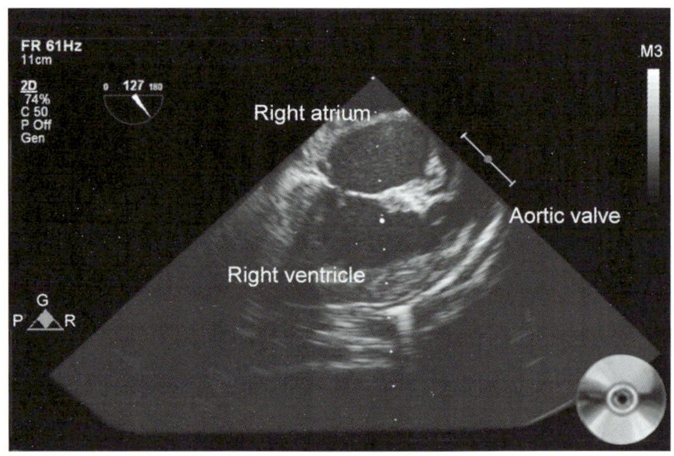

Figure 24 (Video 8) 2D echo for assessment of transposition of great arteries. The midesophageal long axis view showing the connection from right atrium to right ventricle to aorta

CONCLUSION

Transposition of the great arteries may be associated with complex cardiac disease that could be detected on the 4-chamber view of the heart. When the 4-chamber view is normal, it is important to identify the crisscross relationship of the outflow tracts. If this is not done, it is important to document that the pulmonary artery bifurcates and originates from the right ventricle. Five short axis views of the heart may be helpful to detect conotruncal abnormalities.

REFERENCES

1. Joseph D Tobias, et al. Perioperative management following an atrial level switch (Mustard or Senning procedure) for transposition of the great arteries. Anaesthesia Pain and Intensive Care. 2011;15(3):185-94.
2. Miller-Hance WC, Silverman NH. Transesophageal echocardiography (TEE) in congenital heart disease with focus on the adult. Cardiol Clin. 2000;18:861-92.

Chapter 14

TEE for Congenitally Corrected Transposition of Great Arteries

Poonam Malhotra Kapoor, Sarvesh Pal Singh, Jitin Narula, Sachin Talwar

Chapter Outline

INTRODUCTION

In congenitally corrected transposition of great arteries there is structural discrepancy but physiological correction within the heart. The right atrium drains into the morphologic left ventricle or the venous ventricle (Atrioventricular discordance) which in turn ejects into the pulmonary artery (Ventriculoarterial discordance). Similarly on left side, the left atrium drains into the morphologic right ventricle which in turn ejects into the aorta. Because of the physiological correction and a normal series circulation, these patients usually present at advanced age.[1] Since morphologic right ventricle acts as a systemic ventricle it is destined to fail as the age, cardiac output and oxygen demand increases. Associated cardiac abnormalities include **(Fig. 1)**:

- Subpulmonary perimembranous VSD (70% cases).
- LVOT obstruction in the form of pulmonary atresia, pulmonary and subpulmonary stenosis.

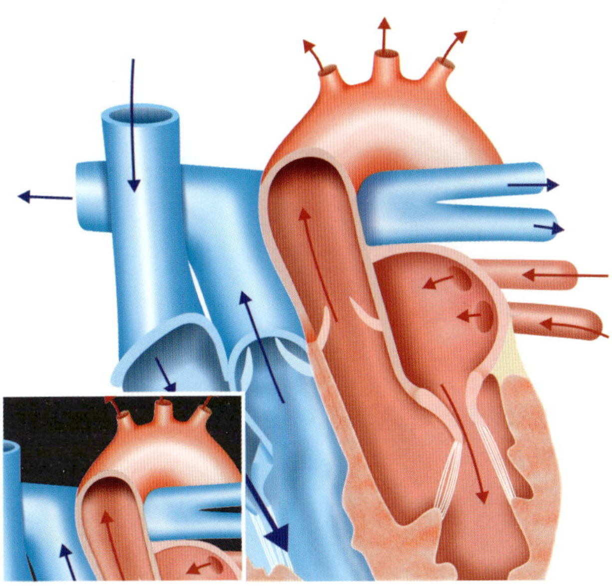

Figure 1 Congenitally corrected transposition of great arteries

- Ebstein-like malformation of the left-sided systemic valve (tricuspid valve).
- Abnormal position of the AV node and disturbances in conduction (AV block).
- Inverted coronary artery anatomy. The right-sided coronary artery gives rise to the left anterior descending coronary artery and circumflex arteries, whereas the left-sided coronary has the course and distribution of a normal right coronary artery.

Associated **clinical features** range from cyanosis in patients in whom pulmonary blood flow is limited (VSD and severe/complete LVOT obstruction) to severe RV dysfunction secondary to tricuspid regurgitation (TR), heart block or systemic afterload by age 45 years leading to clinical CHF in one-third of the patients. The patients with congenitally corrected transposition of great arteries undergo Double Switch Operation (Arterial Switch Operation + Senning repair).

The echocardiography in congenitally corrected transposition of great arteries is very much similar to transposition of great arteries. The identification of the chambers and great vessels should be done systematically. However, surgical options depend on specific echocardiographic findings like severe pulmonary stenosis, juxtaposed appendages as discussed here.[2]

CORRECTED TRANSPOSITION OF GREAT ARTERIES

- In corrected transposition of great arteries there is a atrioventricular discordance and ventriculoarterial discordance, i.e. double discordance **(Figs 2A and B)**
- In effect, right atrium is connected to right-sided morphologic left ventricle which gives rise to pulmonary artery
- Left atrium is connected to left-sided morphologic right ventricle which gives rise to aorta.

PREOPERATIVE TEE ASSESSMENT (FIGS 3 TO 19)

- Identify both atria, valves and ventricles and great arteries and their relation
  - Parallel great vessels with aorta anterior to PA
  - Relation of right ventricle to pulmonary artery in patients destined for Rastelli procedure
  - Pulmonary artery size
  - Pulmonary valve—anatomy (bicuspid or tricuspid), annulus, stenosis.
- Size of both ventricles
- Assessment of mitral and tricuspid valves
  - MV and TV annuli to predict the development of ventricles.

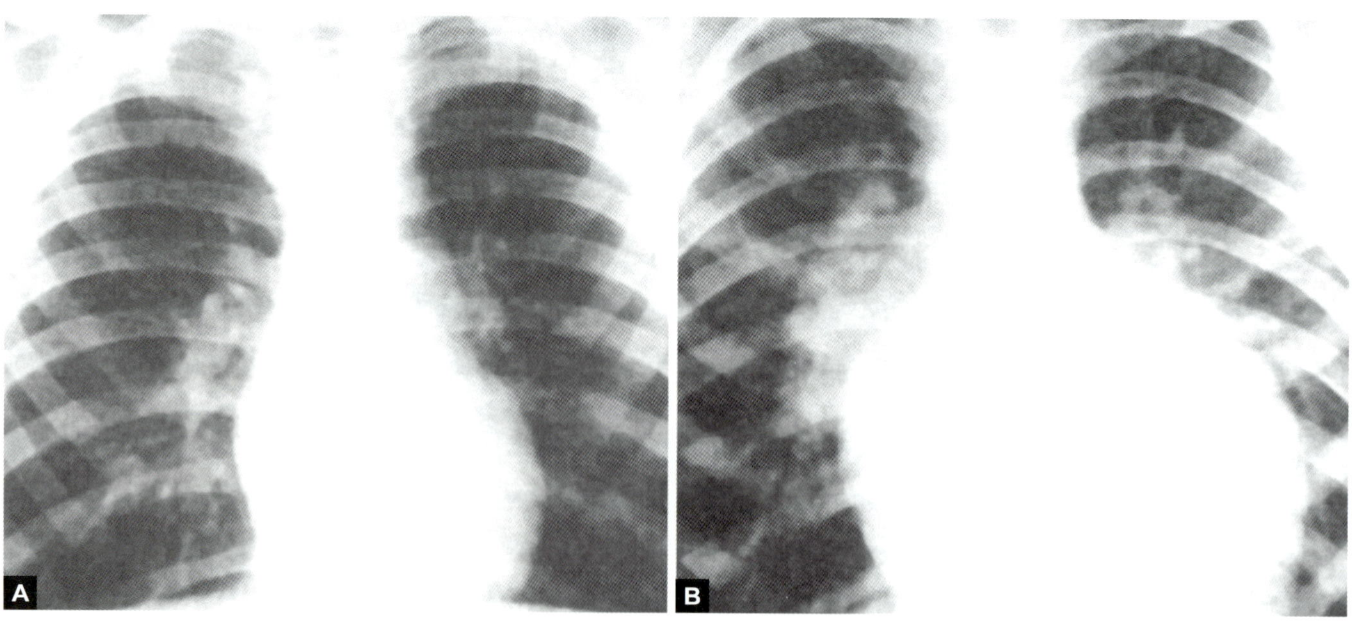

Figures 2A and B Corrected transposition of great arteries in two patients. X-ray (A) is that of a patient with ventricular septal defect and pulmonary stenosis. Left upper border is straight and formed by ascending aorta. X-ray (B) is that of severe atrioventricular valve regurgitation without ventricular septal defect or pulmonary stenosis. Left upper border is concave and is formed by ascending aorta

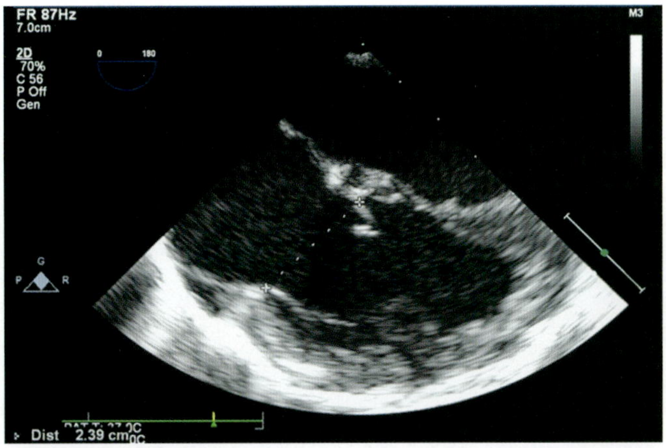

Figure 3 2D echo measuring the mitral valve annulus in midesophageal 4-chamber view. Right atrium is connected to left ventricle through mitral valve

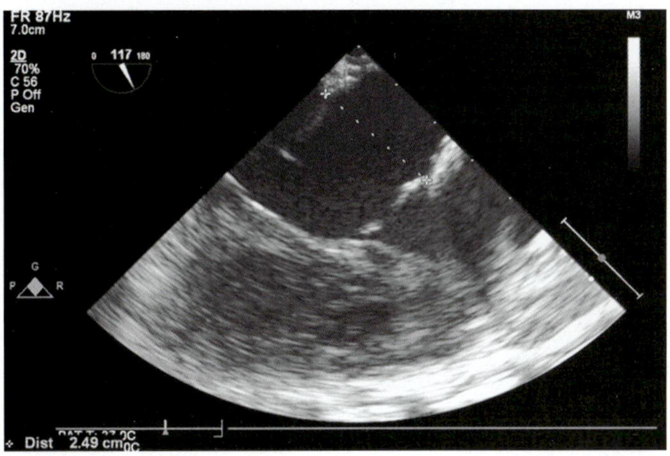

Figure 4 2D echo measuring the pulmonary valve annulus in midesophageal long axis view. Right atrium is emptying into left ventricle which ejects into pulmonary artery

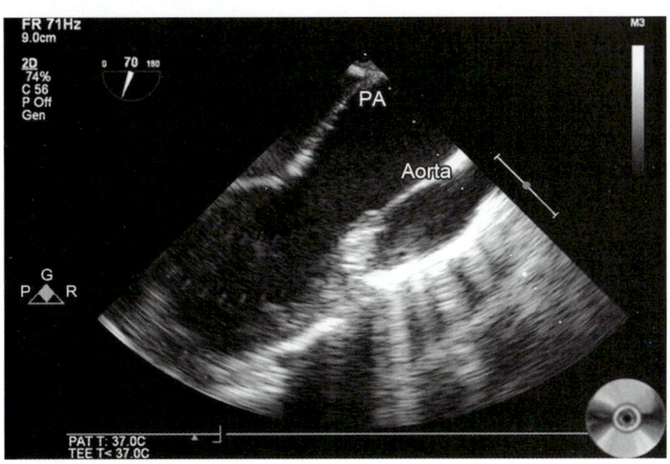

Figure 5 (Video 1) 2D echo in midesophageal long axis view showing the relation between aorta and pulmonary artery. Right ventricle ejects into aorta which is anterior to pulmonary artery

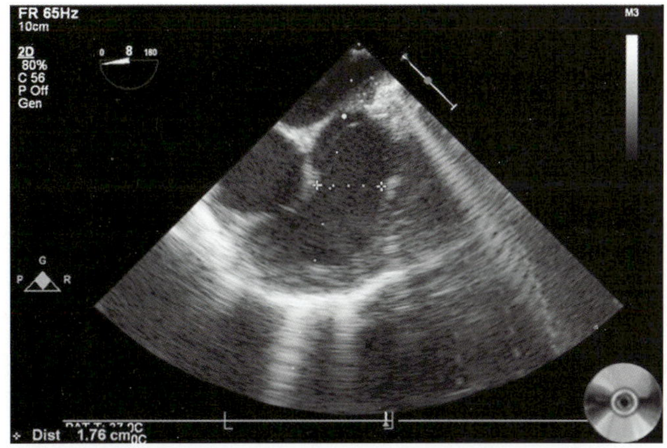

Figure 6 (Video 2) 2D echo in midesophageal 4-chamber view showing perimembranous ventricular septal defect with right atrium opening into left ventricle and left ventricle ejecting into pulmonary artery

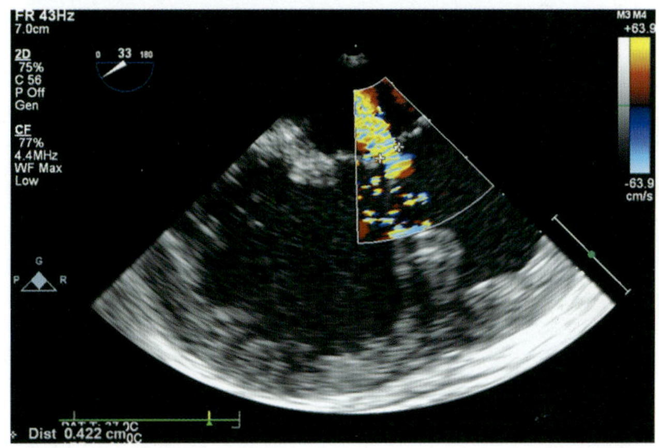

Figure 7 2D echo in midesophageal 4-chamber view showing tricuspid regurgitation in a patient with congenitally corrected transposition of great arteries. Also seen in the ventricular septal defect

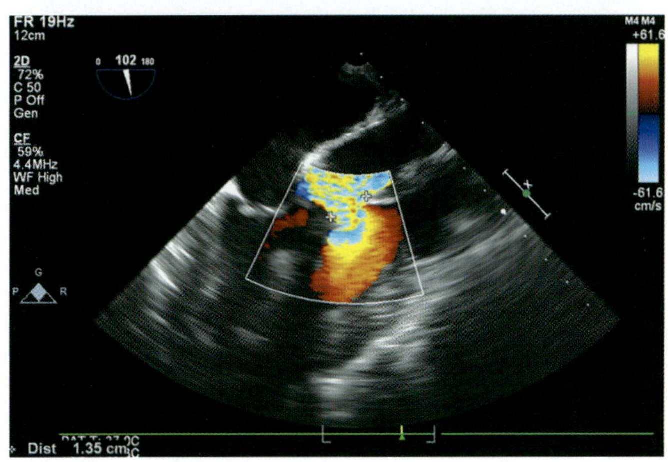

Figure 8 Color Doppler in midesophageal long axis view showing a restrictive ventricular septal defect shunting from morphological left ventricle to morphological right ventricle

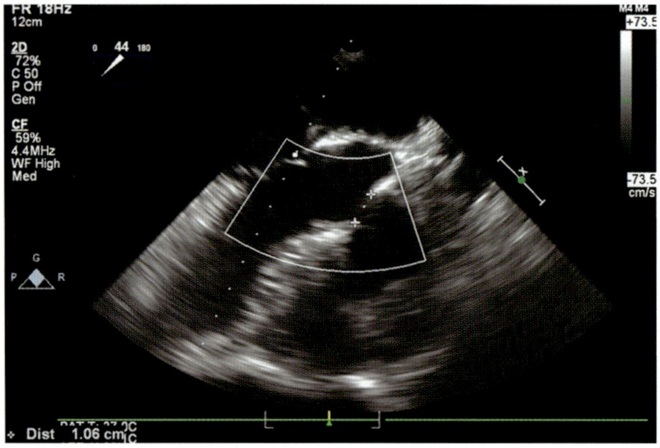

Figure 9 2D echo in midesophageal long axis view showing a restrictive ventricular septal defect

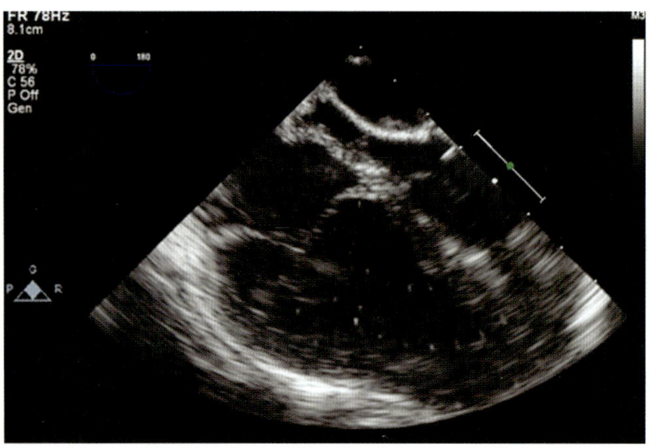

Figure 10 2D echo showing the atrial baffle post Double Switch Operation. Left atrium constructed by pericardium posteriorly is now directed to the left ventricle and the left ventricle now ejects into the aorta (arterial switch done)

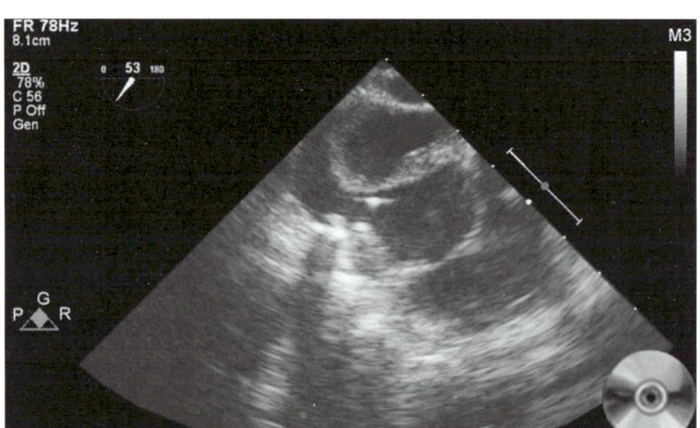

Figure 11 (Video 3) 2D echocardiography in mid esophageal 4-chamber view, of a patient who has undergone "Double Switch Operation", showing an atrial baffle made from atrial wall. The neo left atrium made from pericardium is seen opening into the left ventricle and the left ventricle ejecting into the aorta

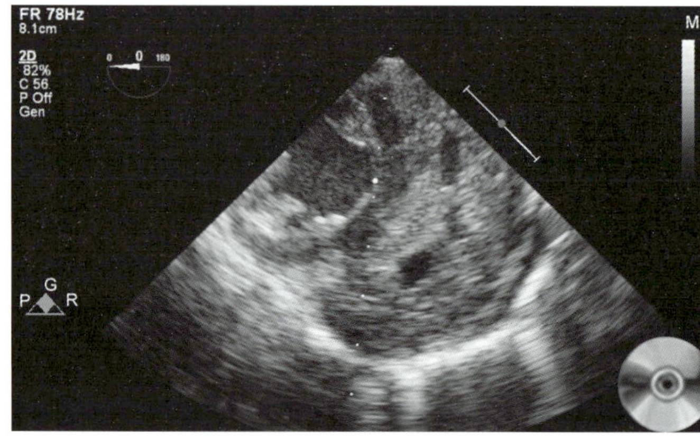

Figure 12 (Video 4) 2D echo in transgastric midpapillary short axis view showing left and right ventricles (crescent-shaped) after a Double Switch Operation. Note the underfilled morphologic right ventricle

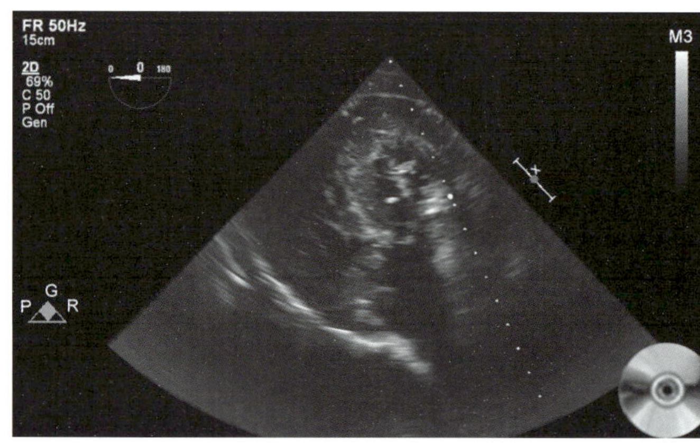

Figure 13 (Video 5) 2D echocardiography in deep transgastric view showing the cross-section of tricuspid valve morphological right ventricle ejecting in the aorta in a patient with congenitally corrected transposition of great arteries

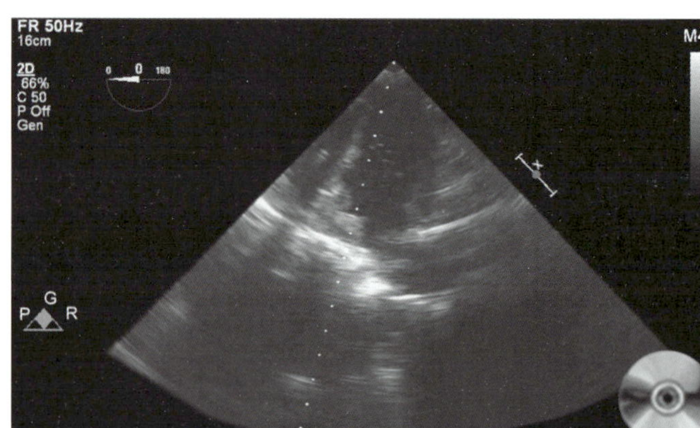

Figure 14 (Video 6) 2D echo post Double Switch Operation (Senning + Rastelli procedure) showing pulmonary artery conduit arising from right ventricle on left side of screen

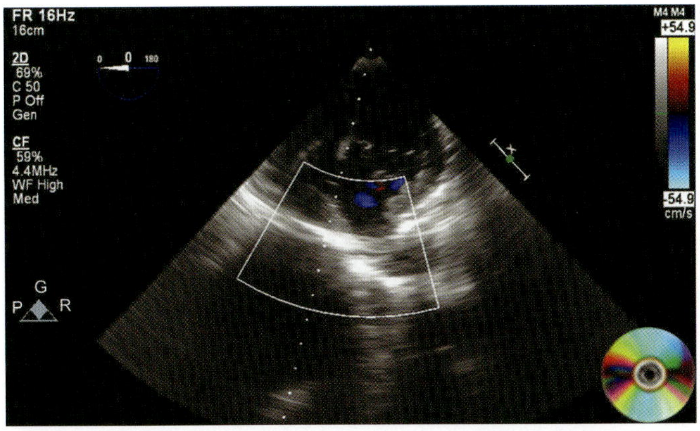

Figure 15 (Video 7) Color Doppler post Double Switch Operation (Senning + Rastelli procedure) showing unobstructed blood flow through pulmonary artery conduit arising from right ventricle on left side of screen

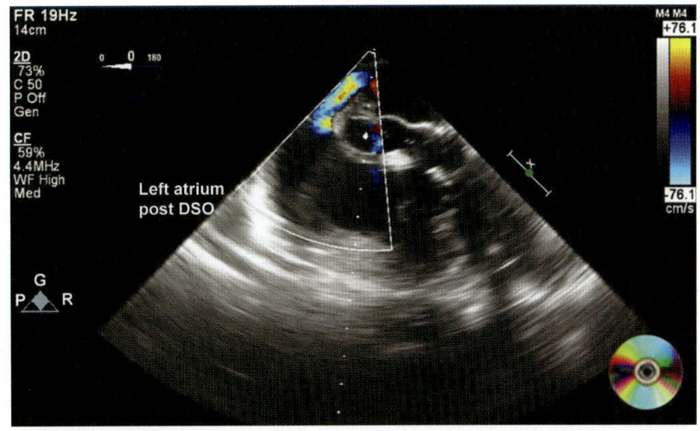

Figure 18 (Video 10) Color Doppler post Double Switch Operation (Senning + Rastelli procedure) showing unobstructed blood flow in the left atrium

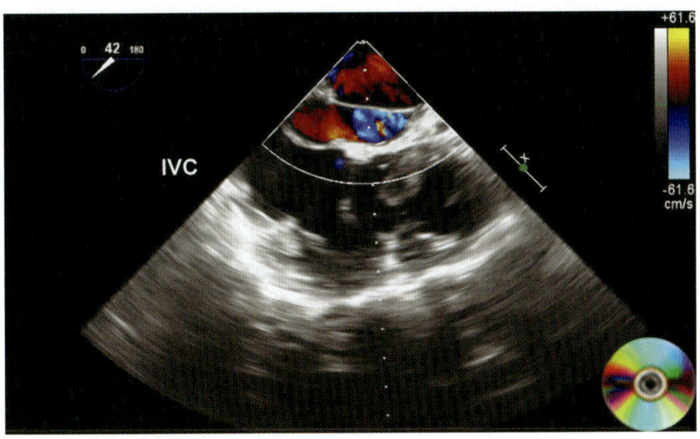

Figure 16 (Video 8) Color Doppler post Double Switch Operation (Senning + Rastelli procedure) showing unobstructed blood flow from inferior vena cava to the right atrium

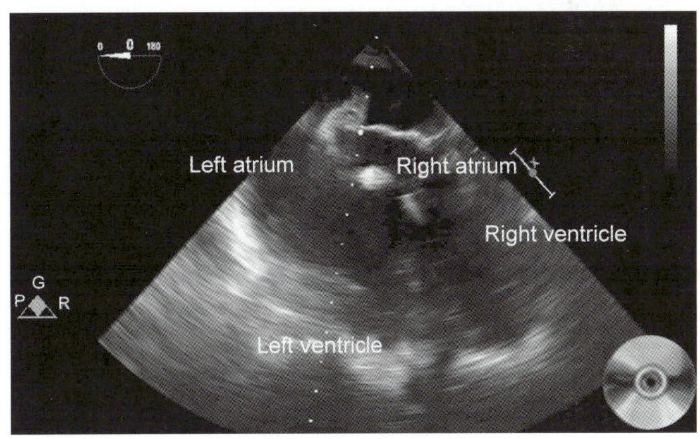

Figure 19 (Video 11) 2D echo in a patient with congenitally corrected transposition of great arteries showing the corrected anatomy after the Double Switch Operation (Senning + Rastelli procedure)

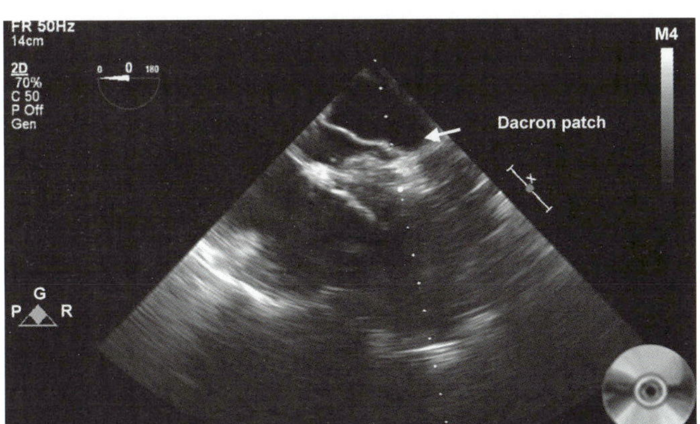

Figure 17 (Video 9) 2D echo post Double Switch Operation (Senning + Rastelli procedure) showing a Dacron patch between the atria used to create the baffle

  - Systemic valve regurgitation, aortic regurgitation
  - Ebstein like/Tricuspid reurgitation.
- VSD/IVS
  - Size and routability of VSD in case of severe PS (Rastelli).
- LA size and RA size (for Senning procedure)
- Juxtaposed appendages (contraindication for performing Senning procedure).
- Severe PS
- ASD.

POSTOPERATIVE TEE ASSESSMENT

- Biventricular function
- Residual gradient across systemic valve

- Regurgitation across mitral/tricuspid valve
  - Mitral regurgitation may occur secondary to papillary muscle dysfunction or to dilation of the mitral valve annulus
- *Functioning of baffle:* Baffle leaks/Baffle obstruction.

CONCLUSION

Patients with CCTGA are increasingly subject to CHF with advancing age; this complication is extremely common by the 4th and 5th decades. Tricuspid (systemic atrioventricular) valvular regurgitation is strongly associated with RV (anatomical right ventricle connected to aorta in CCTGA patients; systemic ventricle in CCTGA) dysfunction and CHF; whether it is causative or a secondary complication remains speculative.

REFERENCES

1. Deepak SM, Royle M, Goode GK. Congenitally corrected transposition of the great arteries (L Transposition). Heart 2003;89:974-6.
2. Hornung TS, Calder L. Congenital heart disease: Congenitally corrected transposition of the great arteries. Heart. 2010;96:1154-61.

Chapter 15

TEE for Ebstein's Anomaly

Poonam Malhotra Kapoor, Sarvesh Pal Singh, Jitin Narula, Pankaj Kumar

Chapter Outline

- Embryology
- Pathophysiology
- Clinical Presentation in Ebstein's Anomaly
- Clinical Implications
- ECG in Ebstein's Anomaly
- X-ray in Ebstein's Anomaly
- Transesophageal Echocardiography for Ebstein's Anomaly
- Echocardiography of Ebstein's Anomaly
- Preoperative TEE Assessment: 2D and 3D
- Postoperative TEE Assessment

INTRODUCTION

Ebstein's anomaly is a rare congenital heart defect that occurs in approximately 1 per 210,000 livebirths.[1] In this structural heart defect, the septal leaflet of tricuspid valve is shifted apically and a large anterior tricuspid leaflet coapts with the posterior and septal leaflets well below the normal coaptation point at the annulus.

EMBRYOLOGY

Embryologically, the tricuspid valve leaflets get formed by exfoliation from the right ventricular myocardium up toward the tricuspid annulus. If this process is arrested or incomplete, the attachment of the leaflets is apically displaced. Ebstein's anomaly can also be left sided in patients with L-TGA, as the tricuspid valve is located in the left-sided ventricle or the morphologic right ventricle.

PATHOPHYSIOLOGY

The primary pathologic finding is abnormal development of the tricuspid valve marked by varying degree of apical displacement of the septal and posterior leaflets into the right ventricle along with leaflet fusion to the ventricular wall.

The apical displacement also leads to the development of an "atrialized ventricle", **(Fig. 1)** portion of heart above the leaflets but below the annulus it has atrial pressure but a ventricular intracardiac electrogram, thus the right atrium can be massively enlarged. The sail-like anterior leaflet is large and redundant. The missing of the inflow portion can lead to an underdeveloped small right ventricle and varying degrees of associated pulmonary stenosis to functional pulmonary atresia may be present **(Figs 3A and B)**.

CLINICAL PRESENTATION IN EBSTEIN'S ANOMALY

This defect is characterized by remarkable morphologic variability and a broadspectrum of clinical presentations, predominant clinical finding being tricuspid insufficiency **(Fig. 2)** leading to variable cyanosis from right-to-left shunting at the atrial level. The degree of cyanosis does not always coincide with the patient's symptoms.[2,3] In fact, a history of relatively good effort tolerance despite cyanosis favors the diagnosis of Ebstein's anomaly.[4]

CLINICAL IMPLICATIONS

Cyanosis may however improve with the normal postnatal decrease in PVR. As time goes on cyanosis may reappear since the inadequate right ventricle, burdened by tricuspid regurgitation, ultimately fails again. Right ventricular end-diastolic pressure rises together with right atrial pressure and a right to left shunt is re-established[5] **(Figs 3A and B)**. Survival into adulthood with minimal symptoms is seen in patients with only mild displacement of the valve leaflets and minimal tricuspid insufficiency.

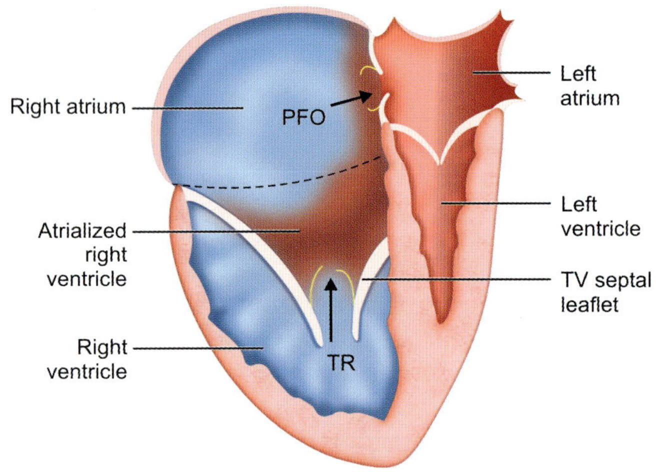

Figure 1 Ebstein's anomaly showing the atrialized ventricle

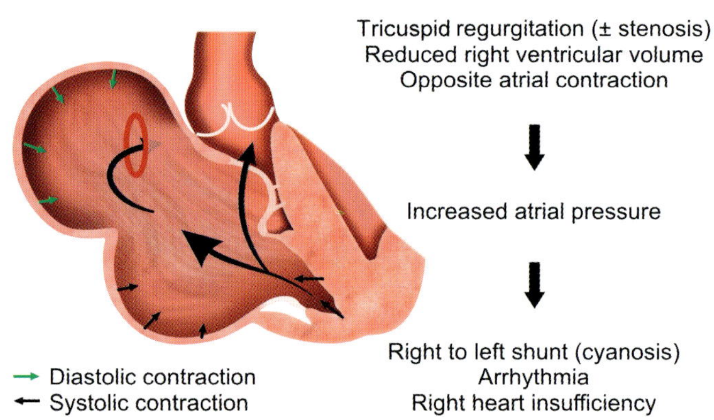

Figure 2 Etiology of tricuspid regurgitation

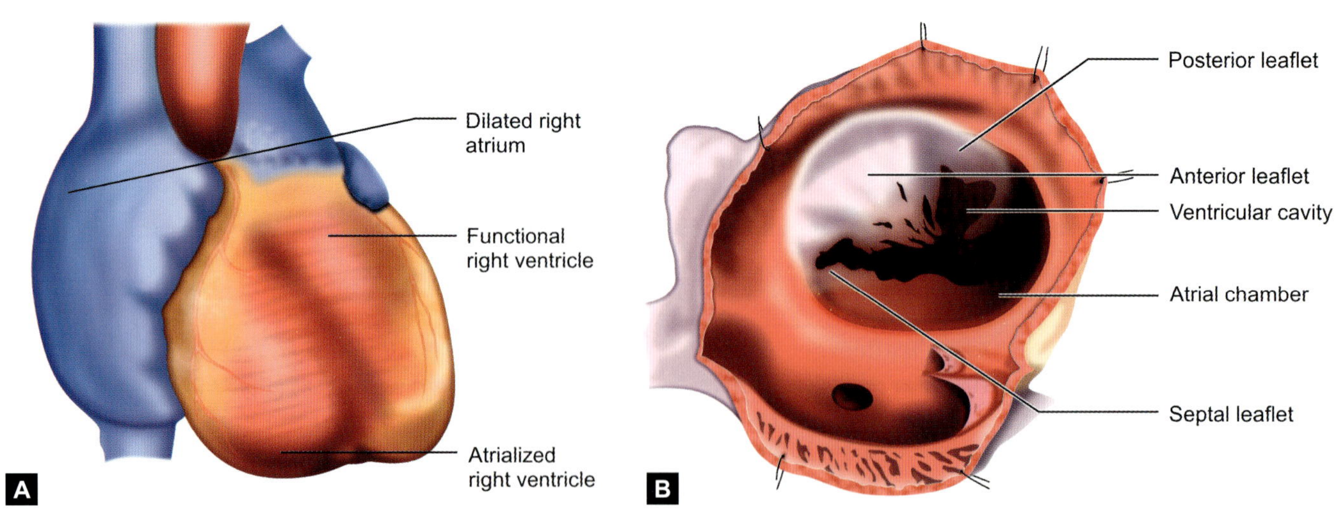

Figures 3A and B Tricuspid anomaly and tricuspid regurgitation in Ebstein's anomaly

ECG IN EBSTEIN'S ANOMALY

- The electrocardiogram is usually abnormal in the adult with Ebstein's anomaly. The P waves may be prominent and the PR interval prolonged **(Figs 4A to C)**.
- Pre-excitation (Wolff-Parkinson-White) has been described in as many as 20–25% of patients with Ebstein's anomaly, and, as would be anticipated, the atrioventricular bypass tracts are usually located on the right.

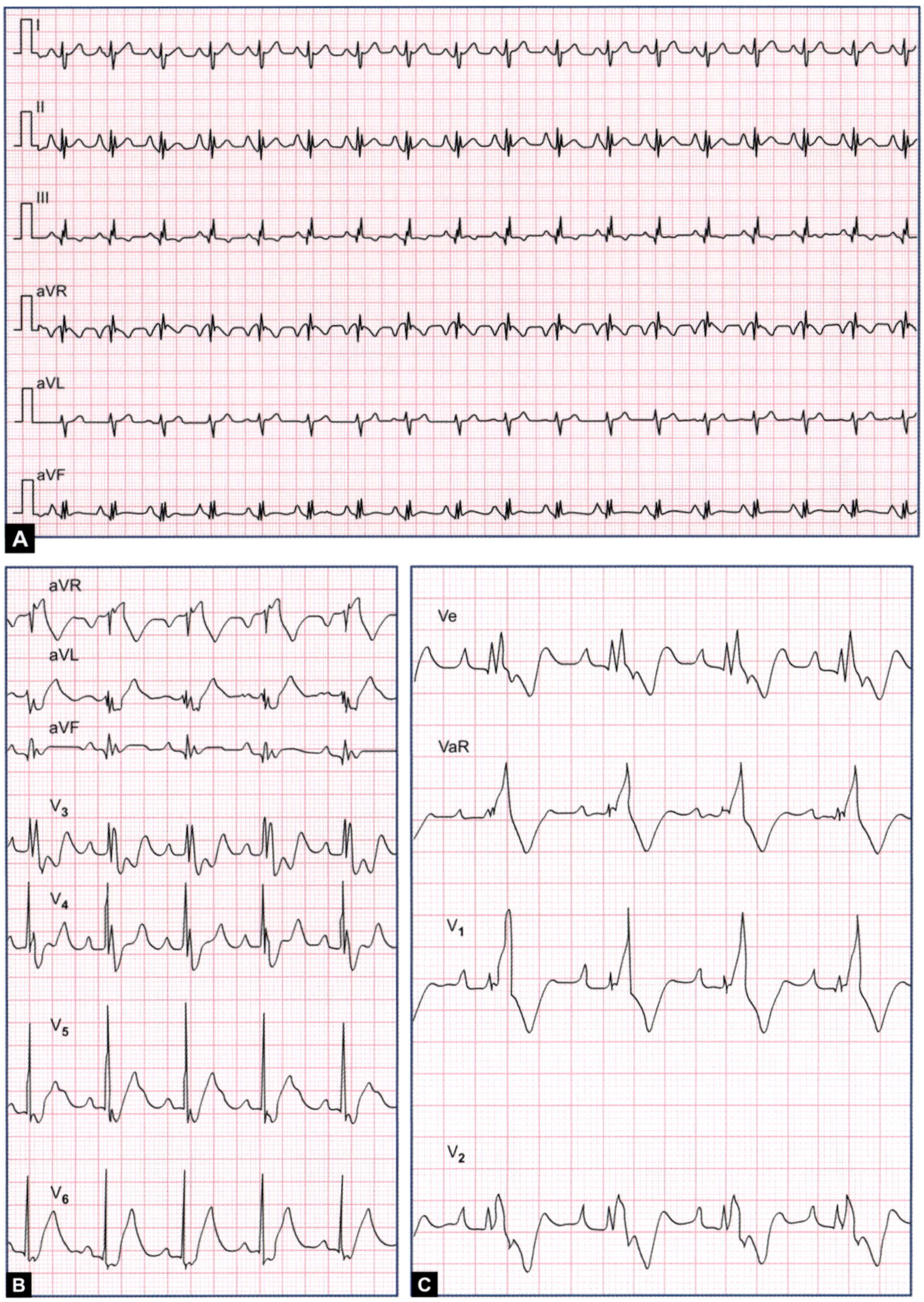

Figures 4A to C The electrocardiogram of a patient with Ebstein's anomaly, showing signs of RA enlargement and tall 'p' (Himalayan) waves (A) in limb leads diagnostic of Ebstein's anomaly, rsR' pattern in chest leads (B) and WPW signs in anterior leads (C)

- Although paroxysmal supraventricular tachycardia occurs from re-entry over the bypass tract, other atrial dysarrhythmias, such as atrial flutter and fibrillation, are also common because of the enlarged right atrium.

X-RAY IN EBSTEIN'S ANOMALY (FIG. 5)

- Cardiomegaly
- Pulmonary oligemia
- SVC and azygos vein distension
- No alveolar edema.
- Dilated RA and RV
- Box like silhouette
- Pericardial effusion may be present
- Homogeneous lesions after mistaken for coin lesions.

TRANSESOPHAGEAL ECHOCARDIOGRAPHY FOR EBSTEIN'S ANOMALY

The diagnosis of Ebstein's anomaly by echocardiography is straightforward as an inadequate delamination of the tricuspid valve (TV) leaflets from the endocardium of the right venticular (RV) results in features that are characteristic of this anomaly, which include apical displacement of the leaflets, particularly the septal leaflet, with associated TR and right ventricular dysfunction **(Figs 6A and B)**.

ECHOCARDIOGRAPHY OF EBSTEIN'S ANOMALY

TEE Views for Evaluation of Ebstein's Anomaly

- Midesophageal (ME) four chamber view
- RV inflow-outflow view
- Transgastric (TG) RV inflow view
- Transgastric (TG) RV outflow view.

PREOPERATIVE TEE ASSESSMENT: 2D AND 3D

- ME 4 chamber view
  - Right ventricular displacement of the leaflet can be visualized.
  - Is the tricuspid valve position normal or its is displaced apically? In Ebstein's anomaly the septal or posterior tricuspid leaflet is displaced towards the **RV apex by at least 0.8 cm/m^2** (in adults, the displacement should be indexed

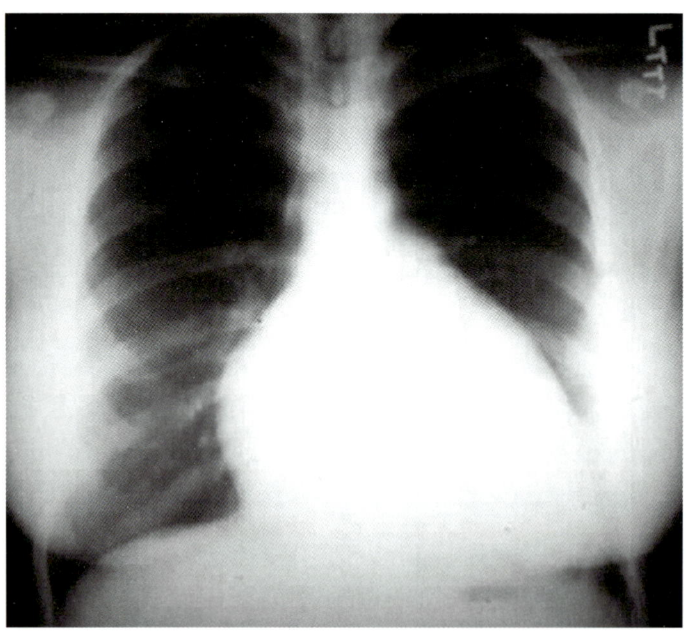

Figure 5 Frontal chest radiograph in an adult with Ebstein's anomaly shows: (i) The abnormal contour associated with distortion of the right ventricle. The pulmonary vasculature is underperfused; (ii) Cardiomegaly due to enlarged RA is always present. The magnitude of right atrial enlargement and arterialized right ventricle depends on measure of displaced attachment of tricuspid valve

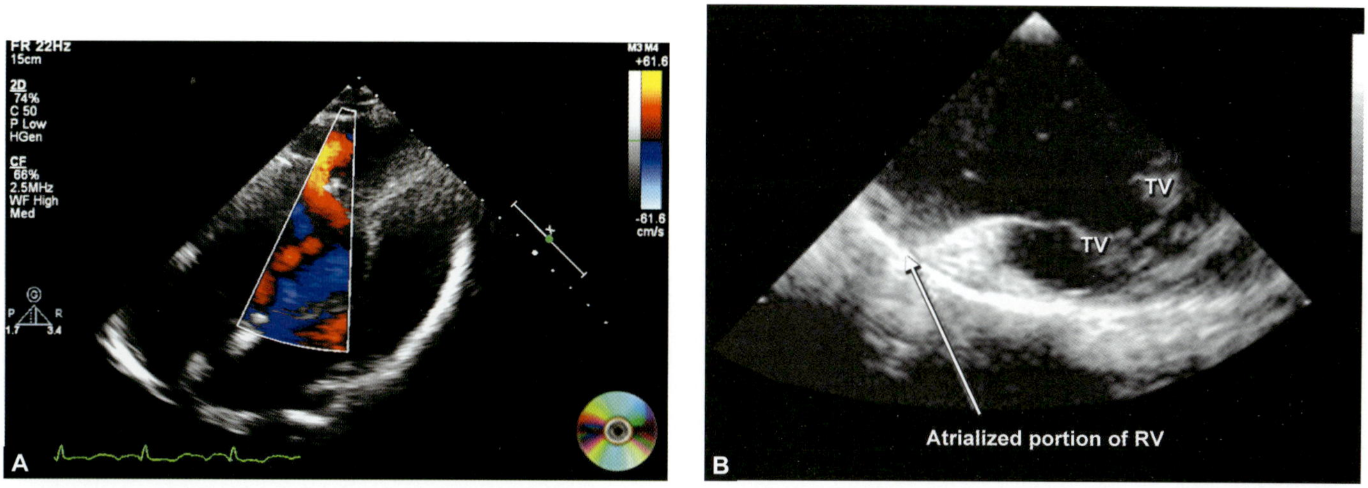

Figures 6A (Video 1) and B TEE image of a patient with Ebstein's anomaly showing apical displacement of the TV leaflet and the thin, "atrialized" portion of the affected right ventricular wall. *Abbreviation:* TV, tricuspid valve

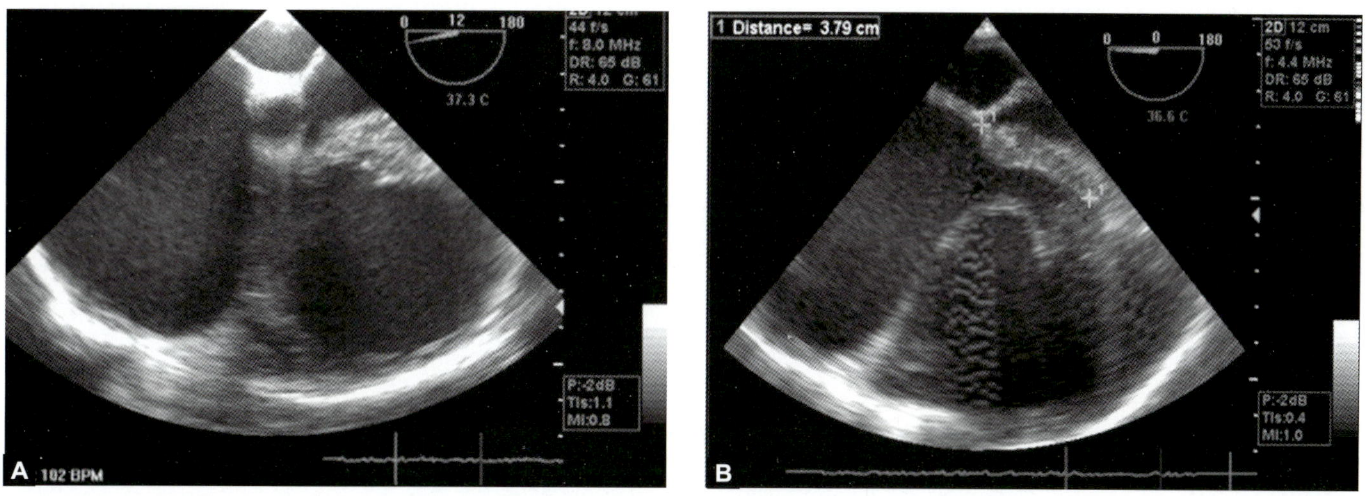

Figures 7A and B Dilated RA, dilated TV annulus—false and true should be measured, atrialization of RV, small functional right ventricle or dilated right ventricle, right heart volume overload may be seen, assessment of RV and LV function

for body surface area), in comparison with the mitral valve plane).
  - Large malformed ATL tethered to the RV wall
  - **Apically displaced STL; distance from MV annulus > 20 mm or > 8 mm/m^2**
- Dilated RA
- Dilated TV annulus—false and true should be measured
- Atrialization of RV **(Figs 7A and B)**
- Small functional right ventricle or dilated right ventricle
- Right heart volume overload may be seen
- Assessment of RV and LV function.
  Use color Doppler to:
  - Assess the severity of tricuspid regurgitation (video)
  - Look for shunts (see 'Associated features' below).
  - Pulmonary stenosis or even functional pulmonary atresia
- *M- mode:*
  - Increased excursion of the tricuspid valve when the echo beam traverses the large anterior leaflet

- The most characteristic M-mode feature is delayed closure (50 ms of more) of the tricuspid valve when compared with that of the mitral valve.
- *Continuous wave (CW) and pulsed wave (PW) Doppler*:
  - Use CW Doppler to obtain a trace of regurgitant flow through the tricuspid valve.
  - Assess the severity of tricuspid regurgitation and calculate pulmonary artery systolic pressure.
- *Other associated anomalies:*
  - Atrial septal defect (ASD)
  - Levo-transposition of the great arteries (L-TGA)
  - Mitral valve prolapsed
  - Patent foramen ovale (PFO).

Surgical Options for Ebstein's Anomaly

- Mobilization of anterior TV leaflet
- Plication of the atrialized right ventricle
- TV repair/annuloplasty preferred over TV replacement.

POSTOPERATIVE TEE ASSESSMENT (FIGS 8 TO 11)

- *After TV repair*: The competence of valve, gradient across valve, functional assessment of the right ventricle.

If after TV repair, the patent is not clinically well then, TV replacement (Bioprosthetic preferred) or addition of bi-directional (BD) Glenn (one-and-half ventricle repair).

- *After TV replacement*: The functioning of prosthetic valve and gradient across it.

KEY POINTS

- Ebstein's anomaly is characterized by an increased apical displacement of the TV annulus caused by failure of delamination of the posterior and septal leaflets.
- The TV is often regurgitant into the atrialized portion of the RV, causing severe right atrial enlargement and right-to-left flow across an ASD.
- The clinical manifestations of Ebstein's anomaly depend largely on the severity of the TV displacement and the resultant physiologic effects. Infants with severe Ebstein's anomaly will present with extreme cyanosis, cardiomegaly, and heart failure.
- The echocardiogram is crucial for accurate diagnosis and prognostic interpretation of disease severity.
- Key features on the echocardiogram include anatomy of the TV leaflets, degree of tricuspid requrgitation (TR) and/or stenosis, degree of right

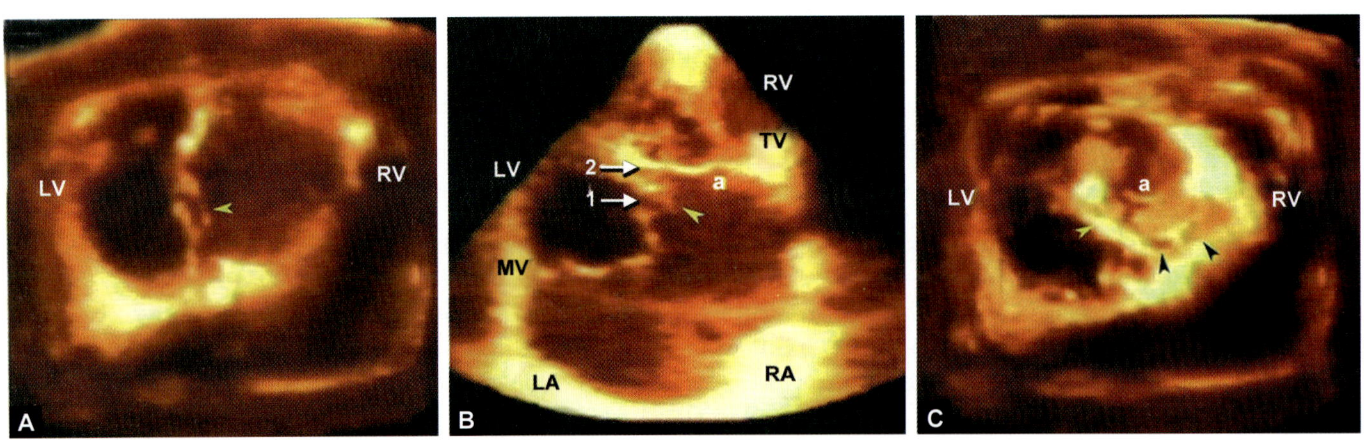

Figures 8A to C Live/real time 3D-transthoracic echocardiography (TTE) in Ebstein's anomaly associated with transposition of the great vessels. (A) Four-chamber view shows apparent displacement of the attachment of the septal leaflet of the tricuspid valve (TV) toward the apex; (B) Tethering of the septal leaflet of the TV results in a bubble-like appearance (yellow arrowhead) in the middle portion of the ventricular septum as the nontethered portion moves toward closure during systole. This transverse section was taken at a level denoted by 1 (B). (C) Transverse section taken at a more inferior level [2 in (B)] demonstrates bubble-like appearance of both septal (yellow arrowhead) and posterior (black arrowheads) TV leaflets produced by tethering[6]

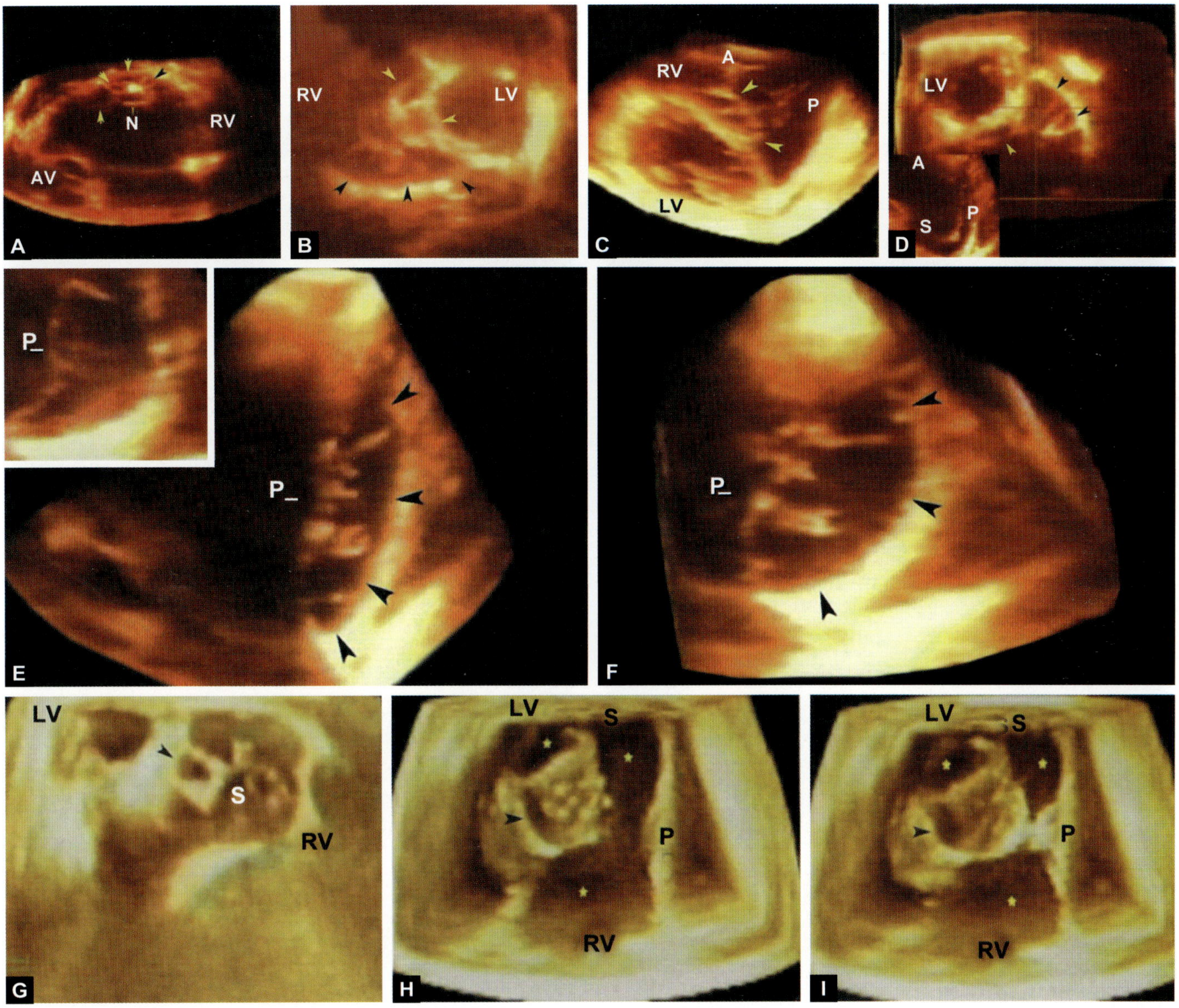

Figures 9A to I Live/real time 3D transthoracic echocardiography in isolated Ebstein's anomaly. (A) Transverse section taken at the apex of tricuspid valve (TV) shows a large area of noncoaptation (N) as well as tethering and bubble-like appearance of anterior (A; yellow arrows) and posterior (P; black arrowhead) TV (Fig. B) (4D) leaflets; (B to D) Transverse sections taken more basally demonstrate multiple "bubbles" in the septal (5; yellow arrowheads) and posterior (P; black arrowheads) TV leaflets. Inset in Figure D shows all three leaflets of the TV in the open position. Oblique section shows multiple "bubbles" (black arrowheads) in the posterior (P) TV leaflet produced by tethering to right ventricular (RV) inferior wall; (E) Inset in Figure E shows a long snake-like posterior (P) TV leaflet; (F) The oblique section shown in Figure E has been rotated to more optimally view the attachment of posterior (P) TV leaflet to the RV inferior wall; (G) The arrowhead in another patient with Ebstein's anomaly shows a bubble-like appearance resulting from tethering of the septal TV leaflet to the ventricular septum; (H and I) The arrowhead points to a large defect in the anterior leaflet of the TV in a different patient with Ebstein's anomaly. Note also small, discrete nodular areas of thickening on the anterior tricuspid leaflet. Asterisks represent loss of TV tissue which is considerable in this patient

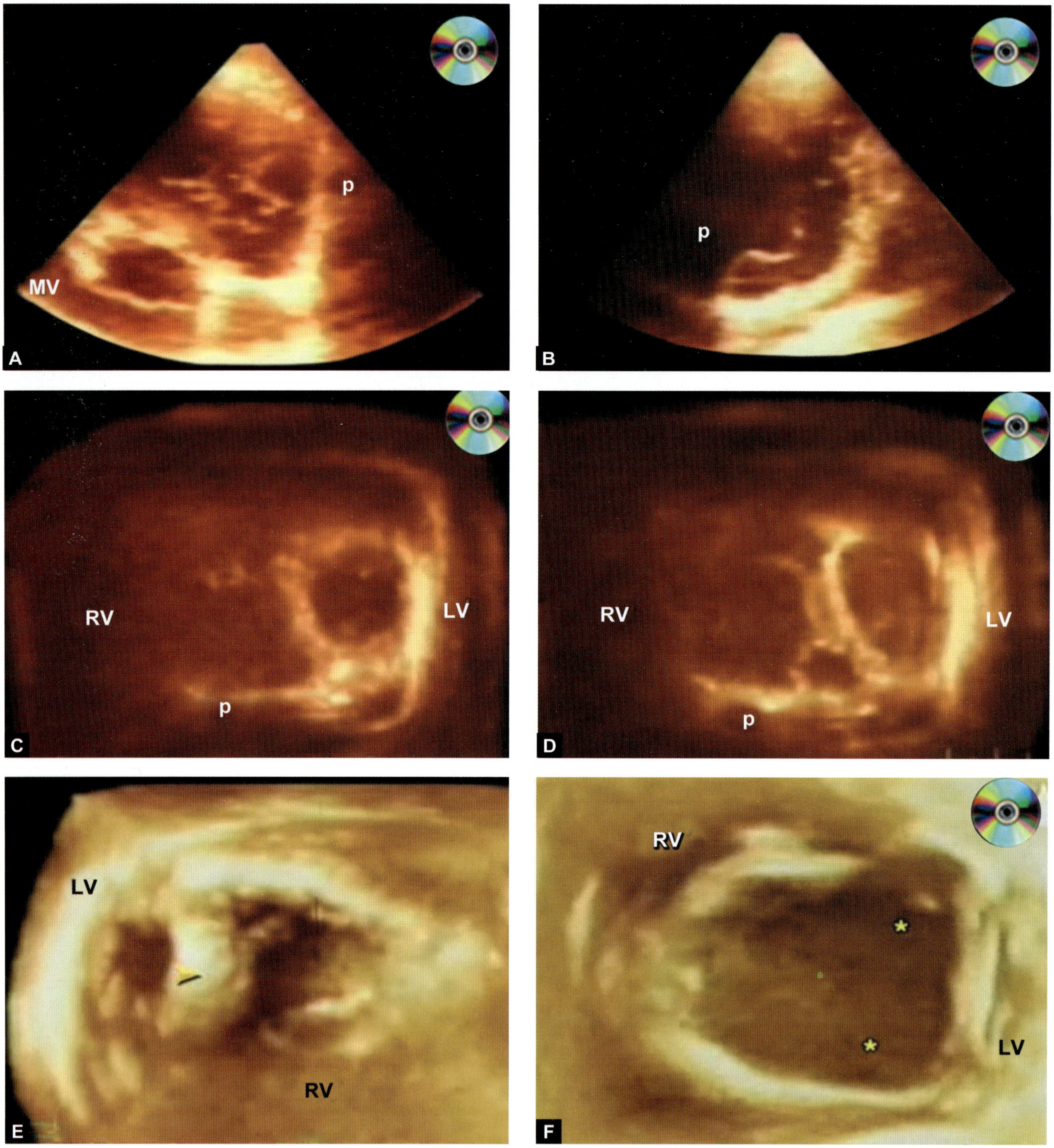

Figures 10A to F (Videos 2 to 6) The septal leaflet of the TV was tethered to the ventricular septum. Showing the dilated RV and "dubble appearance". *Abbreviations:* AV, aortic valve; LV, left ventricle; RV, right ventricle[7]

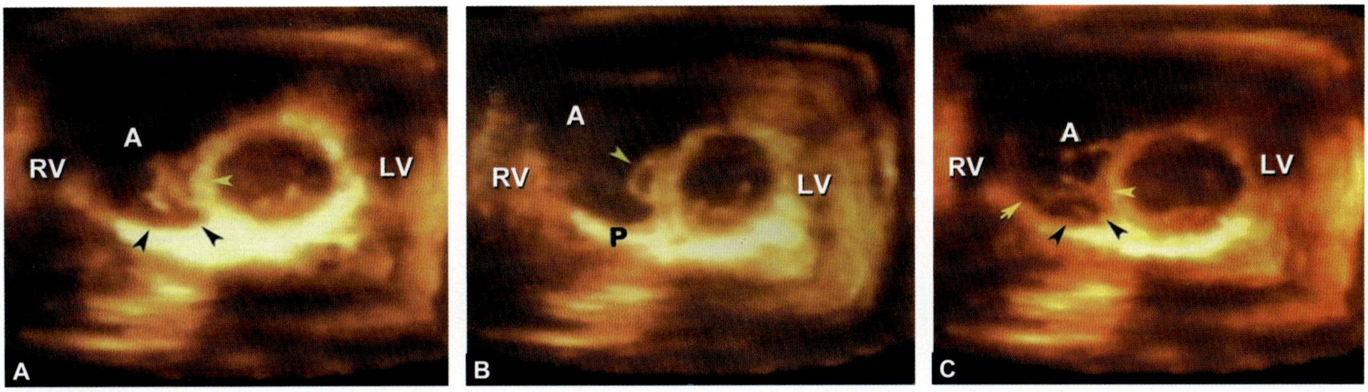

Figures 11A to C Tethering of all three tricuspid valve (TV) leaflets. The resulting "bubbles" are denoted by arrowheads for the septal (yellow) and posterior (P; black) TV leaflets and an arrow for the anterior (A) TV leaflet[8]

atrial enlargement, shunting across the interatrial septum (IAS), patient ductus arteriosus (PDA) flow, ventricular function, and other associated cardiac lesions.

REFERENCES

1. Genton E, Blount SG Jr. The spectrum of Ebstein's anomaly. Am Heart J. 1967;73:395.
2. Kumar AE, Flyer DC, Miettinsen OS, et al. Ebstein's anomaly: clinical profile and natural history. Am J Cardiol. 1971;28:84.
3. Perloff JK. Ebstein's anomaly of the tricuspid valve. In: Perloff JK (Ed). The Clinical Recognition of Congenital Heart Disease, 2nd edn. Philadelphia: WB Saunders, 1978.pp.184-200.
4. Boston US, Dearani JA, O'Leary PW, et al. Tricuspid valve repair for Ebstein's anomaly in young children: a 30-year experience. Ann Thorac Surg. 2006;81:690-5; discussion 695-6.
5. Schiebler GL, Adams PJ, Anderson RC, et al. Clinical study of twenty-three cases of Ebstein's anomaly of the tricuspid valve. Circulation. 1959;19:165-87.
6. Patel V, Nanda NC, Arellano I. Cor triatriatum sinister: assessment by live/real time 3D transthoracic echocardiography. Echocardiography. 2009;23(9):801-2.
7. Pothineni KR, Webb G. Clinical update on adults with congenital heart disease. Lancet. 2003;26:1095-104.
8. Patel V, Nanda NC, Rajdev S. Live/real time three dimensional transthoracic echocardiographic assessment of ebstein's anomaly. Echocardiography. 2005;22:847-54.

Chapter 16

TEE for Double-Inlet Left Ventricle

Poonam Malhotra Kapoor, Sarvesh Pal Singh, Jitin Narula, Suruchi Ladha

Chapter Outline

INTRODUCTION

The double-inlet left ventricle (DILV) is defined as the morphologic arrangement in which more than 50% of both atria are connected to one dominant ventricular chamber. The connection can be either through two separate atrioventricular (AV) valves (one of them may be imperforate) or through a common AV valve. The term '*single ventricle*' is often used in patients with a double-inlet ventricle, although in most instances a rudimentary second ventricle is present.[1]

MORPHOLOGY

Atrial arrangement may be:

- Situs solitus
- Situs inversus
- Atrial isomerism (right or left).

Univentricular atrioventricular connection exists which by definition means that more than 50% of both valves are committed to dominant ventricle. The mode of atrioventricular connection can be in the form of:

- Two patent valves
- One patent valve plus one imperforate valve (right or left)
- One totally committed valve plus one straddling valve (right or left; >50% rule)
- Two straddling valves (>50% rule)
- Common valve (which may or may not straddle).

VENTRICLES

Dominant ventricle in most cases is the left ventricle which has a relatively posterior position, has fine apical trabeculations and has no septal attachment of AV

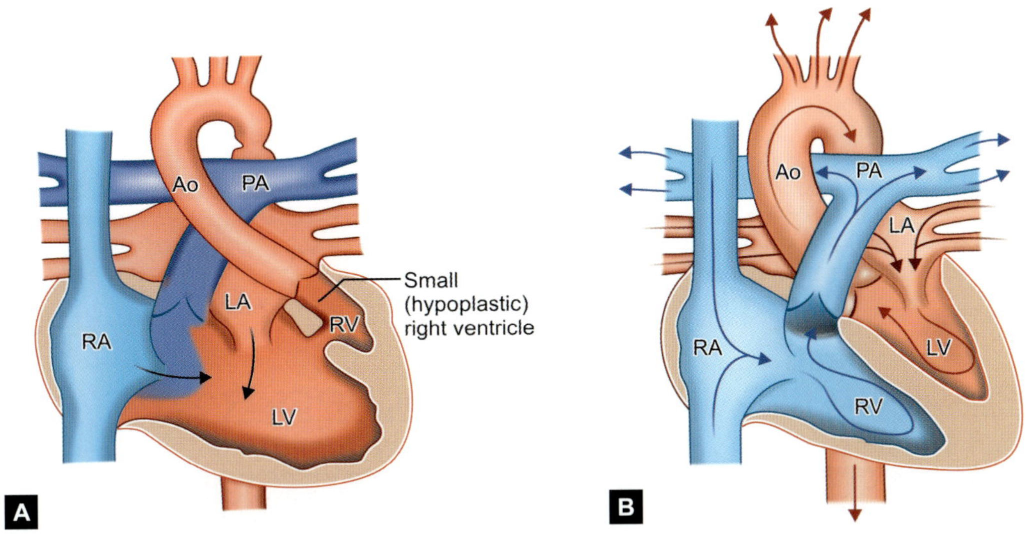

Figures 1A and B (A) Double-inlet left ventricle from right; (B) Left atriums and normal heart

valve leaflet. Right, or very occasionally, indeterminate ventricular morphology may also be present **(Figs 1A and B)**.

Ventriculoarterial connection is most commonly discordant (transposed great arteries). The associated VSD may be restrictive, leading to subaortic stenosis. There may be associated valvular or subvalvular pulmonary stenosis which may protect the pulmonary vascular bed from pulmonary vascular disease.

Holmes heart is a condition characterized by:

- Two atrioventricular valves—tricuspid and mitral
- Both atrioventricular valves opening into single left ventricle
- Normally related great arteries (ventriculoarterial concordance)
- Pulmonary artery arising from hypoplastic right ventricle infundibulum
- May be associated with coarctation of aorta.

ASSOCIATED ANOMALIES WITH DILV

- Coarctation of the aorta
- Arch hypoplasia, or interruption
- Pulmonary atresia
- Pulmonary valve stenosis
- Aortic stenosis.

PATHOPHYSIOLOGY/ NATURAL HISTORY OF DILV

Double-inlet left ventricle occurs in about 5–10 of 100,000 live births and constitutes 1.5% of patients with congenital heart disease. In this defect, pulmonary blood flow through the transposed pulmonary artery to the lungs is excessive and mild obstruction to pulmonary blood flow which may also be present might offer some protection from pulmonary overflow. Systemic blood flow is maintained is across the ventricular septal defect through the aorta to the body and may become restricted if the size of the ventricular septal defect is too small, resulting in serious illness.[2]

CLINICAL PRESENTATION

Neonates may present early after birth with cyanosis if pulmonary obstruction is severe, as seen in patients with severe valvular and subvalvular pulmonary stenosis or in double-inlet left ventricle with ventriculoarterial concordance (Holmes heart) and a severely restrictive VSD.

Patients with DILV with ventriculoarterial discordance and unobstructed pulmonary blood flow on the other hand have a left-to-right shunt, resulting in congestive heart failure with a relative decrease in systemic perfusion. These patients are at risk of developing irreversible pulmonary vascular disease.

Best overall long-term prognosis is however, seen in patients with balanced pulmonary and systemic circulation, moderate to severe pulmonary stenosis, and nonobstructed systemic blood flow. Such patients may then present quite late, with minimal cyanosis and a long ejection systolic heart murmur due to pulmonary stenosis.

TESTS TO DIAGNOSE DILV (TABLE 1)

- Chest X-ray
- Measurement of the electrical activity in the heart (electrocardiogram, or ECG)
- Passing a thin, flexible tube into the heart to examine the arteries (cardiac catheterization)
- Ultrasound exam of the heart (echocardiogram)
- Using magnets to create images of the heart (MRI).

TABLE 1 Tests to diagnosis operability in DILV

Diagnosis/Determination of operability
• Echocardiogram
• Cardiac catheterization
– PVR calculation/transpulmonary gradient calculation
– Qp: Qs calculation
– Aortopulmonary collaterals
– LVEDP
– PA angiography
• CT/MRI

TRANSESOPHAGEAL ECHOCARDIOGRAPHY OF DILV (FIGS 2 TO 7)

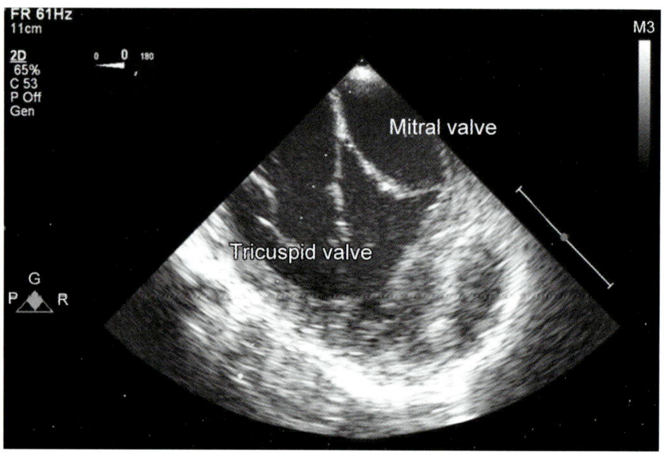

Figure 2 2D echo midesophageal 4 chamber view showing both the atrioventricular valves opening into the single ventricle, in this case morphological left ventricle DILV is a discordant connection of great vessels, best seen by a miniaturized TEE probe in neonates and infants, in which all horizontal, longitudinal and intermediate oblique planes can be obtained with minimal transducer manipulation

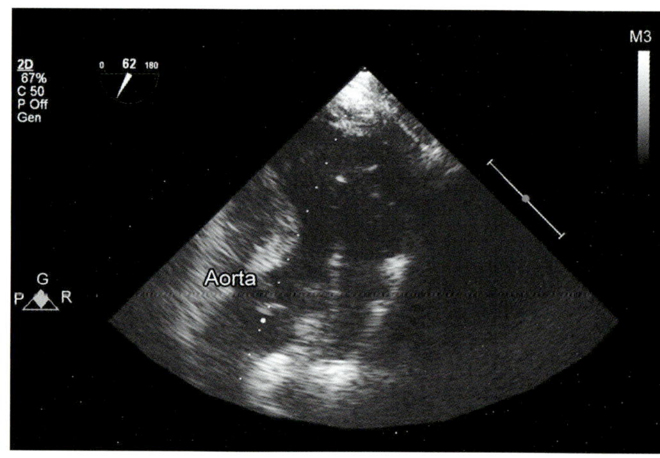

Figure 4 2D echo in deep transgastric long axis view showing aorta arising from the large left ventricle and the pulmonary artery from the rudimentary right ventricle

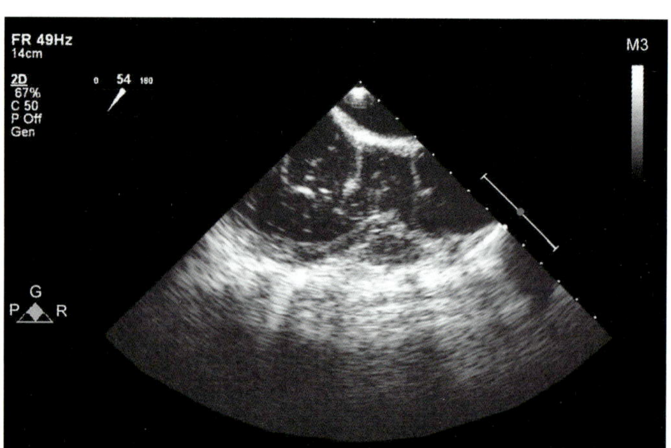

Figure 3 2D echo in midesophageal right ventricle inflow-outflow view showing aorta arising from the large morphological left ventricle

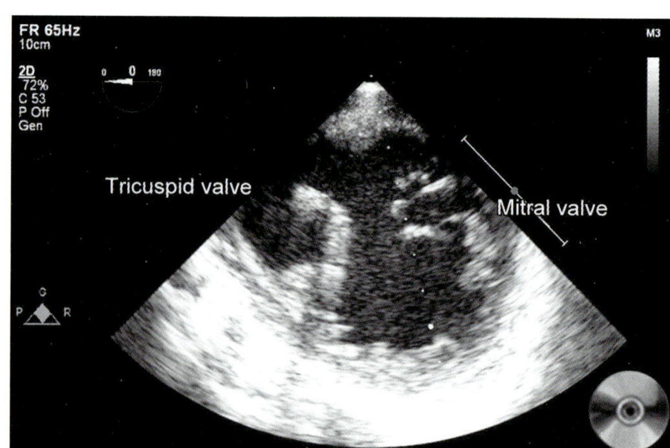

Figure 5 (Video 1) 2D echo in transgastric basal view showing both the atrioventricular valves opening into the single large morphological left ventricle (seen from the apex of heart)

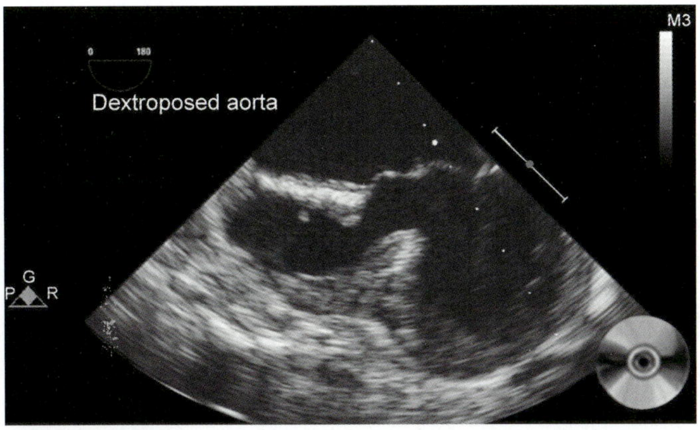

Figure 6 (Video 2) 2D echocardiography in midesophageal 4 chamber view showing a dextroposed aorta from morphological left ventricle in a patient with double-inlet left ventricle

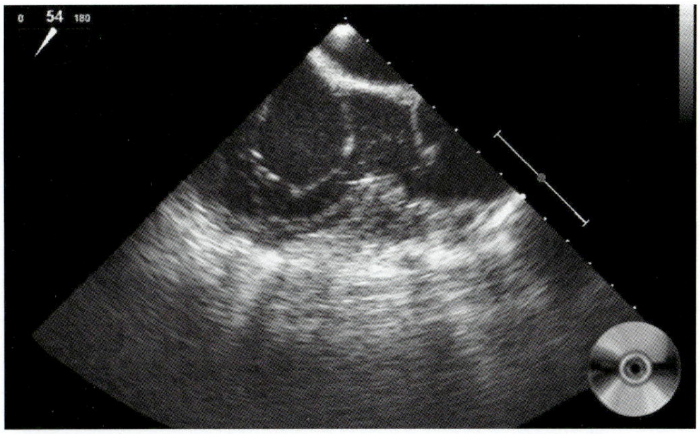

Figure 7 (Video 3) TEE in bicaval view showing discard out LV instead of RV

REFERENCES

1. Elliott LP, Anderson RH, Bargeron LM Jr., et al. Single ventricle or univentricular heart. In: Adams FH, Emmanouilides GC, Riemenschneider TA (Eds): Heart disease in infants and children. Baltimore, MD, Williams and Wilkins; 1989.pp.485-502.
2. Lan YT, Chang RK, Laks H. Outcome of patients with double inlet left ventricle or tricuspid atresia with transposed great arteries. J Am Col Cardiol. 2014; 43:113-9.

Chapter 17

TEE for Univentricular Heart

Poonam Malhotra Kapoor, Ujjwal Chowdhury, Sarvesh Pal Singh, Jitin Narula

Chapter Outline

- Morphology
- Atrioventricular Connections
- Incidence and Significance
- Univentricular Physiology
- Aortopulmonary Shunt
- Bidirectional Glenn Shunt
- Total Cavopulmonary Anastomosis
- Preoperative Assessment
- Obstruction of Anastomosis
- Echocardiography of Univentricular Heart

INTRODUCTION

The univentricular heart refers to a heart in which the atrioventricular connection is predominantly related to a single ventricular chamber that is either morphologically right or left in origin. The heart is incapable of supporting both the pulmonary and systemic circulations and cardiac anomalies do not allow 'in-series' two ventricle circulation. Presence of a second rudimentary or hypoplastic accessory ventricle justifies the term "functional" single ventricle. The univentricular heart encompasses a broad category of congenital cardiac malformations characterized by both atria-related entirely or almost entirely to a functionally single ventricular chamber.

MORPHOLOGY (FIGS 1A AND B)

Left Ventricular Type

The morphologic LV-type univentricular heart is the more common form of single ventricular chamber found in adults. Left ventricle is recognized by the presence of relatively smooth walls, fine trabeculations, and lack septal chordal attachments of the atrioventricular (AV) valve. The rudimentary chamber is usually located at the base, anterior and superior to the ventricle, and often gives rise to the aortic outflow. The orientation of the chambers is most often levo-looped, with the LV somewhat rightward and the rudimentary chamber to the left.

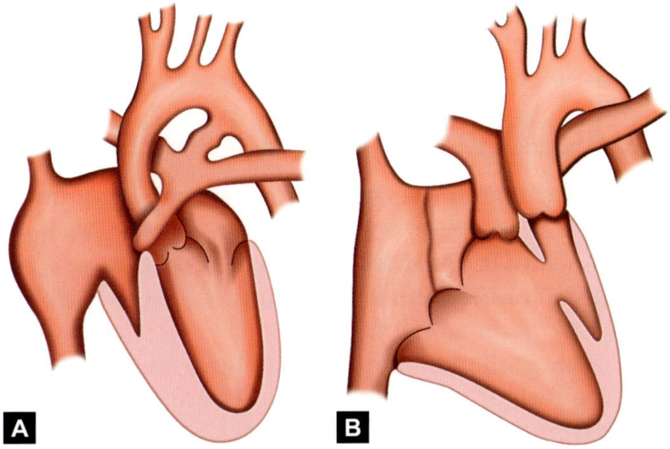

Figures 1A and B Univentricular heart with morphologically left and right ventricular types respectively

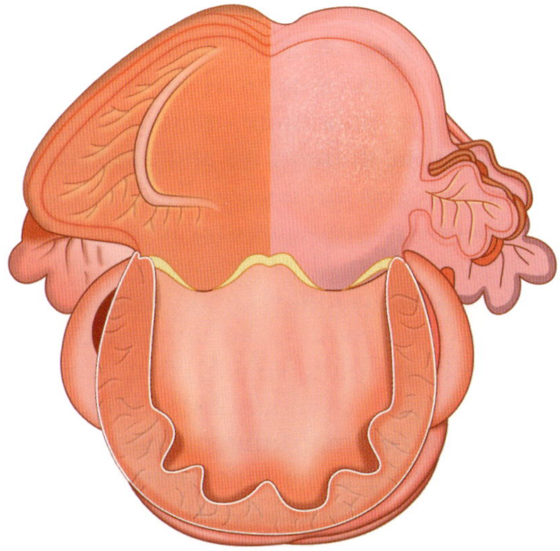
Figure 2 Atrial arrangements in patients with univentricular physiology

Right Ventricular Type

Right ventricles (RVs) are more coarsely trabeculated and commonly have chordal attachments of the AV valve to the septal surface alongwith a more caudally placed. Both great arteries usually arise from the right ventricle. The aorta is characteristically "malposed," as it is anterior to or side-by-side with the pulmonary artery. In this case, the rudimentary chamber is located posterior and inferior to the morphologic and may be present to the right (levo-loop) or to the left (dextro-loop) of the dominant RV.

Indeterminate Type

Occasionally, the morphology of the chamber cannot be determined as these patients most commonly do not possess a second chamber within the ventricular mass and this is referred to as univentricular heart of indeterminate type.

ATRIOVENTRICULAR CONNECTIONS

Atrial arrangement in patients with univentricular physiology may be:

- Usual atrial arrangement
- Mirror imaged arrangement
- Right isomerism
- Left isomerism.

In each of the three morphological types described above, the type of atrioventricular connection may be either absent right, absent left or double inlet (either may be imperforate, stenotic, or regurgitant) type of atrioventricular connection. The mode of connection may be through a common atrioventricular valve or two atrioventricular valves, which may straddle or override the trabecular septum **(Fig. 2)**.

INCIDENCE AND SIGNIFICANCE

The most common form of univentricular heart is the hypoplastic left heart syndrome with an incidence of 2.3 cases per 10,000 livebirths.[1] Tricuspid atresia, is the second most common subtype of univentricular heart occurring once for every 10,000 livebirths.[2] Double inlet left ventricle (DILV) comprises 1% of all congenital heart malformations. Seventy percent with well-formed single left ventricles died before age 16, with an annual attrition rate of 4.8%.[3] For patients with univentricular hearts of right ventricular morphology, natural history and outcome are even worse with only 50% survival 4 years after diagnosis. The common causes of mortality, are arrhythmias, congestive heart failure, and sudden unexplained death.

UNIVENTRICULAR PHYSIOLOGY

Physiology of the univentricular heart is an interplay of various factors like obstruction to outflow, inflow, and/or flow across the atrial septum; AV valve regurgitation; systemic and pulmonary venous return; and pulmonary vascular resistance. Systemic and pulmonary blood flows are interdependent and determined by resistances of the two circulations which in turn determines the direction of flow across the patent ductus arteriosus.[4]

Obstruction to pulmonary venous return in the setting of an atretic mitral valve and a restrictive atrial septal defect (ASD) is physiologically similar to pulmonary venous obstruction and may lead to severe pulmonary hypertension. Unobstructed communication between both venous inflows and the single ventricle in these cases thus requires an unrestrictive ASD. In tricuspid atresia, the physiological effect of a restrictive ASD is akin to systemic venous obstruction.

In short, an optimal univentricular physiology requires a good ventricular function without AV valve regurgitation, an unrestrictive ASD, and well balanced systemic and pulmonary blood flow.

Functionally univentricular heart biventricular repair seems impossible due to the presence of a hypoplastic ventricle, straddling AV valves, severe neonatal AV-regurgitation. Surgical options thus include:

- Aortopulmonary shunt or modified Blalock-Taussig shunt
- Bidirectional Glenn shunt
- Total cavopulmonary anastomosis.

AORTOPULMONARY SHUNT

Modified Blalock-Taussig shunt is difficult to image on transesophageal echocardiography. Right modified Blalock-Taussig shunt may be imaged with repeated sweeping of the structures in the midesophageal ascending aorta short-axis view where the right pulmonary artery can be traced till the junction of polytetrafluoroethylene graft and right pulmonary artery. Left modified Blalock-Taussig shunt cannot be imaged until unless the left pulmonary artery anastomosis is on proximal left pulmonary artery or at the confluence of branch pulmonary arteries as adequate visualization of the left pulmonary artery is not possible due to interposition of the air-filled trachea and bronchi.

Central aortopulmonary shunt is more convenient to image compared to modified Blalock-Taussig shunt.[5]

BIDIRECTIONAL GLENN SHUNT

The imaging of bidirectional Glenn shunt involves the same technique as that in the right modified Blalock-Taussig shunt, only the velocity of blood flow is less compared to modified Blalock-Taussig shunt.

TOTAL CAVOPULMONARY ANASTOMOSIS

The total cavopulmonary anastomosis can be of three types:

1. Extracardiac total cavopulmonary anastomosis
2. Lateral tunnel Fontan operation
3. Classic Fontan operation.

Classic Fontan operation is not done in the present era. The former two operations are performed mostly as destination therapy for patients destined for univentricular repair. Fenestration can be made in both extracardiac total cavopulmonary anastomosis and lateral tunnel Fontan to decompress the Fontan circuit in case there is high pressure in the Fontan circulation.

PREOPERATIVE ASSESSMENT (FIG. 2)

Determination of the morphology of the dominant ventricular chamber should focus on the anatomic landmarks, systemic and pulmonary venous connections, the atrioventricular connections, and the ventriculoarterial connections.

To ascertain the following, before proceeding for a Fontan operation:

- Normally draining systemic veins
- Normal RA or not and following criteria as well.

Pulmonary Anatomy (PA)

- **Nakata index**
  - Diameter of the right and left pulmonary arteries immediately proximal to their first branching. Pulmonary artery size is reported as the sum of the cross-sectional areas of the right and left pulmonary arteries, indexed to body surface area. The normal cross-sectional index is 330 + 30 mm^2/m^2
  - Index > 250 mm^2/m^2 considered adequate for Fontan
- **McGoon's ratio**
  - Dividing the sum of the diameters of RPA (at the level of crossing the lateral margin of vertebral column on angiogram) and LPA (just proximal to its upper lobe branch), divided by the diameter of aorta at the level above the diaphragm

- > 1.5:1 associated with acceptable postoperative RV systolic pressure
- **PASP <15-20 mm Hg**
  - Status of the AV connection
    - Single, double, or common
    - AV valve function
    - Appraisal of straddling and overriding features
    - AV valve stenosis/systemic AV valve regurgitation
- Ventricular function assessment and ejection fraction calculation
- Doppler imaging
- Intracardiac shunt lesions, VSDs; valve abnormalities, such as PS; and residual embryologic vascular connections, such as a left SVC:
  - Identify the direction of flow
  - Quantify flow in intracardiac shunting and valvular abnormalities.

Normally the venous circuit is a low velocity circuit < 1 m/s. It has a biphasic flow—forward flow in diastole and retrograde flow in systole. Also see on TEE:

- Anatomical diagnosis according to the segmental analysis
- Abdominal situs
- Obstructive outflow tract (AS, PS, CoA).

Respiratory variation; increases with inspiration in a spontaneously breathing patient.

OBSTRUCTION OF ANASTOMOSIS

TEE Detected

- Peak velocity > 1 m/s on continuous wave Doppler
- Presence of turbulence
- Loss of respiratory variation
- Flow in inferior vena cava sluggish (Nyquist limit of 15 cm/s may not show any flow in inferior vena cava).

ECHOCARDIOGRAPHY OF UNIVENTRICULAR HEART (FIGS 3 TO 11)

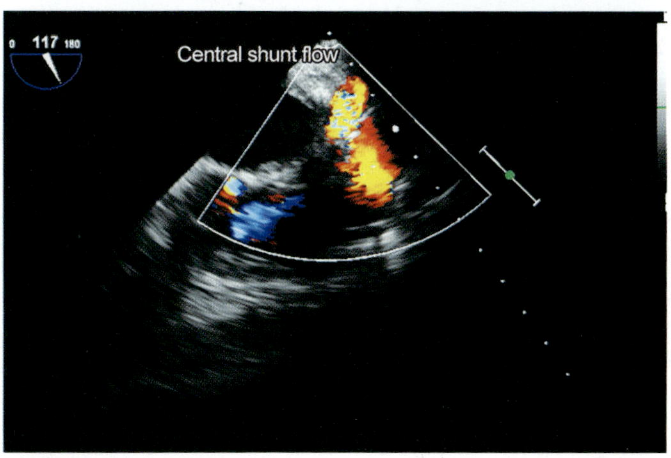

Figure 3 Color Doppler echocardiography in midesophageal ion axis view showing flow through the conduit used to perform the central shunt (connecting ascending aorta with main pulmonary artery)

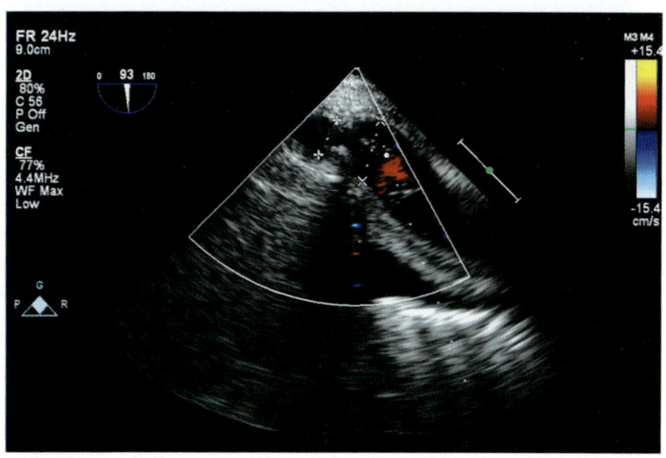

Figure 4 Color Doppler echocardiography, in modified mid-esophageal bicaval view, showing stenosis of the anastomosis between prosthetic conduit and inferior vena cava in a patient who has undergone Fontan operation

CHAPTER 17

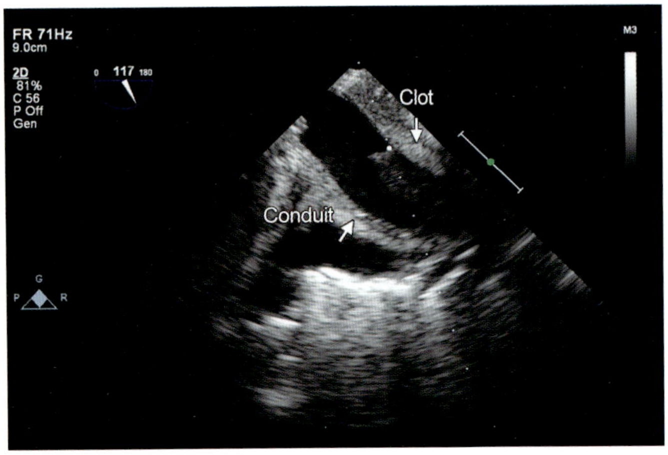

Figure 5 2D echo in midesophageal bicaval view (probe turned to right) showing thrombus in the conduit of the Fontan circulation

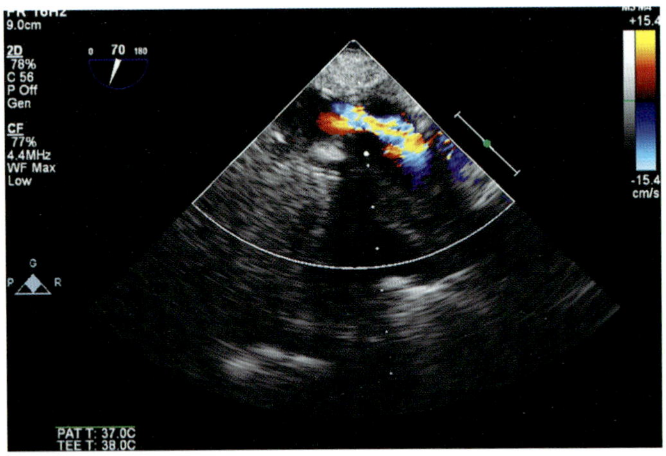

Figure 6 Color Doppler echocardiography, in modified midesophageal bicaval view (probe turned to right), showing stenosis of the anastomosis between prosthetic conduit and inferior vena cava in a patient who has undergone Fontan operation

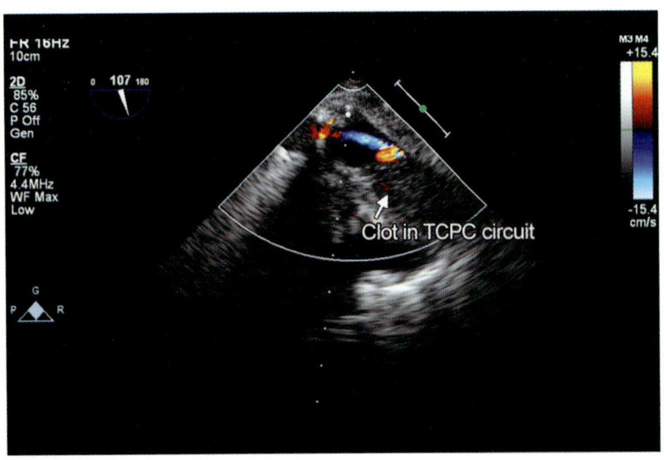

Figure 7 Color Doppler imaging in the midesophageal bicaval view (probe turned to the right) showing both stenosis and thrombus in the Fontan circuit

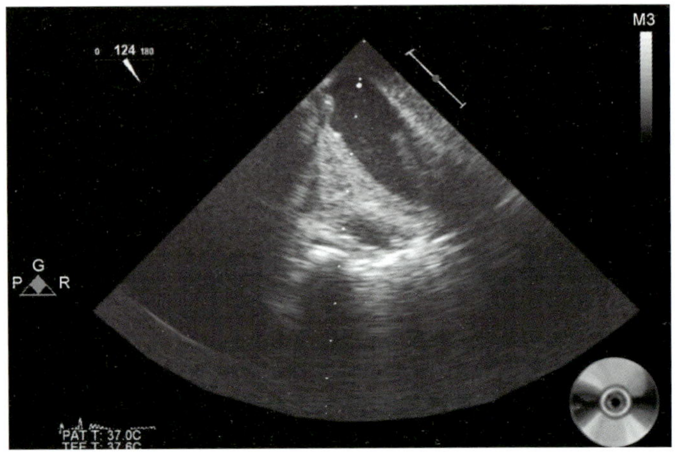

Figure 8 (Video 1) 2D echo in midesophageal bicaval view (probe turned to right) showing thrombus in the conduit of the Fontan circulation. Note the spontaneous echo contrast proximal to the thrombus

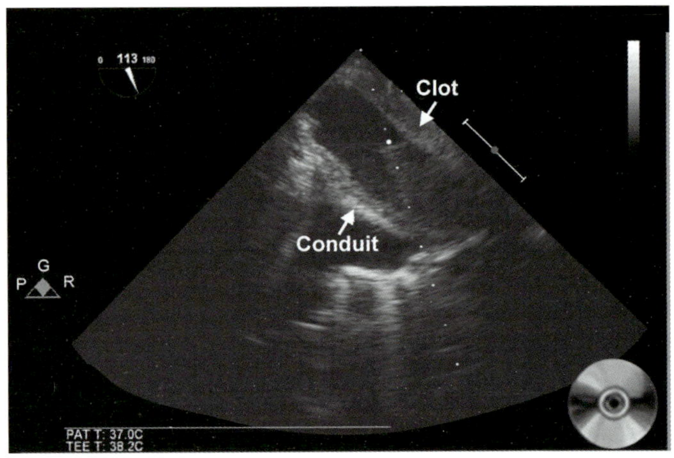

Figure 9 (Video 2) 2D echo in midesophageal bicaval view (probe turned to right) showing thrombus in the conduit of the Fontan circulation

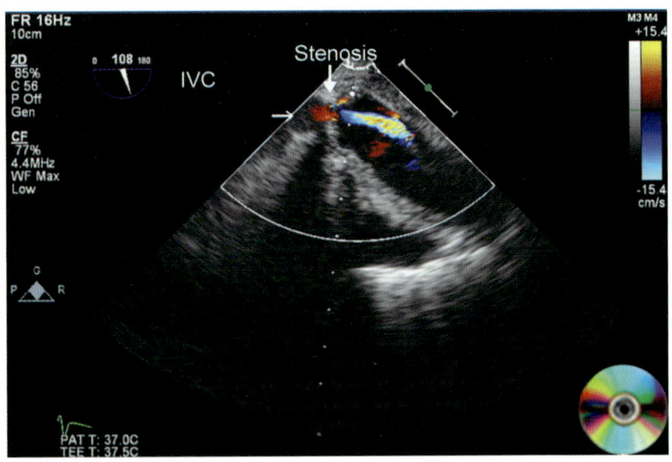

Figure 10 (Video3) Color Doppler echocardiography, in modified midesophageal bicaval view (probe turned to right), showing stenosis of the anastomosis between prosthetic conduit and inferior vena cava in a patient who has undergone Fontan operation

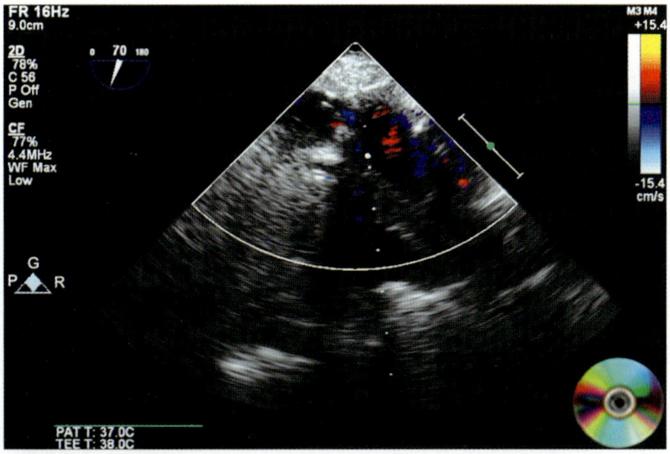

Figure 11 (Video 4) Color Doppler echocardiography, in modified midesophageal bicaval view (probe turned to right), showing stenosis of the anastomosis between prosthetic conduit and inferior vena cava in a patient who has undergone Fontan operation

REFERENCES

1. Hoffman JI, Kaplan S. The incidence of congenital heart disease. J Am Coll Cardiol. 2002;39:1890-900.
2. Rao PS. Tricuspid atresia. Curr Treat Options Cardiovasc Med. 2000;2:507-20.
3. Moodie DS, Ritter DG, Tajik AJ, O'Fallon WM. Long-term follow-up in the unoperated univentricular heart. Am J Cardiol. 1984;53:1124-8.
4. Nelson DP, Schwartz SM, Chang AC. Neonatal physiology of the functionally univentricular heart. Cardiol Young. 2004;14 (Suppl 1):52-60.
5. Chowdhury UK, Mishra PK, Sharma, et al. Postoperative assessment of the univentricular repair by dynamic radionuclide studies. Ann Thorac Surg. 2004;78:658-65.

Chapter 18

TEE for Total Anomalous Pulmonary Venous Connection

Poonam Malhotra Kapoor, Vishwas Malik, Umed Kumar, Kulbhushan Saini

Chapter Outline

- Darling's Modification of Types of TAPVC
- Pathophysiology of TAPVC
- Total Anomalous Pulmonary Venous Connection (Supracardiac)
- X-ray Chest PAV in TAPVC
- X-ray Chest TAPVC
- ECG in TAPVC
- Anesthetic Consideration
- Preoperative Consideration
- Intraoperative Consideration
- Preoperative Assessment of 2D TEE for TAPVC
- Postoperative TEE Assessment
- 3D TEE
- 3D TEE for Surgical Technique

INTRODUCTION

Total anomalous pulmonary venous connection (TAPVC) is a very uncommon cyanotic anomaly comprising 1% of all congenital heart diseases. Since pulmonary veins drain into the systemic venous circulation, TAPVC is incompatible with life unless a communication between the right and left sides of the heart exists; usually via a patent foramen ovale or atrial septal defect. As the right to left shunt is usually small, right heart dilatation and failure ensues owing to a volume overload. Stenosis and obstruction of varying degree at the junction of the anomalous trunk with the vena cava leads to severe pulmonary hypertension which further worsens right heart failure. Patients present in early infancy with bluish discoloration exaggerated by activity and symptoms of heart failure. They are usually severely acidotic and cyanotic. Without surgery most infants die by 12 months of age. However, postoperative mortality is also high owing to increased pulmonary vascular resistance and indequate repair due to obscure anatomy.[1]

DEFINITION

In a normal heart, the blood flows in from the body to the right atrium. It then goes into the right ventricle through the tricuspid valve. The blood travels to the lungs through the pulmonary valve to pick up fresh oxygen. Next, the blood returns to the left atrium, goes into the left ventricle, and goes out to the rest of the body. With TAPVC, the pulmonary veins that return oxygenated blood from the lungs connect to the right side of the heart, instead of the left atrium. This leads to the mixing of oxygenated and deoxygenated blood. The body tissue does not receive as much oxygen as it is supposed to. TAPVC can be mild to severe. There can be a range of connection problems. Other heart problems may be present, as well.[2]

DARLING'S MODIFICATION OF TYPES OF TAPVC

- Type 1, anomalous connection at the supracardiac level - SVC or the innominate vein 50%
- Type 2, anomalous connection at the cardiac level-coronary sinus or directly to the RA 30%
- Type 3, anomalous connection at the infracardiac level-IVC or portal vein 15%
- Type 4, anomalous connection at 2 or more levels (mixed) 5% **(Fig. 1)**.

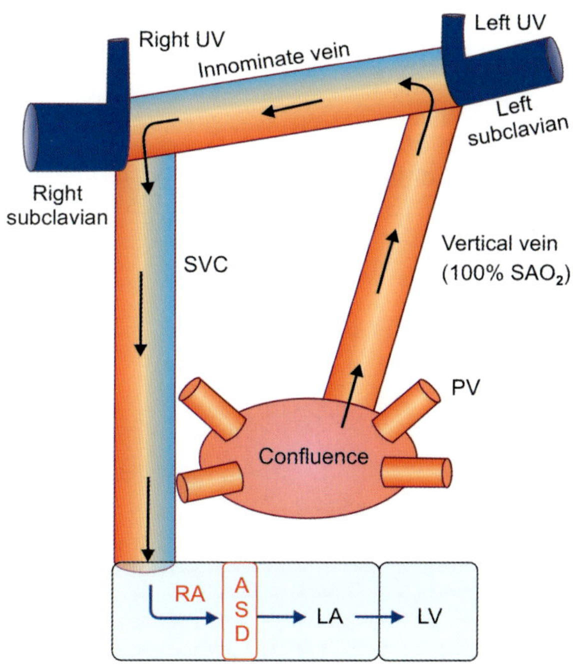

The common types of supracardiac TAPVC:
- There is complete PV-LA discordance
- 100% saturated blood that comes from the lung goes up through vertical vein and mixes with systemic venous flow from left UL and entire head and neck with in SVC
- Further mixing take place in RA with IVC flow. A completely mixed blood then enter LA through ASD and finally reaches LV for systemic circulation
- All four chambers show near equal saturation around 90% with minimal clinical cyanosis

Figure 1 Pathophysiology of TAPVC

- SMITH classification
  - Supracardiac (without pulmonary vein obstruction)
  - Infradiaphragmatic (with pulmonary vein obstruction)
- Burroughs-Edwards classification
  - Long, intermediate, short

PATHOPHYSIOLOGY OF TAPVC

- Pathophysiology of TAPVR depends on obstructed or nonobstructed pulmonary venous return.
- Obstruction will lead to pulmonary venous hypertension and higher back pressures.
- All pulmonary venous blood returns to the right atrium (common mixing chamber)
- A right-to-left shunt at the atrial level (RV complete, ASD size, Rp)
- Increased pulmonary blood flow and pulmonary venous obstruction will eventually result in pulmonary hypertension.
- Infradiaphragmatic draining.

Pulmonary Vein Stenosis

- Obstruction to pulmonary draining with increase in pulmonary venous pressure.
- Capillary leak with interstitial edema.
- Reflex pulmonary vasopressure constriction and progressive increase in Rp = pulmonary hypertension.
- Increased PAP leads to increased RV pressures (sometimes suprasystemic) with RV failure, decreased pulmonary blood flow, decreased Qp: Qs, decreased systemic SAT, peripheral hypoxia and metabolic acidosis with multiorgan failure.
- *PFO obstruction:* Increased LAP, impedes pulmonary venous return, producing pulmonary hypertension.

Supracardiac Type I (TAPVC)

- PA chest radiograph shows mild cardiomegaly
- Increased pulmonary vascular markings
- "Snowman" appearance of supracardiac anomalous drainage.
- *Cardiac TAPVR: There are two types*: The pulmonary veins can directly enter into the right side of the heart, into the right atrium. Alternatively, the pulmonary veins can drain into the coronary sinus.

The coronary sinus normally carries deoxygenated blood from the heart muscle into the right atrium. This vein is usually very small, but becomes quite large with this abnormal amount of blood.

- *Mixed TAPVR:* The pulmonary veins split up and drain partially to more than one of these options.

Cardiac Type—II (TAPVC)

- *Second most common*: 30%
- Drains into coronary sinus or RA
- Coronary sinus more common
- Increased pulmonary vasculature
- Overload of RV leads to CHF after birth
- 20% of I's and II's survive to adulthood
- Remainder expire in first year.

Infracardiac Type—Type III

- *Percent of total*: 12%
- Long pulmonary veins course down along esophagus.

Empty into IVC or portal vein (more common):

- Vein constricted by diaphragm as it passes through esophageal hiatus
- Severe CHF (90%) 2° obstruction to venous return
- Cyanotic 2° right to left shunt through ASD
- Associated with asplenia (80%), or polysplenia
- Prognosis = Death within a few days.

Mixed Type—Type IV

- *Percent of total*: 6%
- Mixtures of types I–III.

TOTAL ANOMALOUS PULMONARY VENOUS CONNECTION (SUPRACARDIAC)

The principle of operative repair is to establish an unobstructed communication between the pulmonary veins and the left atrium, interrupt the connections with the systemic venous circulation, and remove intracardiac shunting.

X-RAY CHEST PAV IN TAPVC (FIGS 2A AND B)

Shape and Size Character

Check the shape:

- Observe the shape of the heart
- If the heart looks like a 'water bottle', it may indicate a pericardial disease or dilatied cardiomyopathy.

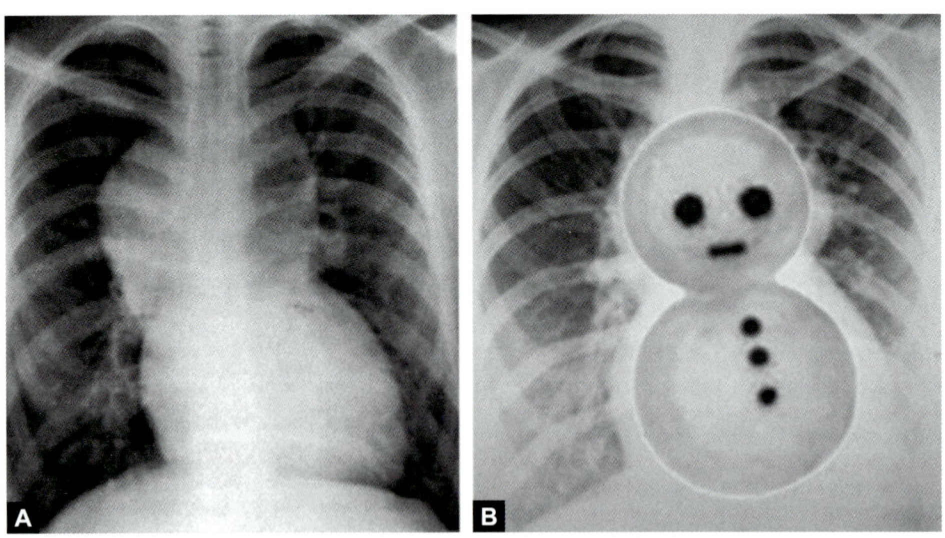

Figures 2A and B TAPVR due to an anomalous connection to left SVC shows the classic "Snowman" or pattern of enlarged supracardiac veins, left SVC, left innominate veins, and right SVC

Chest X-ray is not the means to diagnose TAPVC, but if one is obtained, it can show the classic "snowman pattern".[3]

- Therefore, the clinical history is important, in making the diagnosis.
- This venous pattern is preferentially in the right upper lobe.

X-RAY CHEST TAPVC (FIGS 2A AND B)

- There is cardiomegaly with increased pulmonary arterial markings.
- There is dilation of both the left and right innominate veins.
- The right superior vena cava producing the classical "snowman" or "appearance".
- The superior mediastinum is enlarged secondary to dilation of the right vena cava, innominate vein and ascending vertical vein.
- PA chest radiograph demonstrates increased pulmonary venous pattern with a normal sized heart.
- There is a right sided pleural effusion.
- The end tracheal tube is just above the level of the carina.
- The heart is normal sized with increased pulmonary venous pattern.

ECG IN TAPVC (FIG. 3)

Patient may present with including:

- Supraventricular tachycardia
- Bradyarrhythmia
- Sick sinus syndrome
- Multiform supraventricular
- Ventricular ectopic beats.

These arrhythmias may persist long after TAPVC correction.

ANESTHETIC CONSIDERATION

- Patients with obstructed TAPVR are:
  - Sicker and
  - Will need higher PaO_2
  - Ionotropic support repeated
  - Blood gases to control acidosis

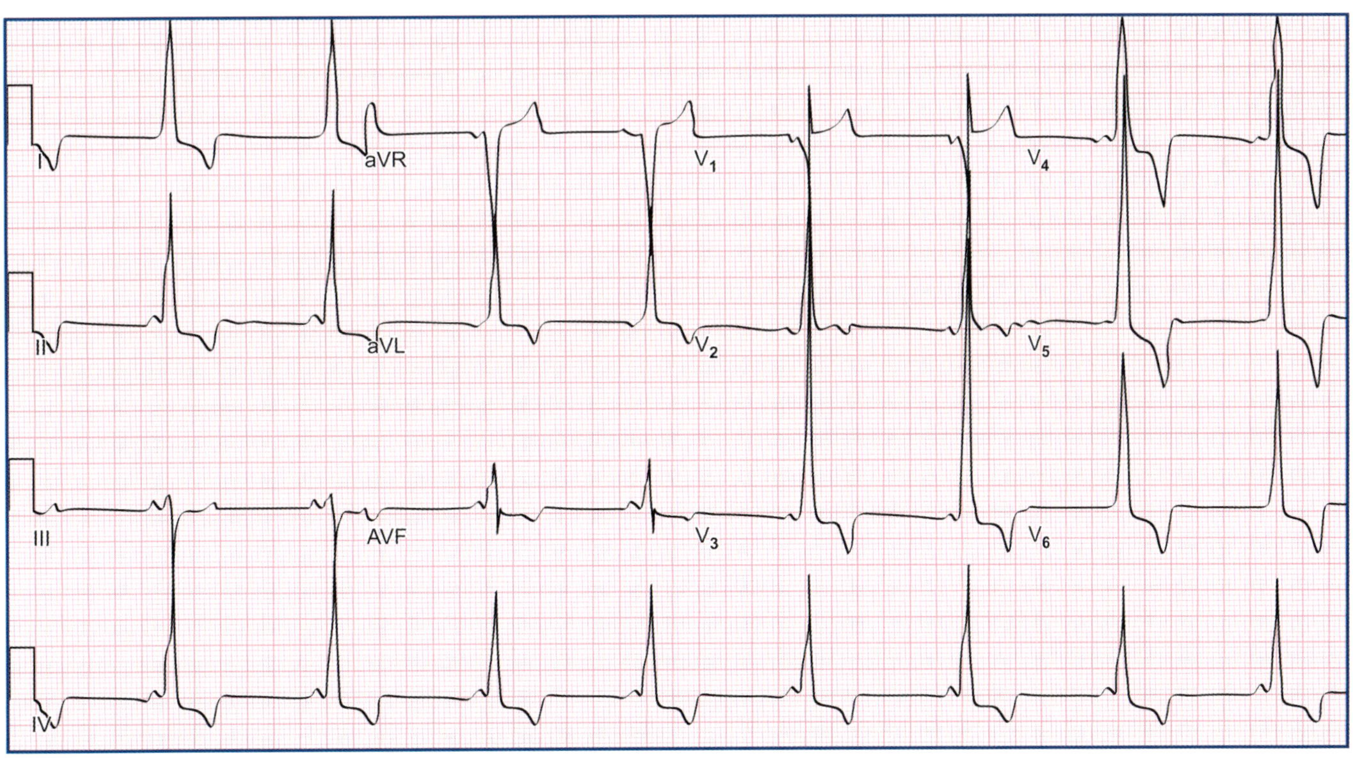

Figure 3 ECG of a patient with TAPVC

- Postbypass period require
  - High PaO_2
  - Hyperventilation
  - Inotropic support
  - Good sedation, paralysis and NO
- TEE usually not done
  - Intraoperative, except in experienced hands
  - TTE and epicardial echo can be performed to look at venous return in the left atrium.

PREOPERATIVE CONSIDERATION

- Neonates typically present with PAH,
  - Cynosis
  - Metabolic acidosis
  - Poor perfusion
- Often already intubated and receiving inotropic support
- PGE may decompress a hypertensive PA system and even open a ductus venosus, relieving a degree of pulmonary venous obstruction.

INTRAOPERATIVE CONSIDERATION

- A technique should be used to minimize myocardial depression
  - Typically with intravenous narcotics and paralytics.
- Inhalational anesthetics are generally not tolerated in the sick neonate but may be
  - Acceptable in the older child without obstruction and minimal symptoms
- Two issues arise when planning therapy for separation from CPB:
  - First, these children have reactive pulmonary vascular beds, and efforts must center around decreasing PVR to improve right heart function
  - Therefore, high oxygen levels, hyperventilation, alkalosis, nitrates, isoproterenol, PGE, and nitric oxide may be considered.

PREOPERATIVE ASSESSMENT OF 2D TEE FOR TAPVC (FIGS 4 TO 6)

Most of the types of TAPVC are difficult to image on TEE due to restriction of movement. Type 2 TAPVC can be imaged on TEE with the indirect evidence of increased coronary sinus flow and absent normal pulmonary venous drainage.

- Increase in the transmitral flow velocities are observed
- Excessive flow across coronary sinus abolished may be able to image one of the pulmonary veins into LA. All four pulmonary veins form a common chamber

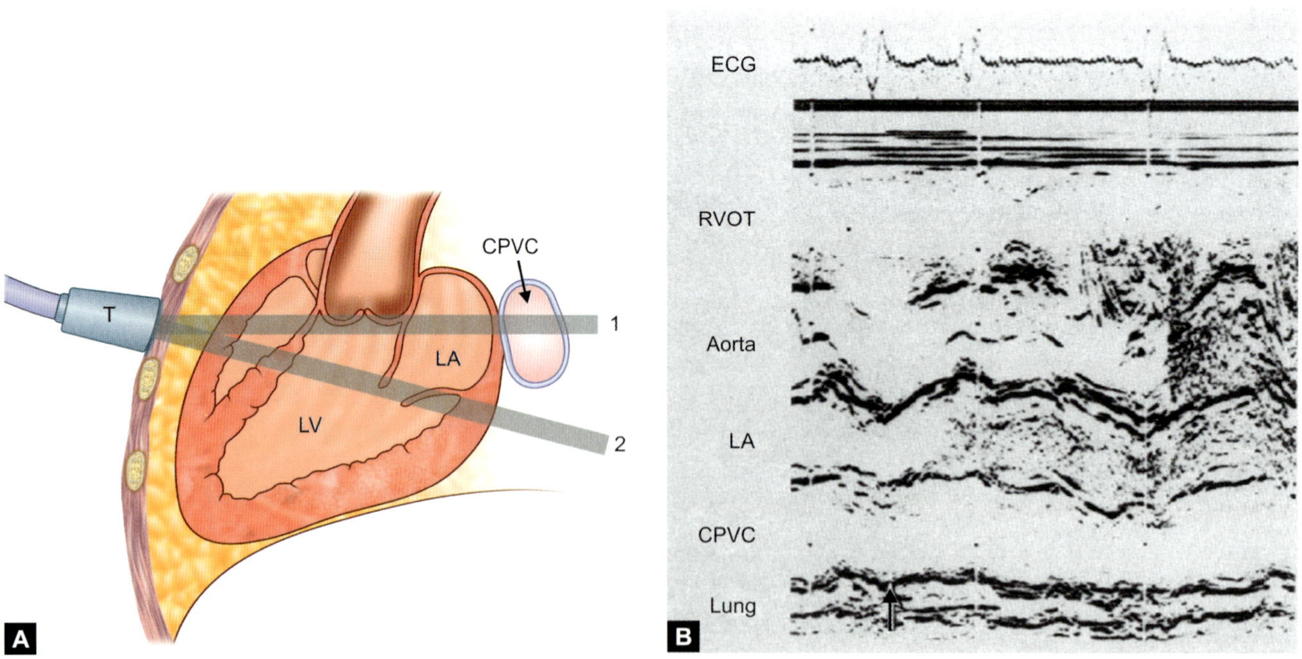

Figures 4A and B (A) Diagram showing the anatomic relation between the left atrium (LA) and the common pulmonary venous chamber in TAPVC; (B) The ejection was made into the LA. After the injection a cloud of echoes fills the LA without pacification of the echo-free space. Note the position of the common chamber (CPVC) behind the LA (LA and CPVC on M-mode)

CHAPTER 18

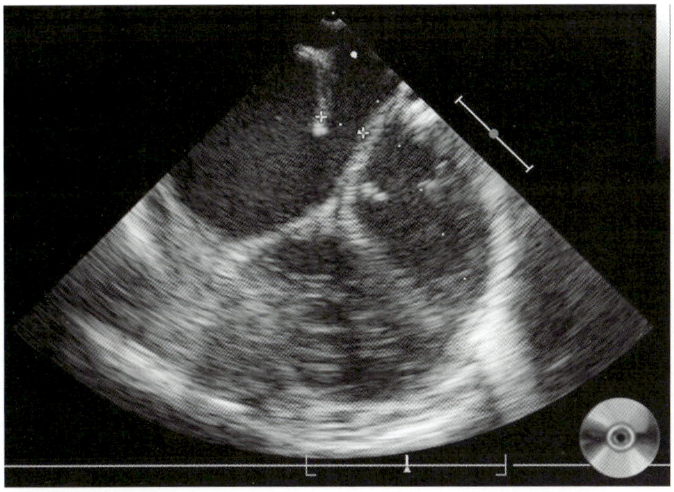

Figure 5 (Video 1) 2D echo in midesophageal 4 chamber view showing a dilated coronary sinus which is present in coronary sinus total anomalous pulmonary vein connection

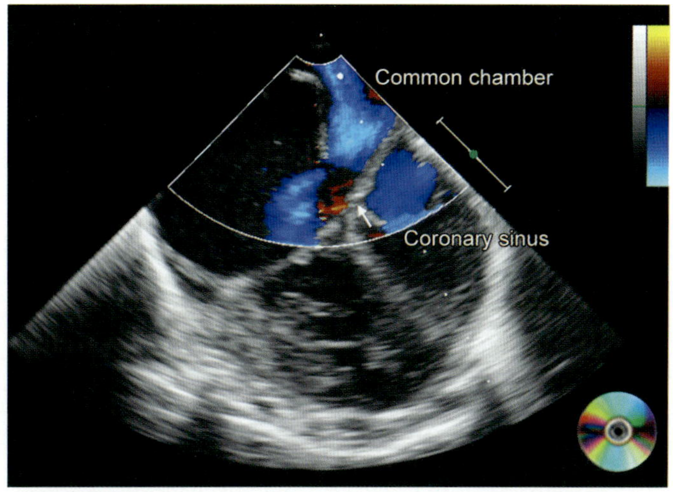

Figure 6 (Video 2) Color Doppler in midesophageal 4 chamber view showing increased blood flow through the coronary sinus indicative of coronary sinus total anomalous pulmonary vein connection

(CPVC) which drains into the SVC via the vertical vein.

- Tajik et al.[4] in 1972 first described the echocardiographic features of right ventricular, diastolic volume overload (RVDVO) in a patient with TAPVC.
- Glaser et al.[5] and later Meyer and Kaplan[6] suggested that a small left atrial size associated with paradoxical motion of the interventricular septum was characteristic of TAPVC. This proposal was challenged by Godman et al.[7] who suggested that in newborns with TAPVC the presence of pulmonary hypertension may prevent the development of abnormal septal motion.
- Paquet et al.[8] showed that the identification of this common chamber (CPVC), combined with echocardiographic evidence of RVDVO, is strongly suggestive of TAPVC irrespective of the site of drainage and this is followed, worldwide.

On 2D TEE

- Most of the types of TAPVC are difficult to image on TEE due to restriction of movement. Type 2 TAPVC can be imaged on TEE with the indirect evidence of increased coronary sinus flow and absent normal pulmonary venous drainage.
- Lack of connection of pulmonary veins to the LA. Delineate the course and site of the anomalous pulmonary venous drainage as well as the obstruction of the pulmonary venous inflow, by ruling out the following:
- Atrial septal defect
- Bowing of interatrial septum towards left
- Right atrium and right ventricle volume overload
- Left ventricle size and mitral valve annulus
- Mitral valve inflow velocities are high
- Dilated coronary sinus
- **Color flow Doppler:** Shows an increased coronary sinus flow
- **On 2D TTE** examination will show an enlarged right atrium (RA)
- A relatively small and septated LA with a solid, thin echogenic membrane (indicating the LA diaphragm) separating the LA into two distinct chambers
- A larger (proximal) LA chamber in the superior aspect; and a small (distal) LA chamber in the inferior aspect.
- The distal LA chamber has a mitral valve (MV) apparatus and communicates with the left ventricle (LV).
- Although intraoperative 2D TEE findings correspond quite well with preoperative TTE findings, they do not provide the detailed information regarding the extent of the LA diaphragm and the shape of the diaphragmatic defect.
- Important information for understanding the intracardiac flow pattern of the systemic and pulmonary circulation cannot be provided by using 2D TEE alone. A 2D TTE is needed to confirm the identification of an ehcofree space behind the LA which is the common chamber, combined with echocardiographic evidence of RVDVO (Right ventricular, diastolic volume overload) which is strongly suggestive of TAPVC irrespective of the site of PA drainage.

- In a supracardiac type of total anomalous pulmonary venous connection (TAPVC), all the four pulmonary veins form a common chamber which drains into the SVC via the vertical vein. During surgery, this common chamber is anastomosed to the left atrium. On TEE (mid-esophageal four-chamber view) this anastomosis has to be assessed for any gradient.

POSTOPERATIVE TEE ASSESSMENT

- LA size (increase in LA size)
- LV with normal how across the mitral and aortic valve
- Increase in the transmitral flow velocities
- Excessive flow across coronary sinus abolished
- May be able to image one of the pulmonary veins into LA
- Biventricular function
- ASD patch for residual shunt.

3D TEE

- Additional real time 3D "en face" image and cropped images from the real time 3D volume images facilitate a complete understanding of the whole features of the complex anomalies of this case, shape and size of the diaphragm in a considerably easier and faster manner.
- 3D TEE shows that the RA dimension is much larger than the LA dimension with a thin membranous diaphragm traversing the whole LA to form a horizontal roof between the proximal and distal LA chambers.
- *The LA diaphragm does not have any holes*: The proximal LA chamber communicate with the RA through a small defect in the interatrial septal area, which allows the drainage of pulmonary venous blood from the proximal LA into the enlarged RA and thus contributed to the role of the RA as a mixing chamber for systemic, pulmonary, and coronary venous blood.
- The mixed blood in the RA then flows through the tricuspid valve to reach the right ventricle, as well as through a ASD to reach the distal LA chamber.
- The relatively small distal LA serves as a functional LA with a left atrial appendage and MV apparatus at the bottom.

3D TEE FOR SURGICAL TECHNIQUE

- Right atriotomy is performed through a median sternotomy after initiation of moderate hypothermic cardiopulmonary bypass. A self-retaining retractor is used to maximize the exposure of all intracardiac structures, including the LA diaphragm, atrioventricular valve apparatus, and coronary and pulmonary venous openings. After confirming the above determinations by surgical perspectives, the following procedures are performed; full resection of the LA diaphragm, tricuspid valve ring annuloplasty, removal of the diaphragmatic defect by constructing of a new interatrial septum using a bovine pericardial patch, and closure of the ASD.
- The newly constructed septum separates the pulmonary and systemic flow which drains into LA and RA, respectively.

CONCLUSION

In Indian circumstances, mortality continues to be high in infants with total anomalous pulmonary venous connection. Severe pulmonary arterial hypertension appears to be the most important predictor of operative mortality. Severe malnutrition, delayed diagnosis and late referrals possibly contribute to the high mortality.[9]

REFERENCES

1. Khanna S. Total anomalous pulmonary venous connection: post operative problems and management. Indian Anaest. 2009;53(1):71-4.
2. American Heart Association. Total anomalous pulmonary venous connection (TAPVC). American Heart, July 8, 2010.
3. TAPVC. European Association for Cardio-thoracic Surgery, 2007.
4. Tajik AJ, Gac GT, Schattenberg TT. Echocardiogram in total anomalous pulmonary venous drainage. Mayo Clin Proc. 1972;47:247.
5. Glaser J, Whitsia V, Liebman J. The differential diagnosis of total anomalous pulmonary venous drainage in infancy by echocardiography. Circulation. 1972;46 (Suppl II):11-38.
6. Meyer RA, Kaplan S. Noninvasive techniques in pediatric cardiovascular disease. Prog Cardiovasc Dis. 1973;15:341.
7. Godnian MJ, Thani P, Langfoid Kidd BS. Echocardiography in the evaluation of the cyanotic newborn infant. Br Heart J. 1974;36:154.
8. Paquet M, Gutgesell H, et al. Echocardiographic features of total anomalous pulmonary venous connection. Circulation. 1975;51:599-605.
9. Choudhary SK. Total-anomalous-pulmonary-venous-connection: surgical experience in Indians. Indian Heart J. 2001;53:754-60.

Chapter 19

TEE for Cor Triatriatum

Poonam Malhotra Kapoor, Neeti Makhija, Sarvesh Pal Singh

Chapter Outline

- Pathophysiology
- Embryological Origin
- Intraoperative TEE
- Congenital Cardiac Lesions Associated with CTS
- Differentiation between Supramitral Ring and Cor Triatriatum

DEFINITION

Cor triatriatum is a rare congenital anomaly, accounting for 0.1% of congenital heart disease. Classic cor triatriatum is characterized by a common pulmonary venous chamber separated from the true left atrium inferiorly by a fibromuscular membrane. The membrane is fenestrated to allow blood flow into the left atrium. The natural history of the defect is dependent on the size of the fenestration. If the opening is small, infants with this defect are critically ill and die at a young age. If the opening is larger, patients may present in childhood or young adulthood with a clinical picture similar to that of mitral stenosis.

PATHOPHYSIOLOGY

Triatrial heart is a rare congenital abnormality, reported by Jeiger at the autopsy, in 0.4% of patients with congenital heart disease,[1] and found in less than 0.1% of clinically diagnosed cardiopathies.[2] Though it was first described by Church in 1868, as a left atrium divided by an abnormal septum, the name "cor triatriatum" was given by Borst in 1905.[3] It involves usually the left atrium (cor triatriatum sinister) and rarely the right atrium (cor triatriatum dexter), in this chapter, we will be discussing cor triatriatum sinister (CTS).

The atrium is divided into two distinct chambers, usually by a thick fibromuscular septum, which could be membranous with transverse or horizontal orientation, band-like or funnel shaped **(Fig. 1)**. The proximal accessory pulmonary venous chamber or superior chamber drains the pulmonary venous blood while the distal inferior chamber (or true atrium) is in contiguity with the atrioventricular valve and contains the atrial appendage and the true atrial septum.

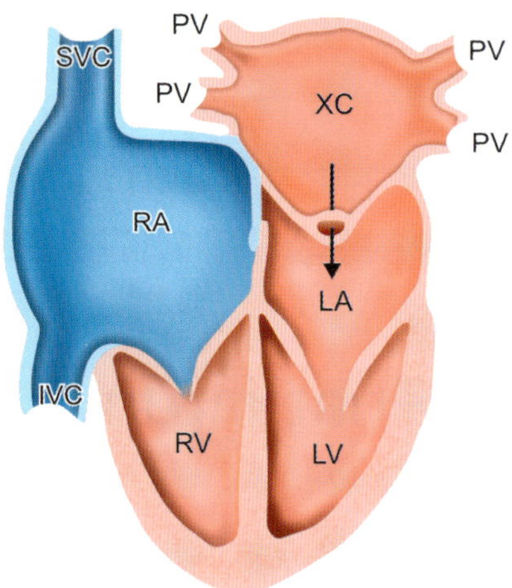

Figure 1 Diagrammatic anatomy of cor triatriatum

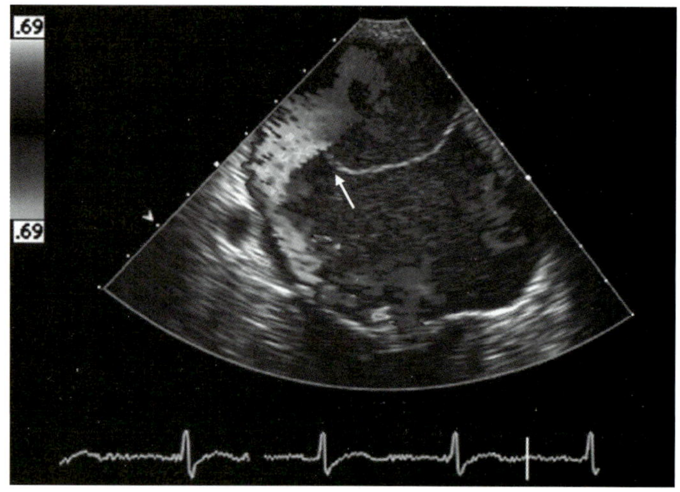

Figure 2 Transesophageal echocardiography showing an isolated membranous cor triatriatum with a single orifice (arrow) and mitral regurgitation

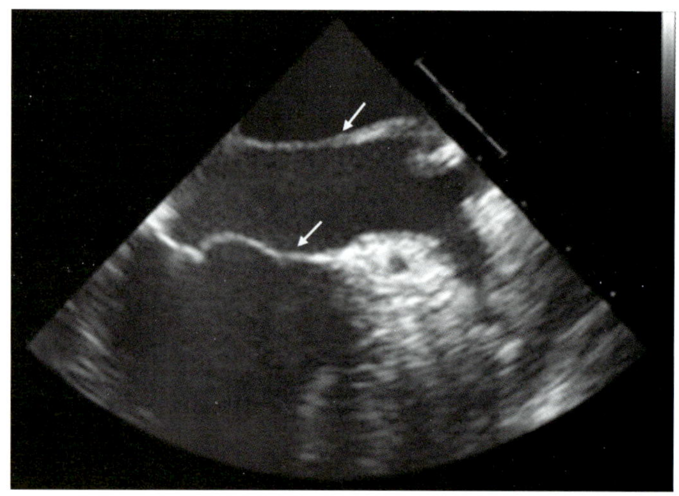

Figure 3 Still image of 2D TEE showing the membrane consistent with cor triatriatum, and its relationship to the left atrial appendage and the left upper pulmonary vein

EMBRYOLOGICAL ORIGIN

- **Malseptation:** The septum subdividing the left atrium is the result of an abnormal overgrowth of septum primum.
- **Entrapment:** The left horn of the sinus venosus entraps the common pulmonary vein and prevents its incorporation into the left atrium.
- **Malincorporation:** Incomplete incorporation of the common pulmonary vein into the left atrium.

INTRAOPERATIVE TEE (FIGS 2 AND 3)

Views for the evaluation of cor triatriatum:

- ME 4 chamber view
- ME 2 chamber view
- ME long axis view
- Transgastric long axis view.

Intraoperative TEE Assessment (Figs 4 and 5)

- Intra-atrial membrane dividing the LA into two parts and inserting into the Coumadin ridge proximal to the left atrial appendage (LAA) seen in multiple views
- Diastolic movement of the membrane towards the MV
- Color flow Doppler showing laminar or turbulent flow
- Pulse wave Doppler showing significant mean gradient >10–12 mm Hg. The grading should follow the same grading as for mitral stenosis.

Figure 3 shows 2D echo in midesophageal 4 chamber view showing a complete membrane in the left atrium with a central inflow into the lower part of left atrium. This central orifice creates a gradient between the upper and lower chambers in the left atrium.

There was almost no change in the mitral valve z-score over time, whereas the z-score for the pulmonary valve decreased to some extent. The aortic and tricuspid valve changes are most likely related to changes in flow and hemodynamics. This is further underlined by the drop in right ventricular pressure, which seems to plateau after five years.

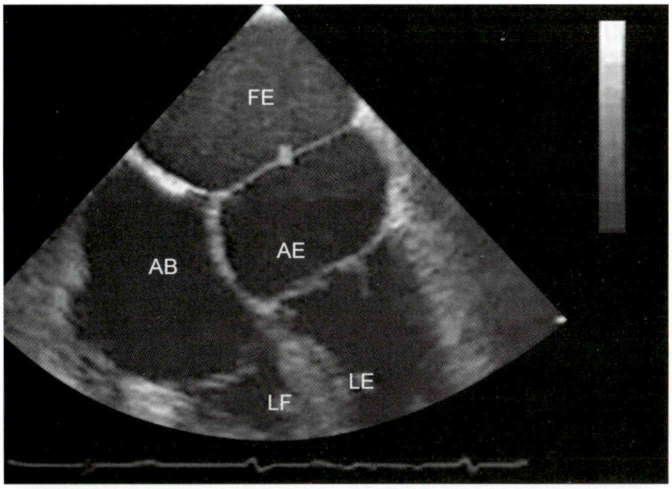

Figure 4 Intra-atrial membrane dividing the LA into two parts and inserting into the Coumadin ridge proximal to the LAA seen in multiple views

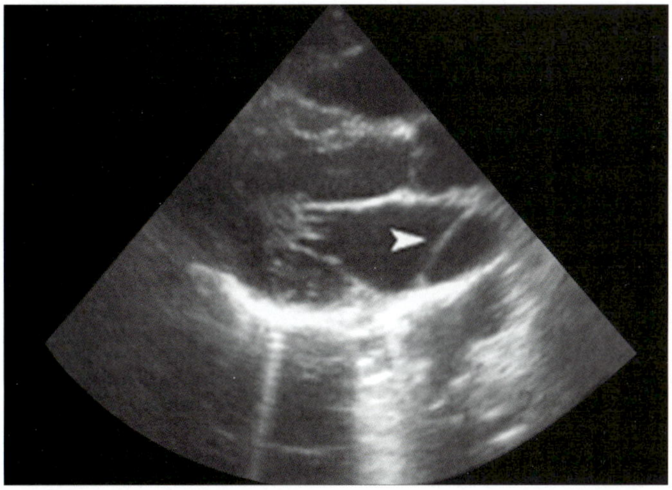

Figure 5 Cor triatriatum sinistrum dividing the left atrium into two components in parasternal long axis view

Spontaneous echo contrast can be seen in the upper part of left atrium due to distal obstruction. Postrepair there shall not be any gradient across the left atrium.

CONGENITAL CARDIAC LESIONS ASSOCIATED WITH CTS[4]

- Atrial septal defect
- Anomalous pulmonary venous return
- Tetralogy of Fallot
- Bicuspid aortic valve
- Double outlet right ventricule
- Coarctation of the aorta
- Persistant left superior vena cava with unroofed coronary sinus
- Ventricular septal defect
- Common atrioventricular canal
- Hypoplastic mitral valve
- Bicuspid right atrioventricular valve.
- Good early and long-term results for classic and atypical cor triatriatum.[5]

DIFFERENTIATION BETWEEN SUPRAMITRAL RING AND COR TRIATRIATUM (FIGS 6A AND B)

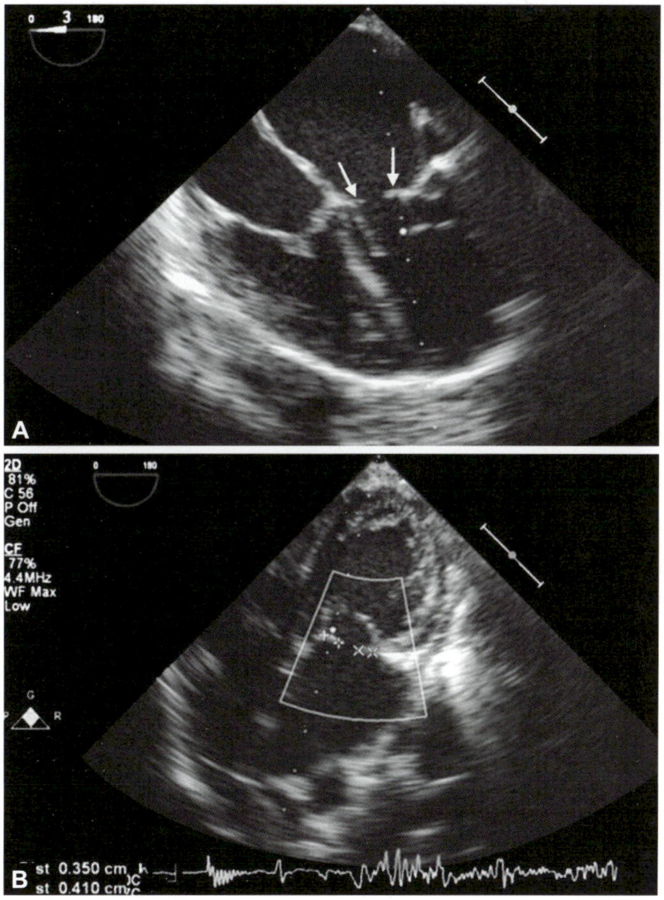

Figures 6A and B TEE view showing LA divided into two parts by the Intra-atrial membrane inserting into the Coumadin ridge proximal to the LA appendage

CHAPTER 19

REFERENCES

1. Jeiger W, Gibbons JE, Wiglesworth FW. Cor triatriatum: clinical, hemodynamic and pathological studies surgical correction in early life. Pediatrics. 1963;31:255-67 [PubMed: 14010411].
2. Talner CN. Report of the New England Regional Infant Cardiac Program, by Donald C Fyler. Pediatrics. 1998;102(1 pt 2):258-9 [PubMed: 9651450].
3. Borst H. Ein cor triatriatum. Zentralble Allg Pathol. 1905; 16:812-5.
4. Humpl T, Reineker K, Manlhiot C, Dipchand AI, Coles JG, McCrindle BW. Cor triatriatum sinistrum in childhood. A single institution's experience. Can J Cardiol. 2010; 26(7):371-6 [PubMed: 20847964].
5. Alphonso N, Nørgaard MA, Newcomb A, et al. Cor triatriatum: Presentation, diagnosis and long-term surgical results. Ann Thorac Surg. 2005;80:1666-71. [PubMed].

Chapter 20

TEE for Left Superior Vena Cava

Sarvesh Pal Singh, Poonam Malhotra Kapoor, Arindam Choudhury

Chapter Outline

- Pathophysiology
- Importance of LSVC to the Cardiac Surgeon
- Identification
- TEE for LSVC Diagnosis
- LSVC Presence in CHD

DEFINITION

The left superior vena cava (LSVC) is the anatomical variant that results when the left anterior cardinal vein fails to involute in embryologic development. The persistent left SVC can drain into the right atrium or coronary sinus, the left atrium, left pulmonary veins, or a deroofed coronary sinus. Sometimes both right and left venae cavae drain to the left atrium.[1] LSVC is associated with the presence of other congenital cardiac anomalies (e.g. ASD, VSD, cor triatriatum, mitral atresia).

PATHOPHYSIOLOGY

Persistent left superior vena cava (PLSVC) is the most common thoracic venous anomaly. Isolated persistence of the left superior vena cava (SVC) (Duplication of SVC) affects up to 0.5% of the population, but in patients with congenital cardiopathy it has a prevalence that ranges from 3% to 10%.[2,3] When present, it drains more commonly into the coronary sinus that might present varying degrees of dilation and in most cases leads to the diagnostic suspicion. Transesophageal echocardiography (TEE) shows the left SVC as a hypoechoic image between the left atrial appendage and the left superior pulmonary vein. In longitudinal views, left SVC is seen as a vascular structure anterior to the left atrium and draining into the coronary sinus.

Almost 40% of patients with LSVC can have a variety of associated cardiac anomalies, such as:

- Atrial septal defect
- Bicuspid aortic valve
- Coarctation of aorta
- Coronary sinus ostial atresia
- Cor triatriatum.
- Absence of the hepatic portion of the IVC

The presence of associated anomalies is more common with concomitant absence of right SVC the notation of which warrants appropriate investigation to rule out other anomalies. The PLSVC has been associated with anatomical and architectural abnormalities of the sinus node and conduction tissues (Mahaim fibers, Kent bundles) being noted ten times more frequently. Both sinus and AV node can have persistent fetal dispersion in the central fibrous body in subjects with PLSVC. AV node and His bundle dysfunction secondary to the dilation of the coronary sinus opening into which the entire SVC flow drains may occur. A systemic venous connection to the right atrium is associated with only an abnormality in the site of connection and is associated with little functional consequences. Varying degrees of systemic arterial desaturation can be seen in patients with SVC drainage to the left atrium secondary to right-to-left shunting as one-third of venous return occurs through the SVC.

IMPORTANCE OF LSVC TO THE CARDIAC SURGEON

- Bilateral bidirectional Glenn shunt
- During a left BT shunt will come in the way
- Transvenous pacing from the left side will be impossible
- Cannulation/occlusion during CPB
- Cannot give retrograde cardioplegia
- Difficult for robotic cardiac surgery
- Incidence higher with single ventricle physiology, atrioventricular canal, tricuspid atresia, and tetralogy of Fallot.

IDENTIFICATION

- Color flow Doppler will show left superior vena cava as a distinct entity with blood flow velocity (color difference) different form than in the left atrial appendage and left superior pulmonary vein.
- Continuous wave Doppler may be used to measure velocity in the left superior pulmonary vein and left superior vena cava. The left superior pulmonary vein will have higher velocity (45–80 cm/s).
- Saline contrast can be injected from a peripheral vein in the left hand and the contrast seen emerging from the left superior vena cava.

TEE FOR LSVC DIAGNOSIS (FIGS 1 TO 6)

- Choose the TEE view that permits the best vantage point to simultaneously assess the SVC and coronary sinus

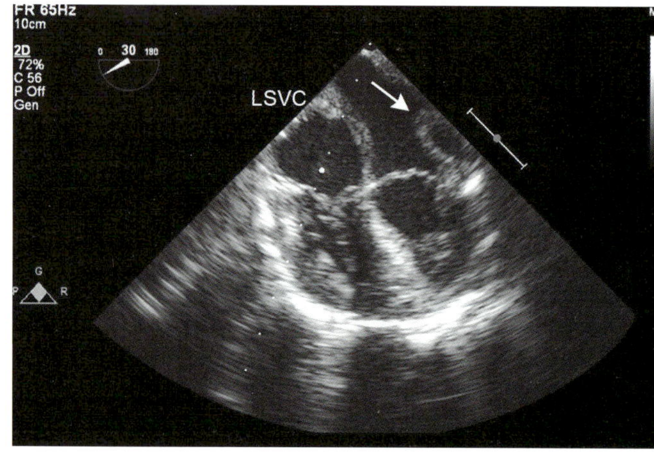

Figure 1 2D echo in midesophageal four chamber view showing a distinct vessel near the lateral annulus of mitral valve. Left superior vena cava is seen (arrow) and should always be ruled out by the echocardiographer preoperatively

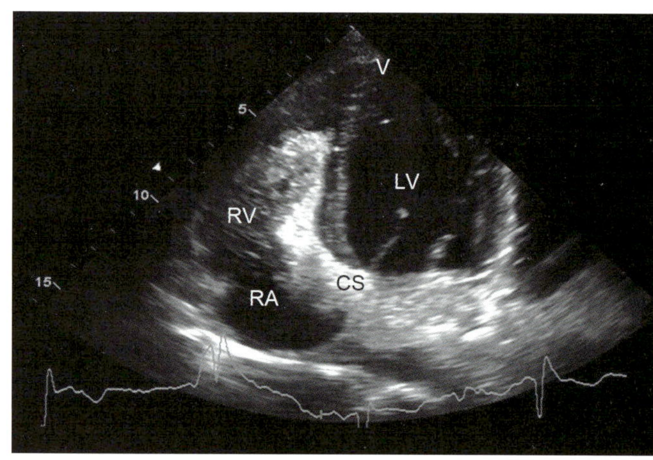

Figure 2 Concomitant persistent left superior vena on transthoracic ECHO

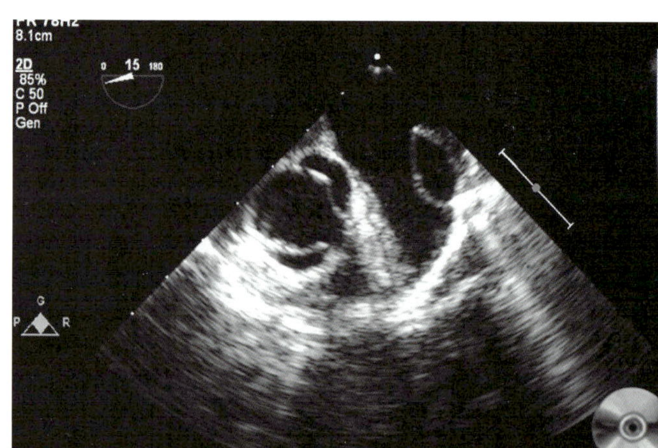

Figure 3 (Video 1) 2D echo in midesophageal modified aortic valve short axis view (probe rotated to left) showing left superior vena cava as a distinct entity near the left atrial appendage

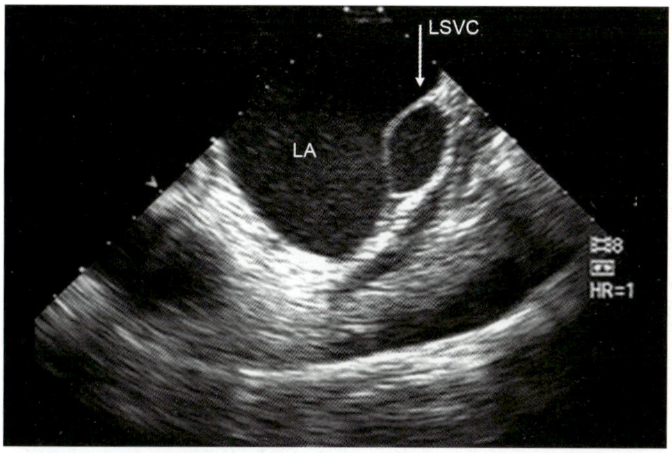

Figure 4 LSVC in TEE of 3 cm^2 size

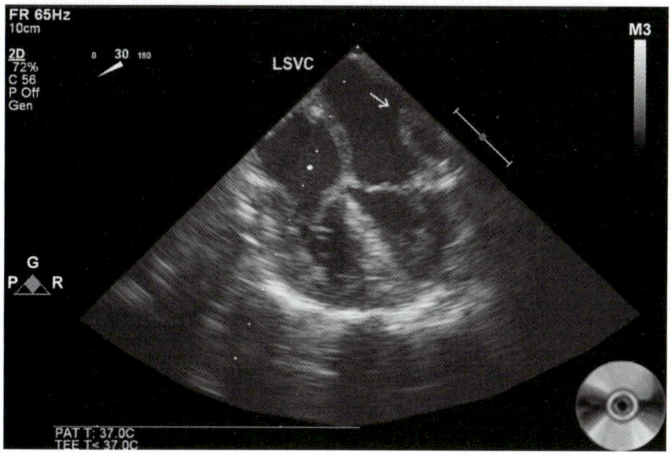

Figure 5 (Video 2) 2D echo in midesophageal 4 chamber view showing a distinct vessel near the lateral annulus of mitral valve. Left superior vena cava is seen (arrow)

- Inject your 10 mL of contrast medium and flush it in while the intraoperative sonographer waits at the ready to capture the image
- If contrast exits the SVC first then a LSVC is less likely (i.e. it could still be present but emptying into the left atrium or the left upper pulmonary vein)
- If contrast exits the dilated coronary sinus first then a LSVC is likely

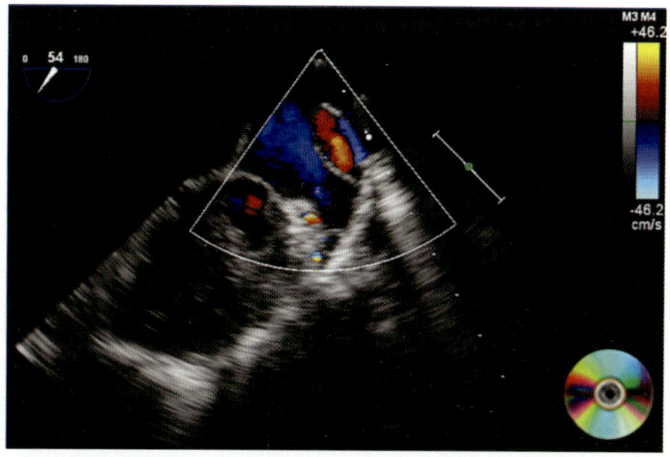

Figure 6 (Video 3) Color Doppler in midesophageal modified aortic valve short axis view (probe rotated to left) showing blood flow in left superior vena cava near the left atrial appendage

- If contrast exists both the SVC and the coronary sinus simultaneously then a LSVC is likely in the setting of an intact innominate vein.

The role of noninvasive diagnosis of PLSVC has been recently reviewed. Echographic finding of dilated CS is suggestive of PLSVC, and when associated with a right sided SVC, dilatation is maximal, in the range of 30 mm diameter and 3 cm^2 area (as in the present case) vs 20 mm and 1,8 cm^2 area in the patients with both venae cavae as normal. Further, intravenous agitated saline injected in left antecubital vein visualizing dilated coronary sinus draining into right atrium provides a rapid demonstration of the presence of PLSVC, and the same is true for right antecubital vein injection to demonstrate ARSVC.

LSVC PRESENCE IN CHD

Persistent LSVC is an anomaly of the systemic venous system that has been described to occur in 0.3–0.5% of the general population. In patients with congenital heart disease, the incidence increases to 4.3% when present; it usually drains via the coronary sinus into the right atrium. It has also been described as draining into both the left atrium and pulmonary veins. When large, they

Persistent LSVC is an anomaly of the systemic venous system that has been described to occur in 0.3–0.5% of the general population. In patients with congenital heart disease, the incidence increases to 4.3% when present; it usually drains via the coronary sinus into the right atrium. It has also been described as draining into both the left atrium and pulmonary veins.

can cause systemic desaturation. They can also serve as a pathway for paradoxical embolism that can occur secondary to right-to-left shunting. This is air embolism after injection of flush solution through the peripheral intravenous line can be diagnosed. An air embolus could have coursed through the persistent left superior vena cava into the patient's left upper pulmonary vein and left atrium, subsequently causing a TIA.

The TEE demonstrates the presence of micro bubbles in the left atrium. Careful and complete evaluation of all four pulmonary veins demonstrate micro bubbles coursing through the left upper pulmonary vein into the left atrium. While it is certainly serendipitous that the bubble study was performed through a left arm peripheral IV line, it certainly is possible to miss the diagnosis of persistent LSVC-to-left upper pulmonary vein if the bubble study had been performed through a right arm peripheral IV line. Based on the information it is recommend that saline bubble injection be performed through both a right arm and left arm peripheral IV line so as not to miss anomalous systemic-to-pulmonary venous communications, which can serve as pathways for both air and thromboembolism. Once the diagnosis of possible anomalous systemic-to-pulmonary venous anomaly is suspected, these patients will need to undergo cardiac catheterization to better delineate their systemic and pulmonary venous anatomy.[4]

REFERENCES

1. Goor DA, Lillehei LW. Congenital malformations of the heart. New York: Grune and Stratton; 1975.pp.400-4.
2. Winter FS. Persistent left superior vena cava, survey of world literature and report of thirty additional cases. Angiology 1954;5:90-132.
3. James T, Marshall T. XVIII. Persistent fetal dispersion of the atrioventricular node and His bundle within the central fibrous body. Circulation 1976;53(6):1026-34.
4. Rare Case of Persistent Left Superior Vena Cava to Left Upper Pulmonary Vein: Pathway for Paradoxical Embolization and Develop. Volume 19 - Issue 10 - October, 2007.

Chapter 21

TEE for Pulmonary Artery Hypertension

Poonam Malhotra Kapoor, Minati Choudhury, SN Das, Sarvesh Pal Singh

Chapter Outline

- Causes of Pulmonary Artery Hypertension
- Chest X-ray Features of PAH
- Echocardiographic Features in Pulmonary Arterial Hypertension
- Preoperative 2D TEE Assessment
- Evaluation with Color Flow Doppler

INTRODUCTION

Pulmonary arterial hypertension (PAH) is a rare and serious disease, characterized by increased pulmonary vascular resistance leading to right heart failure and death. PAH is defined as mean pulmonary artery pressure (PAP), 25 mm Hg at rest (measured during heart catheterization).[1]

Echocardiography should be an investigation of choice for both screening and management of this disease, because of its reliability, harmlessness, and ability to reveal echocardiographic parameters that are predictive of mortality. Although several authors have drawn attention to the key role of echocardiography in the management of PAH,[2,3] its present role is still a restricted one.

To date, five echocardiographic parameters have been described in the literature as associated with mortality in PAH—degree of pericardial effusion,[4-6] right atrial area indexed to body surface area,[6] end-diastolic eccentricity index,[6] right ventricular (RV) Tei index,[7] and tricuspid annular plane systolic excursion (TAPSE).[8] Other clinical, biological, hemodynamic, and MRI parameters have also been described.[9-14] Although numerous treatments have been introduced with subtle improvements in echocardiographic parameters,[15,16] the prognosis of the disease remains somber. The clinician needs objective parameters to detect worsening of the patient's condition as early as possible and initiate optimal treatment.

In this study, we sought to identify new echocardiographic prognostic factors for mortality and so to define the place of echocardiography in the management of patients with PAH.

CAUSES OF PULMONARY ARTERY HYPERTENSION

- L → R shunt
- Pulmonary embolism
- Cor pulmonale
- Mitral stenosis
- Idiopathic pulmonary artery hypertension.

CHEST X-RAY FEATURES OF PAH (FIGS 1A AND B)

- Enlarged, well-defined hilar vessels arise from hilum with or without calcification.
- Rapid tapering of vessels. The lower lobe vessels are larger than the upper lobe vessels. There is a rapid decrease in the size of the peripheral vessels from which they come (pruning).
- Very few peripheral vascular markings
- No effusions or Kerley lines, i.e. no signs of LVF
- Cardiomegaly—RV and RA
- Prominent IVC and SVC
- CXR changes are late.

Precapillary PAH

It may be due to pre-existing left to right shunt going for Eisenmenger's syndrome like atrial septal defect, ventricular septal defect, patent ductus arteriosus and aortopulmonary window **(Figs 1C and D)**.

Sometimes precapillary PAH may result from primary pulmonary hypertension, acute or chronic cor pulmonale, or acute or chronic thromboembolic phenomenon.

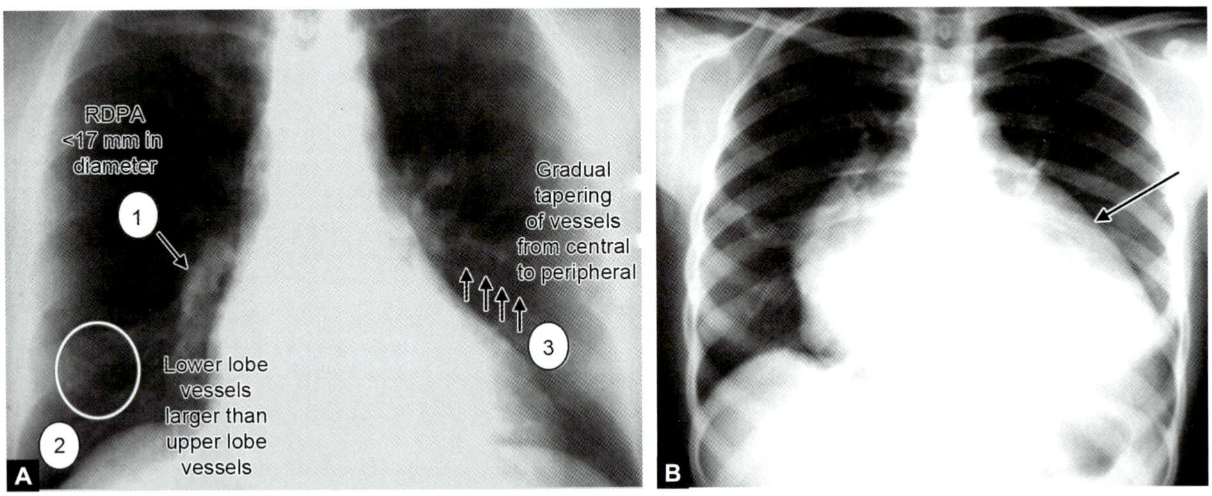

Figures 1A and B Chest X-ray of PAH with cardiomegaly and pruning. (A) 1–RDPA<17 mm in diameter; 2—Lower lobe vessels larger than upper lobe vessels; 3—Gradual tapering of vessels from central to peripheral

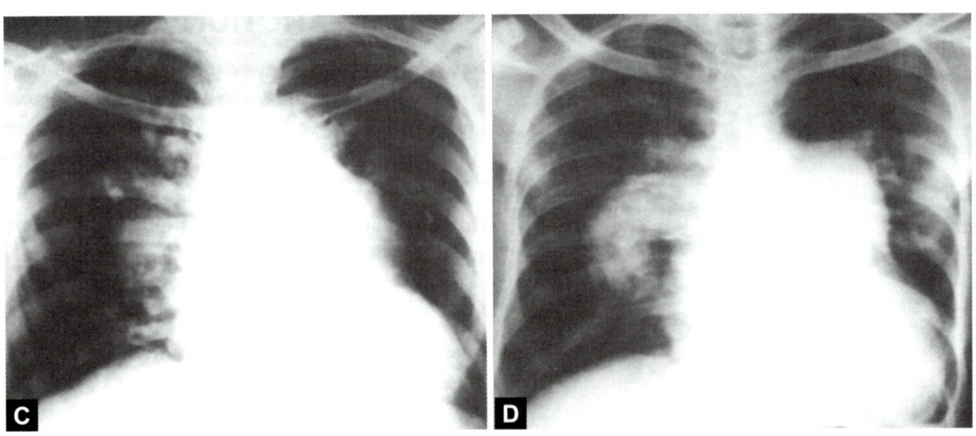

Figures 1C and D Precapillary pulmonary hypertension. (C) shows X-ray of a patient with patent ductus arteriosus. (D) shows X-ray of a patient with atrial septal defect

Dominant Right Ventricle with Pulmonary Hypertension

Eisenmenger's atrial septal defect, ventricular septal defect, patent ductus arteriosus and aortopulmonary window **(Figs 2 and 3)**.

All features of primary pulmonary hypertension will be present.

Eisenmenger's atrial septal defect (ASD): Right pulmonary artery will be more prominent than left pulmonary artery. Small left ventricle and ascending aorta.

Eisenmenger's ventricular septal defect (VSD): Both pulmonary arteries are equally prominent with left ventricular enlargement and small aorta.

Eisenmenger's patent ductus arteriosus (PDA) and aortopulmonary (AP) window: Both pulmonary arteries are prominent with left ventricular enlargement and prominent ascending aorta.

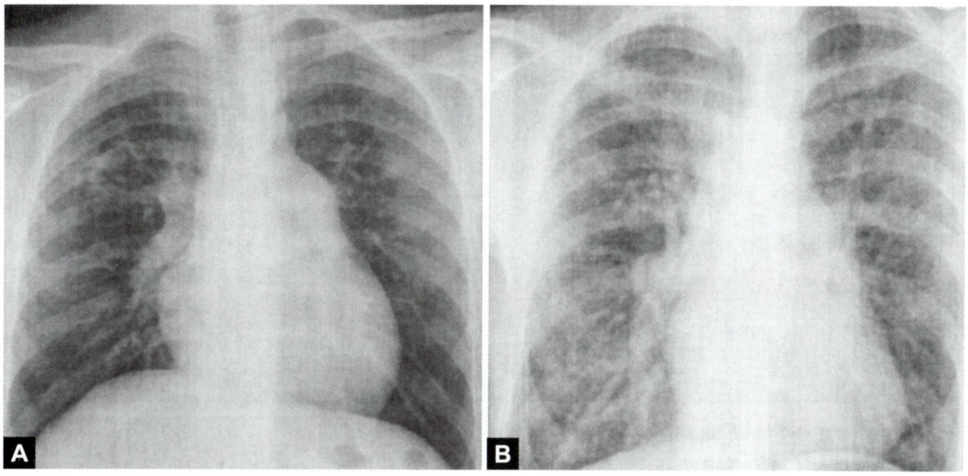

Figures 2A and B Chest films of different patients with Eisenmenger's complex and PAH

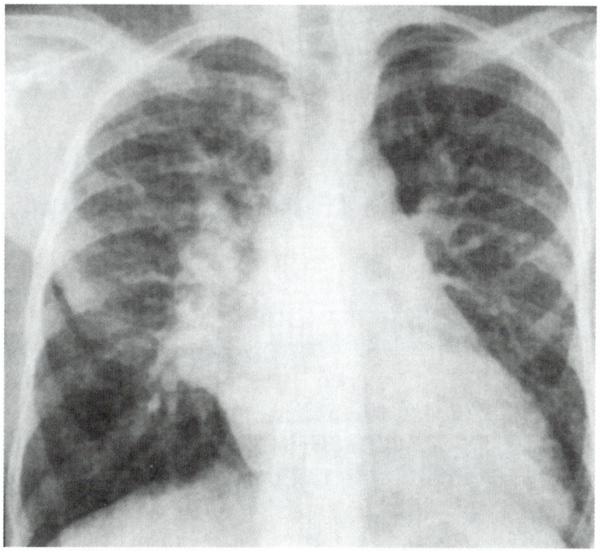

Figure 3 Chest film of a patient with patent ductus arteriosus with severe pulmonary hypertension

ECHOCARDIOGRAPHIC FEATURES IN PULMONARY ARTERIAL HYPERTENSION

Figures 4A to D and **Table 1** describe echocardiographic features in PAH. Because of chronic RV pressure overload, at the time of diagnosis, most patients present with enlarged right-side chambers, RV hypertrophy, increased interventricular septal thickness, an abnormal interventricular septum/posterior left ventricular (LV) wall ratio (>1), and reduced global RV systolic function. Furthermore, the abnormal pressure gradient between the left and right ventricles results in shape distortion and motion of the interventricular septum (''flattening''), which persists throughout the cardiac cycle.[17] As a consequence, the left ventricle appears D-shaped, with reduced diastolic and systolic volumes but preserved global systolic function.[18] Pericardial effusion and mitral valve prolapse have also been described in patients with PAH; the former may be a manifestation of impaired venous and lymphatic drainage secondary to elevated RAP, and the latter is related to a small left ventricle and the possible involvement of valve leaflets affected by associated connective tissue disorders.[19]

At the time of definitive diagnosis, most patients with PAH show at least moderate TR, with SPAP more than 60 mm Hg. TR is usually caused by tricuspid annular dilation, altered RV geometry, and apical displacement of the tricuspid leaflets. The degree of TR cannot be used as a surrogate for the degree of PAP elevation.[20] Significant pulmonic valvular regurgitation is common in PAH.

Pulsed-wave Doppler interrogation of the RV outflow tract usually reveals an acceleration time of <100 msec, which reflects abnormal MPAP.[21] Finally, as a result of altered RV-LV interaction, LV diastolic dysfunction may be characterized by a marked dependence of LV filling on atrial contraction.[22,23]

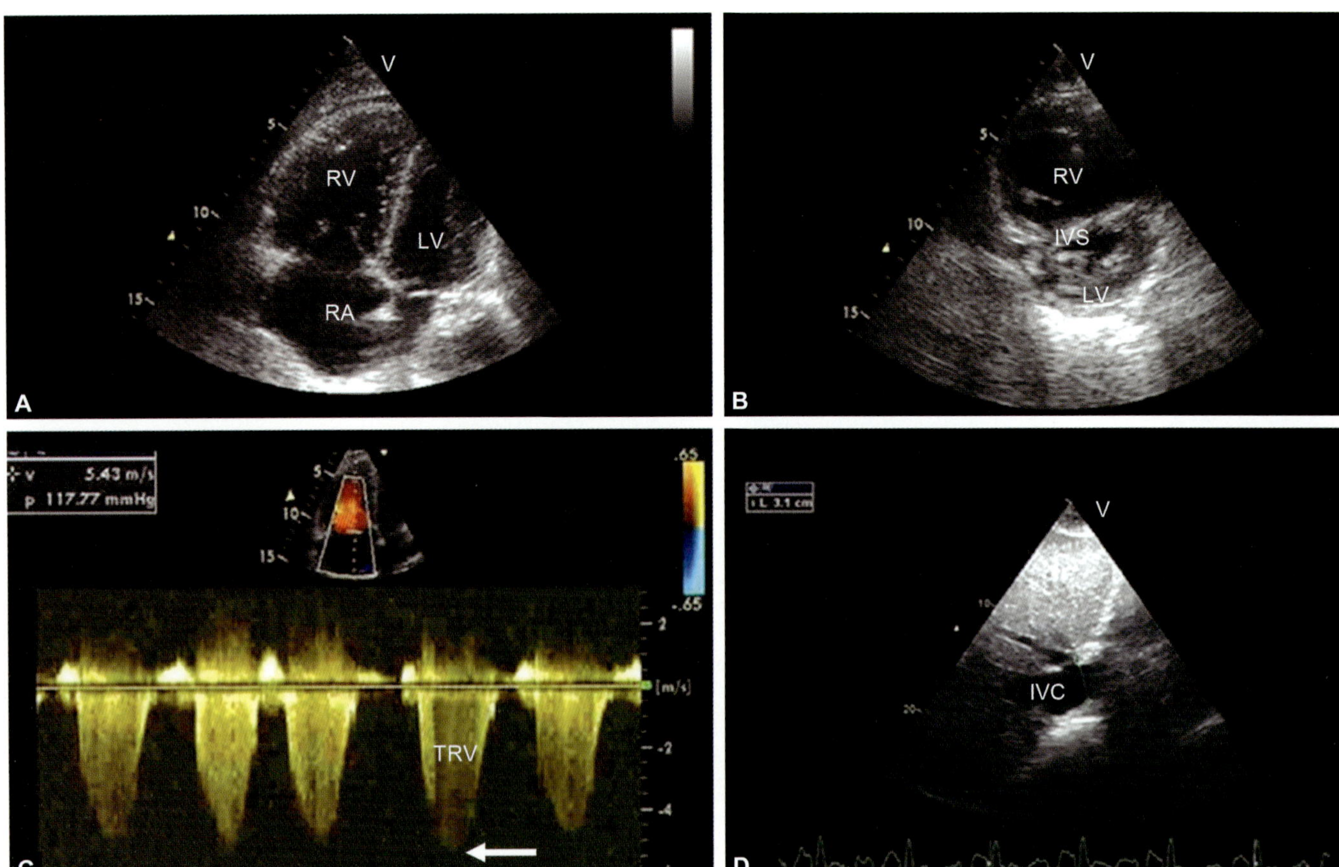

Figures 4A to D A young patient with IPAH. (A and B) Apical four-chamber and parasternal short-axis views, showing severe right ventricular enlargement and dislocation of the interventricular septum (IVS) towards the left ventricle (LV); (C) Doppler tracing of TR, showing severe PH (TRV >5 m/sec) (arrow); (D) Dilated inferior vena cava (IVC) from the subcostal view. *Abbreviations:* RA, right atrium; RV, right ventricle

PREOPERATIVE 2D TEE ASSESSMENT

- Two-dimensional (2D) echocardiography shows features of long standing RV pressure overload. Most patients present with enlarged right-side chambers, RV hypertrophy, increased interventricular septal thickness and, an abnormal interventricular septum/posterior LV wall ratio (>1), IVC diameter >20 mm, enlarged main pulmonary artery trunk and reduced global RV systolic function.
- The abnormal pressure gradient between the left and right ventricles results in shape distortion and motion of the interventricular septum ("flattening"), which persists throughout the cardiac cycle.
- The left ventricle thus appears D-shaped, with reduced diastolic and systolic volumes but preserved global systolic function. Small pericardial effusion may be seen secondary to impaired venous and lymphatic drainage due to elevated RAP.
- LV diastolic dysfunction may occur due to altered RV-LV interaction be characterized by a marked dependence of LV filling on atrial contraction.

EVALUATION WITH COLOR FLOW DOPPLER (TABLE 1)

- Significant tricuspid and pulmonary valve regurgitation commonly seen in pulmonary artery hypertension.

TABLE 1 Doppler echocardiographic indices for the evaluation of patients with clinical suspicion of PH

Key indices (cut-off)	*Additional indices (cut-off)*	*Complementary indices (cut-off)*
Pulmonary hemodynamics $SPAP = 4 \times TRV^2 + RAP$[9-12] (TRV > 2.8–2.9 msec: SPAP 36 mm Hg)	$MPAP = TVI_{TR} + RAP$[13] (≥ 25 mm Hg)	AT_{RVOT} (<100 msec $\log_{10}(EPSPAP) = -0.004\,(PAAT) + 2.1$[15]
RAP = IVC size and collapsibility[16] (>2.1 cm, collapse <50%: RAP 15 mm Hg)		RV IVRT' (by DTI; > 65 msec: SPAP > 40 mm Hg; <59 msec: RAP > 8 mm Hg)
$MPAP = 4 \times PRV^2 + RAP$[17,18] (≥ 25 mm Hg)	$MPAP = 0.61 \times SPAP + 2$ mm Hg[19]	$MPAP = 90 - 0.62 \times AT_{RVOT}$[20] $MPAP = 79 - 0.45 \times AT_{RVOT}$
$DPAP = 4 \times (PRV\ ED)^2 + RAP$		
$PVR = TRV/TVI_{RVOT}\,(cm) \times 10 + 0.16$[21] (>0.2: PVR > 2 WU; <0.15: normal PVR)	$PVR = SPAP/(HR \times TVI_{RVOT})$[22] (>0.076: indexed PVR > 15 RU)	FVE_{RVOT}[23] = (midsystolic "notch")
$PCWP = 1.9 + 1.24 \times E/E$ (E/E' >15: PCWP > 15 mm Hg)	LAVi (>31 mL/m^2)	
Impaired RV systolic function		
TAPSE (<16 mm)	Tei index: (IVRT + IVCT)/ET (>0.40 by PW Doppler; >0.55 by DTI	
RV FAC (<35%)		
S'-wave velocity by DTI (<10 cm/sec)		

Guidelines for PAH

- The European Society of Cardiology guidelines for the diagnosis and treatment of PAH suggest considering
- Pulmonary hypertension (PH) unlikely for TRV < 2.8 m/sec, SPAP <36 mm Hg (assuming RAP of 5 mm Hg), and no additional echocardiographic signs of PH.
- PH possible for TRV 2.8 m/sec and SPAP 36 mm Hg but the presence of additional echocardiographic signs of PH or TRV of 2.9 to 3.4 m/sec and SPAP of 37 to 50 mm Hg with or without additional signs of PH.
- PH likely for TRV > 3.4 m/sec and SPAP > 50 mm Hg with or without additional signs of PH.

- TR seen is usually caused by tricuspid annular dilation, altered RV geometry, and apical displacement of the tricuspid leaflets.
- The degree of TR however cannot be used as a surrogate for the degree of PAP elevation.
- Pulsed-wave Doppler interrogation of the RV outflow tract usually reveals an acceleration time of <100 msec, which reflects abnormal MPAP.
- Peak early diastolic and the end-diastolic velocities of pulmonary regurgitation correlate with mean PAP (PAPm) and pulmonary artery end-diastolic pressure (PEDP)

$$PAPm = 79\text{-}0.45\ (RVOT\ AT)$$

$$PAPm = 4 \times (\text{peak pulmonary regurgitation velocity})^2$$

$$PEDP = 4 \times (\text{pulmonary regurgitation end-diastolic velocity})^2 + \text{right atrial pressure}$$

- Tricuspid regurgitation jet velocity (TRV) is used in daily practice to determine RV systolic pressure (RVSP), which is considered equal to systolic PAP (SPAP) in the absence of pulmonary outflow tract obstruction and/or pulmonic valve stenosis. This is done by calculating the systolic trans tricuspid gradient using the modified Bernoulli equation. The peak pressure gradient of tricuspid regurgitation = 4 × (tricuspid regurgitation velocity)^2

  RVSP = Tricuspid regurgitation pressure gradient + estimated right atrial pressure

- As velocity measurements are angle dependent, TRV should be taken from multiple views searching for the best envelope and maximal velocity. Additionally, the use of color flow Doppler is recommended to obtain the best alignment between regurgitant flow and the Doppler signal.

Estimation of PVR

Pulmonary vascular resistance may be estimated by dividing TR peak velocity (in meters per second) by the time-velocity integral of the RV outflow tract (in centimeters) (*See* **Table 1** for values).

CONCLUSION

Echocardiography is an essential component of the diagnostic algorithm of PAH insofar as it makes it possible to confirm the diagnosis. It may also help to exclude PH related to congenital systemic to pulmonary shunts or secondary to pulmonary venous hypertension, thromboembolic disease or obstructed pulmonary vessels, predict the prognosis, monitor the efficacy of specific therapeutic interventions, and detect the preclinical stage of the disease.

REFERENCES

1. Galie N, Hoeper MM, Humbert M, Torbicki A, Vachiery JL, Barbera JA, et al. Guidelines for the diagnosis and treatment of pulmonary hypertension: The Task Force for the Diagnosis and Treatment of Pulmonary Hypertension of the European Society of Cardiology (ESC) and the European Respiratory Society (ERS), endorsed by the International Society of Heart and Lung Transplantation (ISHLT). Eur Heart J. 2009;30:2493-537.
2. Bossone E, Bodini BD, Mazza A, Allegra L. Pulmonary arterial hypertension: the key role of echocardiography. Chest. 2005;127:1836-43.
3. Bossone E, Citro R, Blasi F. Echocardiography in pulmonary arterial hypertension: an essential tool. Chest. 2007;131:339-41.
4. Eysmann SB, Palevsky HI, Reichek N, et al. Two-dimensional and Doppler-echocardiographic and cardiac catheterization correlates of survival in primary pulmonary hypertension. Circulation. 1989;80:353-60.
5. Hinderliter AL, Willis PWt, Long W, Clarke WR, Ralph D, Caldwell EJ, et al. Frequency and prognostic significance of pericardial effusion in primary pulmonary hypertension. PPH Study Group. Primary pulmonary hypertension. Am J Cardiol. 1999;84:481-4, A410.
6. Raymond RJ, Hinderliter AL, Willis PW, Ralph D, Caldwell EJ, Williams W, et al. Echocardiographic predictors of adverse outcomes in primary pulmonary hypertension. J Am Coll Cardiol. 2002;39:1214-9.
7. Yeo TC, Dujardin KS, Tei C, Mahoney DW, McGoon MD, Seward JB. Value of a Doppler-derived index combining systolic and diastolic time intervals in predicting outcome in primary pulmonary hypertension. Am J Cardiol. 1998;81:1157-61.
8. Forfia PR, Fisher MR, Mathai SC, Housten-Harris T, Hemnes AR, Borlaug BA, et al. Tricuspid annular displacement predicts survival in pulmonary hypertension. Am J Respir Crit Care Med. 2006;174:1034-41.
9. McLaughlin VV, Presberg KW, Doyle RL, Abman SH, McCrory DC, Fortin T, et al. Prognosis of pulmonary arterial hypertension: ACCP Evidence-based Clinical Practice Guidelines. Chest. 2004;126:78S-92S.
10. McLaughlin VV, Shillington A, Rich S. Survival in primary pulmonary hypertension: the impact of epoprostenol therapy. Circulation. 2002;106:1477-82.
11. Miyamoto S, Nagaya N, Satoh T, Kyotani S, Sakamaki F, Fujita M, et al. Clinical correlates and prognostic

significance of six-minute walk test in patients with primary pulmonary hypertension. Comparison with cardiopulmonary exercise testing. Am J Respir Crit Care Med. 2000;161:487-92.
12. Paciocco G, Martinez FJ, Bossone E, Pielsticker E, Gillespie B, Rubenfire M. Oxygen desaturation on the six-minute walk test and mortality in untreated primary pulmonary hypertension. Eur Respir J. 2001;17:647-52.
13. Wensel R, Opitz CF, Anker SD, Winkler J, Hoffken G, Kleber FX, et al. Assessment of survival in patients with primary pulmonary hypertension: importance of cardiopulmonary exercise testing. Circulation. 2002;106: 319-24.
14. Van Wolferen SA, Marcus JT, Boonstra A, Marques KM, Bronzwaer JG, Spreeuwenberg MD, et al. Prognostic value of right ventricular mass, volume, and function in idiopathic pulmonary arterial hypertension. Eur Heart J. 2007;28:1250-7.
15. Hinderliter AL, Willis PWt, Barst RJ, Rich S, Rubin LJ, Badesch DB, et al. Effects of long-term infusion of prostacyclin (epoprostenol) on echocardiographic measures of right ventricular structure and function in primary pulmonary hypertension. Primary Pulmonary Hypertension Study Group. Circulation. 1997;95:1479-86.
16. Galie N, Hinderliter AL, Torbicki A, Fourme T, Simonneau G, Pulido T, et al. Effects of the oral endothelin-receptor antagonist bosentan on echocardiographic and Doppler measures in patients with pulmonary arterial hypertension. J Am Coll Cardiol. 2003;41:1380-6.
17. Armstrong WF, Ryan T. Feigenbaum's Echocardiography, 7th edn. Philadelphia, PA: Lippincott Williams and Wilkins; 2009.
18. Oh JK, Seward JB, Tajik AJ. The Echo Manual, 2nd edn. Philadelphia: Lippincott Williams and Wilkins; 1999. p. 222.
19. Hinderliter AL, Willis PW IV, Long W, Clarke WR, Ralph D, Caldwell EJ, et al. PPH Study Group. Frequency and prognostic significance of pericardial effusion in primary pulmonary hypertension. Am J Cardiol. 1999; 84:481-4.
20. Hinderliter AL, Willis PV IV, Long WA, Clarke WR, Ralph D, Caldwell EJ, et al. PPH Study Group. Frequency and severity of tricuspid regurgitation determined by Doppler echocardiography in primary pulmonary hypertension. Am J Cardiol. 2003;91:1033-7.
21. Dabestani A, Mahan G, Gardin JM, Takenaka K, Burn C, Allfie A, et al. Evaluation of pulmonary artery pressure and resistance by pulsed Doppler echocardiography. Am J Cardiol. 1987;59:662-8.
22. Louie EK, Rich S, Brundage BH. Doppler echocardiographic assessment of impaired left ventricular filling in patients with right ventricular pressure overload due to primary pulmonary hypertension. J Am Coll Cardiol. 1986;8:1298-306.
23. Stojnic BB, Brecker SJ, Xiao HB, Helmy SM, Mbaissouroum M, Gibson DG. Left ventricular filling characteristics in pulmonary hypertension: a new mode of ventricular interaction. Br Heart J. 1992;68:16-20.

Chapter 22

TEE for Eisenmenger's Syndrome

Poonam Malhotra Kapoor, Sameer Taneja

Chapter Outline

INTRODUCTION

Eisenmenger's syndrome is defined as severe pulmonary arterial hypertension (PAH) in conjunction with congenital heart disease and reversal of shunt with ensuing cyanosis.[1] Eisenmenger's syndrome frequently occurs in patients with large, nonrestrictive intracardiac or extracardiac communications, including atrial septal defects, ventricular septal defects, atrioventricular septal defects, and patent ductus arteriosus (PDA). It has been suggested that up to 10% of patients with congenital heart disease may develop Eisenmenger's syndrome,[2] although this may reflect a different era of late diagnosis and suboptimal care.[3,4] Advanced therapies targeting PAH have been shown to improve hemodynamics, symptoms, quality of life, and possibly survival in patients with Eisenmenger's syndrome.[5,6] The timing of initiation of such therapies in Eisenmenger's patients remains controversial but is based primarily on subjective assessment of disease severity and progression of symptoms.

PATHOPHYSIOLOGY OF EISENMENGER'S SYNDROME

Eisenmenger's syndrome is described as a chronic, uncorrected right to left shunt, right ventricular hypertrophy (RVH), elevated pulmonary artery pressure, and right ventricular dysfunction. The primary lesion may be an ASD, VSD or PDA **(Fig. 1)**. The pulmonary and the RV musculature undergoes remodeling in response to chronic pulmonary volume overload, the high fixed pulmonary artery pressure limits flow through

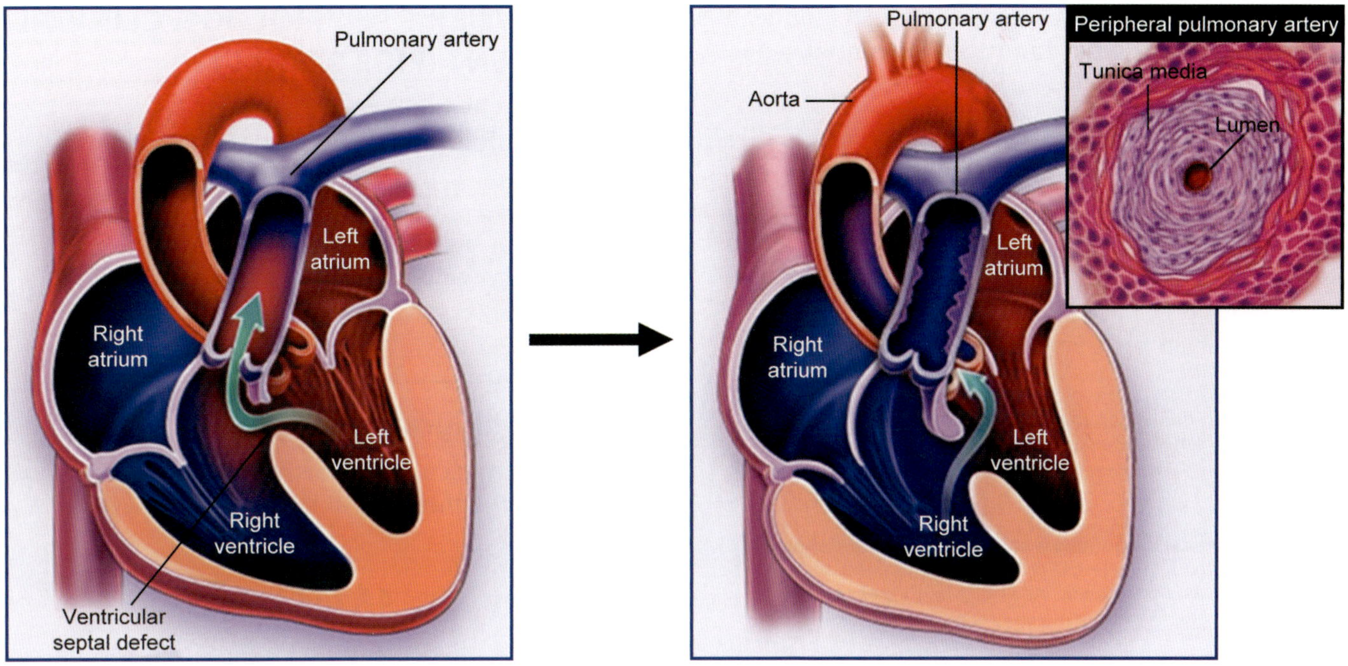

Figure 1 Eisenmenger's syndrome

the pulmonary vasculature and when pulmonary artery pressure exceeds the level of systemic pressure, reversal of shunt flow occurs. The initial left to right shunt becomes a right to left shunt, ultimately leading to the Eisenmenger's syndrome, which includes the sequelae of arterial hypoxemia, and RV failure. Clinical manifestations include dyspnea, clubbing of nails, polycythemia and peripheral edema and cyanosis. In an established case of Eisenmenger's syndrome, pulmonary hypertension when permanent, surgical correction of the defect at this stage is unhelpful and may increase mortality.

Examination in Eisenmenger's Syndrome

- Central cyanosis with digital clubbing
- May have differential cyanosis and clubbing
- Hypoxemia with resting oxygen saturation <90%
- Lungs are usually clear
- RV heave, palpable P2, right sided S4, and occasionally pulmonary ejection click
- Murmurs likely to be heard include a high-pitched diastolic decrescendo murmur of pulmonic insufficiency and a holosystolic murmur of TR
- Murmurs related to the defects connecting the systemic and pulmonary circulations are not usually heard.

Diagnostic testing: It should be done in all patients suspected of pulmonary artery hypertension to know that PAH exists or not and to identify its underlying causes.

- *Goals:*
  - For the diagnosis of heart defect
  - For evaluating the severity
  - For stratification, predictable prognostic factors? For surgery?

CLINICAL IMPLICATIONS

Cardiac physiology and chronic adaptation to long-standing advanced pulmonary vascular resistance with underlying congenital heart disease and cyanosis (Eisenmenger's syndrome) is strongly predictive of mortality in this adult population. Easily acquired and widely available echocardiographic indices, such as tricuspid annular plane systolic excursion (TAPSE), ratio of RV effective systolic to diastolic duration, RA area, and ratio of RA to LA area, are predictive of mortality, both independently and even more so in a composite score, and should therefore be incorporated routinely in the periodic assessment of Eisenmenger's patients. A more aggressive management approach could be encouraged for patients identified as high risk on the basis of these criteria, including advanced therapy, particularly because recent evidence has suggested that the latter improves functional capacity and possibly survival.

EISENMENGER'S SYNDROME: A PROGRESSIVE DISEASE

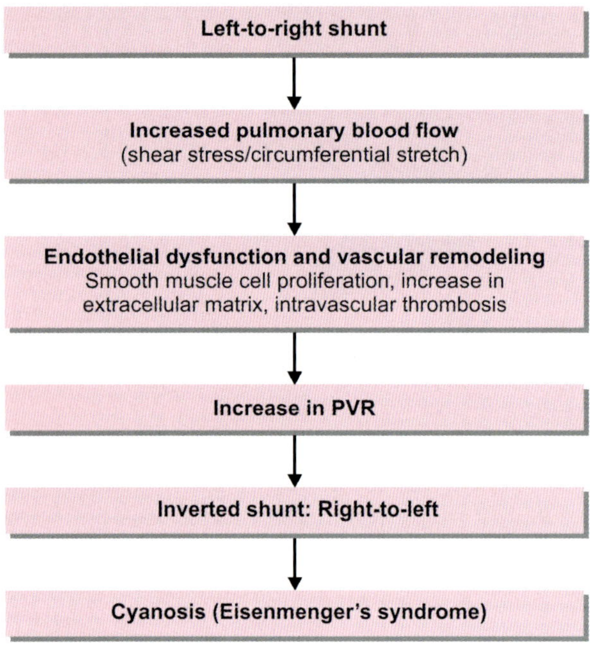

EISENMENGER'S PHYSIOLOGY: CLINICAL ASSESSMENT (FIGS 2A TO C)

- *Cyanosis:* Generally mild
- Absence of cardiomegaly, heart failure
- Minimal left parasternal lift
- Constant ejection click of PAH
- Absence of significant shunt murmurs
- Pulmonary regurgitation murmur may be audible.

CHOICES

Electrocardiography (Fig. 3)

RAE, right ventricular hypertrophy (RVH), right axis deviation, arrhythmia, nost-Twave changes.

Chest X-ray (Figs 4A to C)

Cardiomegaly, dilated pulmonary arteries, pulmonary artery calcification.

- Central pulmonary artery dilatation **(Fig. 4A)**
  - "Pruning" of the peripheral pulmonary vasculature **(Figs 4A and C)**
  - RA/RV dilatation **(Figs 4B and C)**
  - Other lung pathologies like oligemia of peripheral lung fields
  - Small aortic shadow.

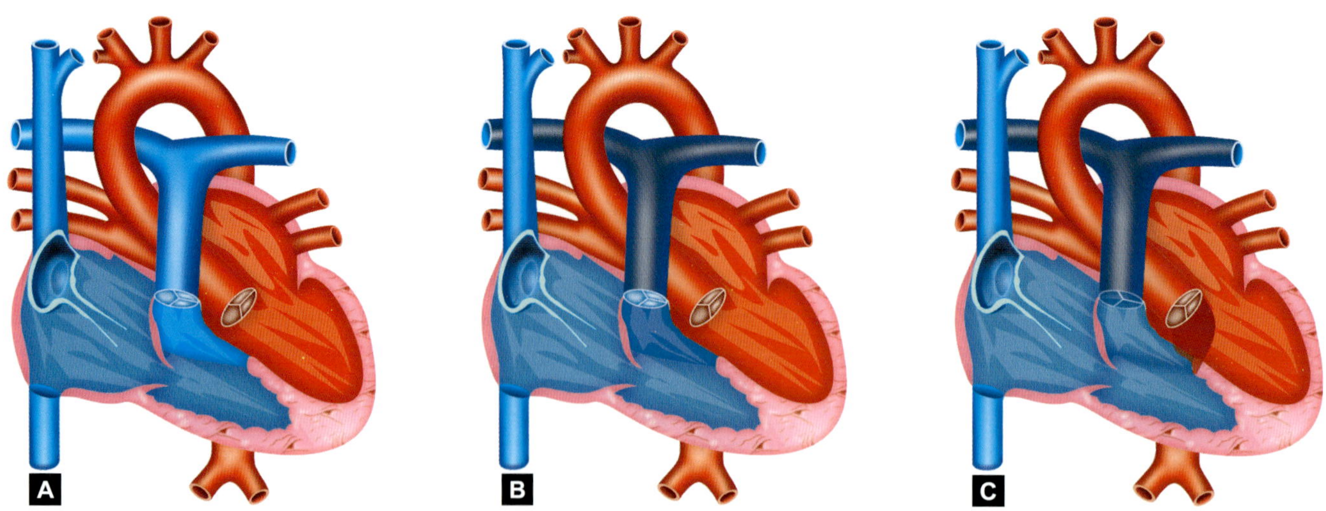

Figures 2A to C (A) Low pulmonary pressure left to right shunt increased pulmonary saturation; (B) Systemic pulmonary pressure small bidirectional shunt no saturation changes; (C) Suprasystemic pulmonary pressure, right to left shunt cyanosis

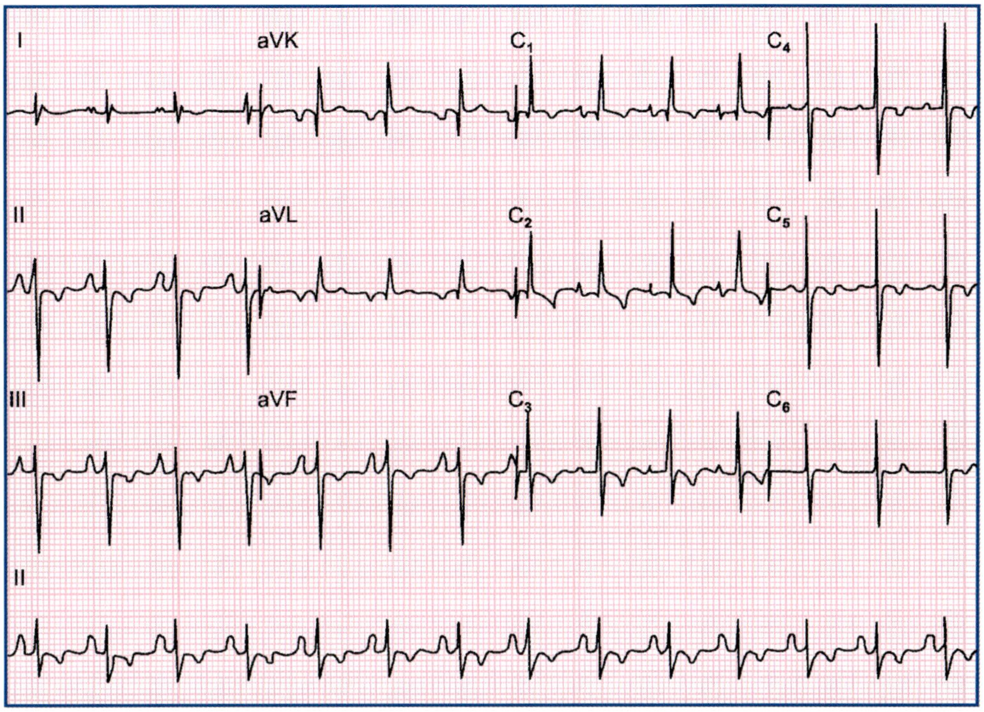

Figure 3 12-lead resting electrocardiogram from the same patient with Eisenmenger's syndrome and a large VSD. Note extreme right axis deviation with RV hypertrophy and first-degree heart block. T wave inversion across the left and precordial leads suggests possible ischemia

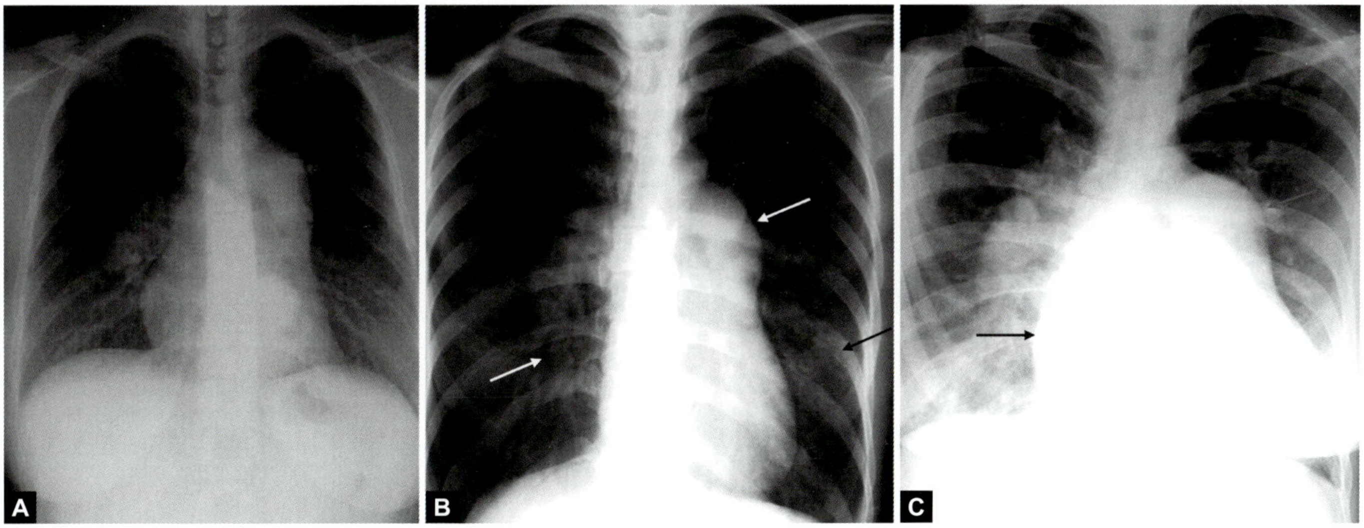

Figures 4A to C X-ray of a patient with Eisenmenger's syndrome

Echocardiography

TEE is preferred and accurate for the diagnosis of SVD should be undertaken in any patient with unexplained dilatation of the right side of the heart. The best view on TEE for recognition of ASD sinus venosus (SVC type) is bicaval view **(Figs 5A and B)**.

- Heart defect, ↓ in TAPSE <15 mm, RV dilatation, duration of TR, direction of shunting, pulmonary hypertension
- Cardiac catheterization
- Open lung biopsy.

Exercise Testing with Pulse Oximetry Most Useful

Decrease in oxygen saturation at pulse oximetry after exercises. Patients with little or no pulmonary vascular disease should continue to shunt left to right during exercise, and thus their pulse oximetry should be normal throughout. Patients with bidirectional shunting may have normal resting pulse oximetry but typically it will fall during exercise, reflecting shunt reversal. Those with advanced pulmonary vascular disease will have hypoxemia at rest, which should worsen significantly with any level of exercise activity.[7]

2D ECHO: EISENMENGER'S SYNDROME (FIGS 6A TO D)

Primary imaging modality in Eisenmenger's syndrome is TEE. It helps:

- Identify underlying cardiac diagnosis and cause of R→L shunting
- Estimate the pulmonary artery pressure **(Fig. 6A)**
- Assessment of RV function/risk
- *For pulmonary artery pressure (PAP)*: Use following calculations
  - Right ventricular systolic pressure (RVSP) = 4 $(\text{TR jet velocity})^2$ + RA pressure
  - In the absence of a gradient across right ventricular outflow tract (RVOT) or PV, RVSP = SPAP
  - PADP = 4 $(\text{end-diastolic pulmonary regurgitant velocity})^2$ + RA pressure
- *Echocardiographic predictors of outcome for mortality*: Strong predictors of all cause mortality
  - TAPSE <15 mm
  - Ratio of RV effective systolic to diastolic duration ≥ 1.5
  - RA area ≥ 25 cm^2
  - Ratio of RA to LA area ≥ 1.5
- *RV systolic function*: It is good if following calculated are within the range shown
  - TAPSE (>15 mm) **(Fig. 6B)**
  - RIMP/MPI/ TEI Index **(Fig. 6C)**
    - Pulsed Doppler MPI (<0.4)
    - Tissue Doppler MPI (<0.55)
  - Tissue Doppler Imaging
    - RV S'(> 10 cm/s)
  - RV FAC (Fractional area change) (>35%) **(Fig. 6D)**.

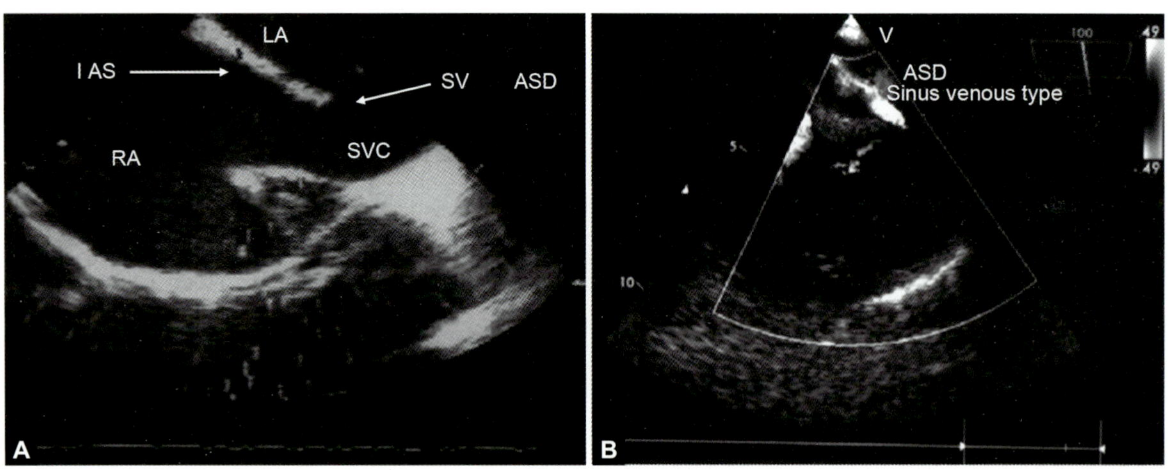

Figures 5A and B (A) Longitudinal plane of interatrial septum showing the typical appearance of sinus venosus defect which may lead to Eisenmenger's syndrome with L → R shunting (SV ASD). *Abbreviations*: IAS–interatrial septum, LA–left atrium, RA–right atrium, SVC–superior vena cava; (B) Sinus venosus type ASD with bidirect

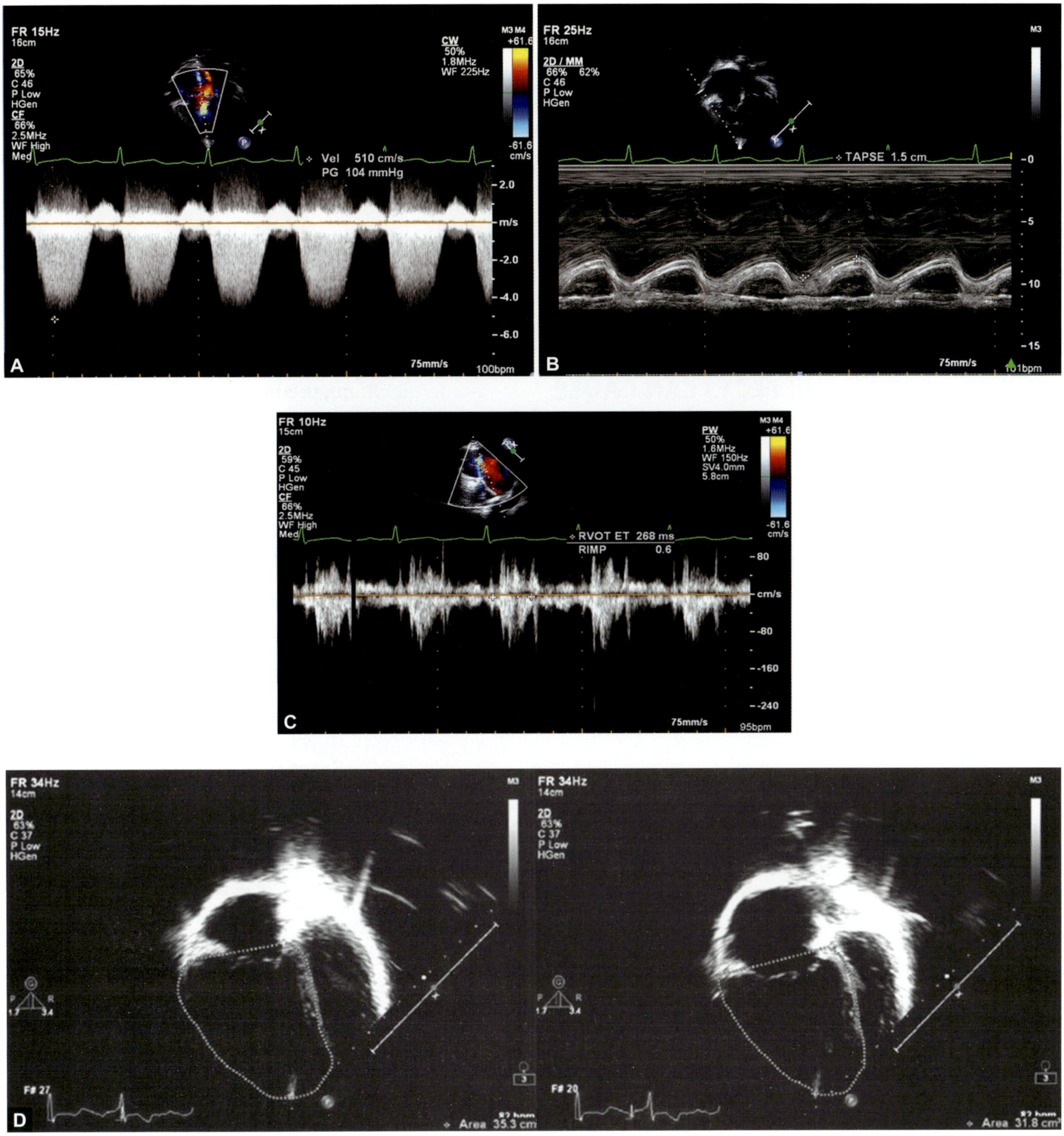

Figures 6A to D (A) Measurement of pulmonary artery pressure (PAP); (B) Measurement of tricuspid annular plane systolic (TAPSE) on M mode echocardiogram (ECHO); (C) Measurement of right ventricular outflow tract (RVOT)/RMP/TEI INDEX; (D) Measurement of RV FAC. *Abbreviation*: RV FAC–(end-diastolic area—end-systolic area)/end-diastolic area × 100 on transthoracic echo

Course in Adulthood

- Many individuals with Eisenmenger's syndrome survive into adulthood with 80% survival at 10 years, 77% survival at 15 years and 42% at 25 years after diagnosis
- Variables associated with poor prognosis include:
  - Syncope
  - Elevated RA pressure
  - Severe resting hypoxemia (<80% transcutaneous oxygen saturation)
  - CCF (25%↓).

DIFFERENT CONGENITAL INTRACARDIAC OR EXTRACARDIAC DEFECTS CAN CAUSE EISENMENGER'S SYNDROME

Following Three Account for 70–80% of Cases: To Rule Out on TEE

Presence of:

1. VSD
2. Atrioventricular septal defect
3. PDA.

Other Congenital Heart Diseases which can Cause Eisenmenger's Syndrome

- ASD especially the sinus venosus type
- Truncus arteriosus
- Aortopulmonary window
- Univentricular heart without PS
- D-transposition of the great vessels with VSD
- Surgically created aorto-pulmonary connections
- RA and RV dilated with TR and PAH.

The Causes of Death in Eisenmenger's Patients

- Sudden death (30%)
- Congestive heart failure (25%)
- Hemoptysis (15%)
- Pregnancy
- Perioperative following noncardiac surgery
- Infective endocarditis
- Brain abscess
- Noncardiac causes.

Expected Abnormalities

- A number of abnormal findings are expected in Eisenmenger's syndrome patients and should not raise undue concern unless they represent a significant change from past values
- Oxygen saturation at rest usually ranges in 80s
- If checked shortly after exertion, it will be lower (mid 70% range)
- The baseline value should be established after a few minutes of rest
- Hct ↑, PLt ↓ (Platelets decrease)
- INR and APTT are mildly prolonged
- Uric acid and bilirubin are elevated
- Proteinuria, usually less than 1 G/24 hours (this is glomerular in origin and related to the hypoxemia)
- Mildly elevated serum Cr and hematuria can also be found.

Effect of Eisenmenger's Syndrome on Pregnancy

Eisenmenger's syndrome is a complex combination of cardiovascular abnormalities. It consists of pulmonary hypertension, a right to left extra cardiac shunt and arterial hypoxemia. Pregnancy is not well tolerated by patients with this condition. When pregnancy occurs in women with Eisenmenger's syndrome, medical termination is considered safer than any mode of delivery. Acute arrhythmias are particularly dangerous as these patients have little or no cardiac reserve and need a normal sinus rhythm to keep up with the increased workload. Maternal mortality rate is estimated at 30–50%.

Salient Points to be Kept in Mind for the Administration of Safe Anesthesia for Cesarean Section

Anesthetic management of patients with Eisenmenger's syndrome is challenging. If the patient does reach full term, a multidisciplinary approach with close communication between obstetrician, cardiologist and anesthesiologist is essential. Anesthetic consideration centers on the avoidance of any decrease in the SVR.

Hypotension from any cause can progress to insufficient RV pressure required to perfuse the hypertensive pulmonary arterial bed and may result in sudden death of the patient. The anesthetist must be aware of the maternal anticoagulation. If there are no contraindications to regional block, a titrated epidural anesthesia is probably the technique of choice.[8] A slow induction of epidural allows compensation for sympathectomy below the level of block, a dilute solution of phenylephrine may be given as needed to maintain maternal SVR. Oxygen (O_2) should be administered to all patients undergoing surgery under regional anesthesia, as O_2 reduces pulmonary vascular resistance, which benefits the patient with Bisenmenger syndrome. The blood loss should be promptly replaced by crystalloids, colloids, or packed cells. Postpartum auto transfusion may cause intravascular volume overload in these patients. Regional anesthesia may reduce the risk of postoperative deep vein thrombosis.

Drawbacks of Administering General Anesthesia to Parturients with Eisenmenger's Syndrome

Cesarean section can also be conducted under general anesthesia, but there several disadvantages associated with general anesthesia,[8] e.g. effects of IPPV on venous return, ventilation/perfusion mismatch, high pulmonary artery pressure, increased shunt through the anatomic defect and myocardial depression by halogenated agents. If slow induction of anesthesia is used, there is a risk of maternal aspiration. Monitoring includes invasive blood pressure monitoring (A-line), and central venous pressure (CVP) monitoring. Pulmonary artery (PA) catheter use is controversial. It is difficult to position the balloon tipped flow directed catheter into the pulmonary artery and risk of pulmonary artery rupture is always present.

Echocardiography is very useful:

- Defines the large defect (PDA may be difficult)
- Estimates PA pressure by TR/PR jets
- Contrast echo demonstrates R to L shunting
- TEE is safe and may be required in adults for precise delineation of the abnormality.

ECHO PREDICTORS

- A composite score based on the strongest echocardiographic predictors of outcome, including 1 point for each of the following:
  - TAPSE < 15 mm
  - Ratio of right ventricular effective systolic to diastolic duration > 1.5
  - RA area > 25 cm^2
  - Ratio of RA to left atrial area > 1.5
- This score was strongly related to mortality (odds ratio, 3.69; 95% confidence interval, 2.31–5.91 by bootstrap analysis).

CONCLUSION

Echocardiographic parameters of RV function and RA area predict mortality in Eisenmenger's patients.

A new composite echocardiographic score, described herewith, may be incorporated into the noninvasive, periodic assessment of these patients.

POINTS TO BE REMEMBER

- Eisenmenger's syndrome is a pulmonary hypertensive disease caused by left-to-right shunting of blood
- The severity of pulmonary vascular resistance is a important prognostic factor
- Corrective surgery may cause pulmonary crisis. It should be performed in selected patients
- The principle of intervention is nonintervention
- For quality of life, complications must be managed
- *Pregnancy, noncardiac surgery, traveling*: Be cautious
- Transplantation is an effective choice of treatment.

REFERENCES

1. Wood P. The Eisenmenger's syndrome or pulmonary hypertension with reversed central shunt. BMJ. 1958;2:755-62.
2. Engelfriet PM, Duffels MG, Moller T, Boersma E, Tijssen JG, Thaulow E, et al. Pulmonary arterial hypertension in adults born with a heart septal defect: the Euro Heart Survey on adult congenital heart disease. Heart. 2007;93:682-7.

3. Cantor WJ, Harrison DA, Moussadji JS, Connelly MS, Webb GD, Liu P, et al. Determinants of survival and length of survival in adults with Eisenmenger's syndrome. Am J Cardiol. 1999;84:677-81.
4. Niwa K, Perloff JK, Kaplan S, et al. Eisenmenger's syndrome in adults: ventricular septal defect, truncus arteriosus, univentricular heart. J Am Coll Cardiol. 1999;34:223-32.
5. Beghetti M, Galie N. Eisenmenger's syndrome: a clinical perspective in a new therapeutic era of pulmonary arterial hypertension. J Am Coll Cardiol. 2009;53: 733-40.
6. D'Alto M, Romeo E, Argiento P, Sarubbi B, Santoro G, Grimaldi N, et al. Bosentan-sildenafil association in patients with congenital heart disease-related pulmonary arterial hypertension and Eisenmenger's physiology. Int J Cardiol. 2012;155:378-82.
7. Pascoe RD, Oh JK, Warnes CA, Danielson GK, Tajik AJ, Seward JB. Diagnosis of sinus venosus atrial septal defect with transesophageal echocardiography. Circulation. 1996;94:1049-55.
8. Ghai B, Mohan V, Khetarpal M, et al. Epidural anaesthesia for C Section patients with Eisenmenger's syndrome. Int I Obstet Anaesthesia. 2002;11:44-7.

Chapter 23

TEE for Patent Foramen Ovale

Poonam Malhotra Kapoor, Arin Choudhury, Jitin Narula, Sanjay Kumar

Chapter Outline

- Structure of Patent Foramen Ovale
- Clinical Features of Patent Foramen Ovale
- Detection of a Right-to-Left Shunt through a PFO
- Transesophageal Echocardiogram
- Preoperative TEE Assessment of Patent Foramen Ovale
- Postoperative Echo Assessment Following Repair

INTRODUCTION

Patent foramen ovale (PFO) is common in the general population and there is a probe-patent PFO in 15–35% of the population based on a review of over 9000 autopsy studies.[1] Patent foramen ovale has been implicated in the etiology of a number of different pathologies, including cryptogenic stroke, decompression sickness in divers, platypnea orthodeoxia, and migraine with aura **(Fig. 1)**. It has been a matter of controversy for some time whether PFO has a direct causal role in stroke or whether the relationship found in existing case-control studies is merely an association. In support of the causal relationship, there have been numerous case reports of the direct visualization of thrombus in migration through a PFO.[2] There is a direct relationship between the size of a shunt through a PFO and the risk of first stroke **(Fig. 1)**.[3] Moreover, the risk of stroke appears to be increased in the presence

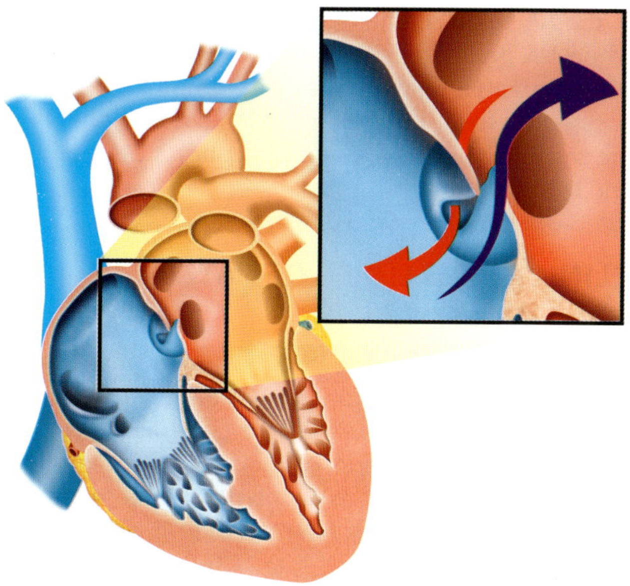

Figure 1 Patent foramen ovale

of defects that direct flow towards a PFO, for example in patients with a prominent Eustachian valve.[4] In addition, hemodynamic changes that increase right-sided pressure (such as a large pulmonary embolism) promote R–L shunting and are associated with increased rates of stroke.[5] Patients with a residual shunt following device closure have a higher rate of recurrent stroke, whereas those with effective closure have a very low rate of further events.[6] Finally, the association between PFO and stroke not only persists but also becomes more pronounced with increasing age, which is likely to reflect the age-related exponential increase in the risk of venous thromboembolism.[7] As a result of these data and a number of case series assessing the efficacy of secondary prevention of thromboembolic events, the procedure has become established—although definitive studies of long-term outcome are still needed. Closure is not without risk however, with death, major hemorrhage, cardiac tamponade, and fatal pulmonary emboli occurring in 1.5% and minor complications including atrial arrhythmia, device embolization, device thrombus, and AV fistula formation occurring in up to 7.9%.[8] This chapter aims to summarize the imaging techniques required in accurate diagnosis and careful assessment of device closure of PFO in order to optimize patient outcomes.

STRUCTURE OF PATENT FORAMEN OVALE

In utero, the foramen ovale is a flap-like structure that permits shunting of blood directly from the RA to the LA **(Fig. 1)**. The flap normally closes after birth, when LA pressure rises, and becomes sealed within 12 months. However, in around 25% of the general population the foramen does not close completely and the resulting PFO is a potential conduit between right and left atria.

CLINICAL FEATURES OF PATENT FORAMEN OVALE

In the majority of people PFO causes no problems and no direct clinical findings, but in a small number it can be a cause of stroke (allowing a clot to pass from the venous to the arterial side of the circulation: 'paradoxical embolism') and is also associated with decompression illness in scuba divers (paradoxical gas embolism). There is also a higher incidence of PFO among patients with migraines.

DETECTION OF A RIGHT-TO-LEFT SHUNT THROUGH A PFO

Several echocardiographic techniques can be utilized in the detection of a PFO shunt, including transthoracic echocardiogram (TTE), TEE, and transcranial Doppler ultra sonography. Because of its superior image resolution and ability to differentiate the location of shunting, TEE is most commonly used for PFO diagnosis. However, TEE is usually preceded by TTE.

TRANSESOPHAGEAL ECHOCARDIOGRAM

A PFO may also be detected by imaging it directly with a TEE probe. In this way, the PFO can be seen very easily. This test is somewhat uncomfortable and a mild intravenous sedative is used to ensure patient comfort and cooperation.

The heart action is viewed "live" and the atrial septum and PFO (if present) is visualized. **Figure 2** shows the right atrium (RA) and left atrium (LA). The arrow points to the trapdoor of the patent foramen ovale (PFO).

Saline solution is injected and the bubbles are easily seen in the right atrium (RA). The presence of a PFO is confirmed by seeing bubbles pass to the left atrium (LA) through the PFO as shown in **Figure 3**.

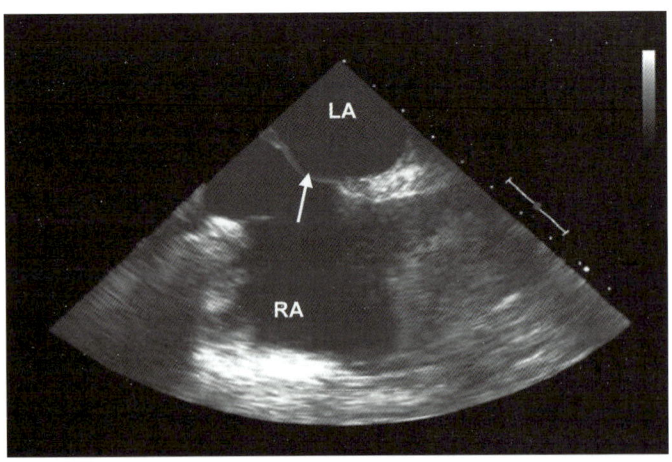

Figure 2 The right atrium (RA) and left atrium (LA) in PFO (Shown with an arrow)

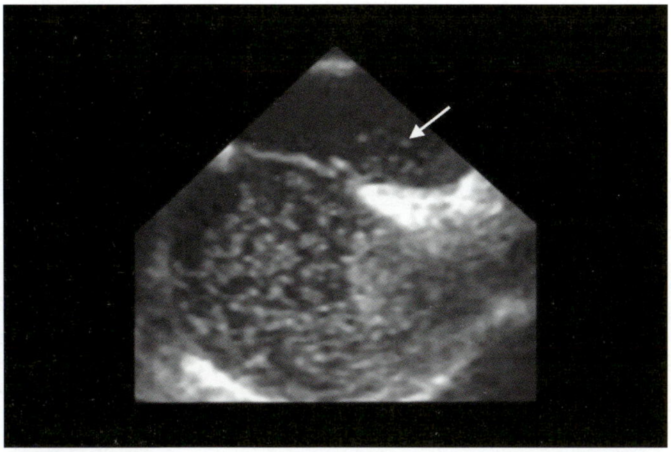

Figure 3 Patent foramen ovale is confirmed by seeing bubbles pass to the left atrium (LA) through the PFO

As with transcranial Doppler the injection is repeated while the patient takes a deep breath and then exhales forcefully as these maneuvers may be required to "open" the PFO.

The results of the transesophageal echocardiogram are also available immediately and are discussed with the patient before he/she goes home. A copy of the results are forwarded to the primary care physician the same day.

PREOPERATIVE TEE ASSESSMENT OF PATENT FORAMEN OVALE

With the echo probe in the midesophageal position, obtain a 4-chamber view and visualize the interatrial septum.

Use color Doppler to check for the presence of any flow across the interatrial septum. Asking the patient to perform and then release a Valsalva maneuver (deep breath in and 'bear down') can momentarily open up a PFO and reveal a brief jet of right-to-left flow.

It may be necessary to go on to perform an 'agitated' saline bubble contrast study. Although TTE can sometimes detect a PFO, TOE is regarded as the investigation of choice (**Fig. 3**).

POSTOPERATIVE ECHO ASSESSMENT FOLLOWING REPAIR

Using the same views as for unrepaired PFO:

- Comment on the presence of a septal device or patch
- Check for any residual shunt
- Flow across the IAS.

REFERENCES

1. Homma S, Sacco RL. Patent foramen ovale and stroke. Circulation. 2005;112:1063-72.
2. Kessel-Schaefer A, Lefkovits M, Zellweger MJ, Brett W, Ruter F, Pfisterer ME, et al. Migrating thrombus trapped in a patent foramen ovale. Circulation. 2001;103:1928.
3. Stone DA, Godard J, Corretti MC, Kittner SJ, Sample C, Price TR, et al. Patent foramen ovale: association between the degree of shunt by contrast transoesophageal echocardiography and the risk of future ischemic neurologic events. Am Heart J. 1996;131:158-61.
4. Schuchlenz HW, Saurer G, Weihs W, et al. Persisting eustachian valve in adults: relation to patent foramen ovale and cerebrovascular events. J Am Soc Echocardiogr. 2004;17:231-3.
5. Lapostolle F, Borron SW, Surget V, Sordelet D, Lapandry C, Adnet F. Stroke associated with pulmonary embolism after air travel. Neurology. 2003;60:1983-5.
6. Wahl A, Meier B, Haxel B, Nedeltchev K, Arnold M, Eicher E, et al. Prognosis after percutaneous closure of patent foramen ovale for paradoxical embolism. Neurology. 2001;57:1330-2.
7. Handke M, Harloff A, Olschewski M, et al. Patent foramen ovale and cryptogenic stroke in older patients. N Engl J Med 2007;357:2262-8.
8. Khairy P, O'Donnell CP, Landzberg MJ. Transcatheter closure versus medical therapy of patent foramen ovale and presumed paradoxical thromboemboli: a systematic review. Ann Intern Med. 2003;139:753-60.

TEE is the investigation of choice in detecting a PFO.

Chapter 24

TEE for Tricuspid Atresia

Poonam Malhotra Kapoor, Sachin Talwar, Parag Gharde, Sameer Taneja

Chapter Outline

INTRODUCTION

Tricuspid valve (TV) atresia is a cyanotic congenital heart lesion that is characterized by congenital agenesis or absence of the tricuspid valve, resulting in no direct communication between the right atrium and ventricle.[1] If untreated, TV atresia has a high mortality rate with a survival rate as low as 10% at one year of age, depending on the type of TV atresia and the presence of other cardiac lesions.[2,3]

DEFINITION

Tricuspid atresia is a cardiac defect present at birth (congenital) in which one of the valves (tricuspid valve) between two of the cardiac chambers is not formed. Instead, there's solid tissue between the chambers.

ANATOMY

Although TV atresia is characterized by the absence of the tricuspid valve, there is a spectrum of anatomic variants based on the morphology of the atresia and the presence of other cardiac structural lesions (**Fig. 1**).

ETIOLOGY AND CLINICAL FEATURES

- Progressive cyanosis as PDA closes
- 30% transposition of great arteries
- 70% some degree of pulmonic stenosis
- Tachypneic, single S2
- Systolic murmur along left lower sternal border (VSD)
- ECG reveals left ventricular hypertrophy.[4]

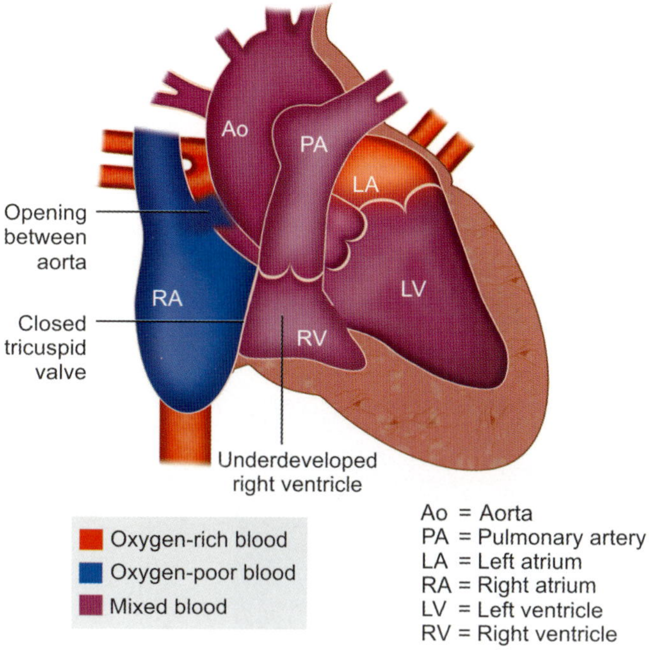

Figure 1 Anatomy of tricuspid atresia

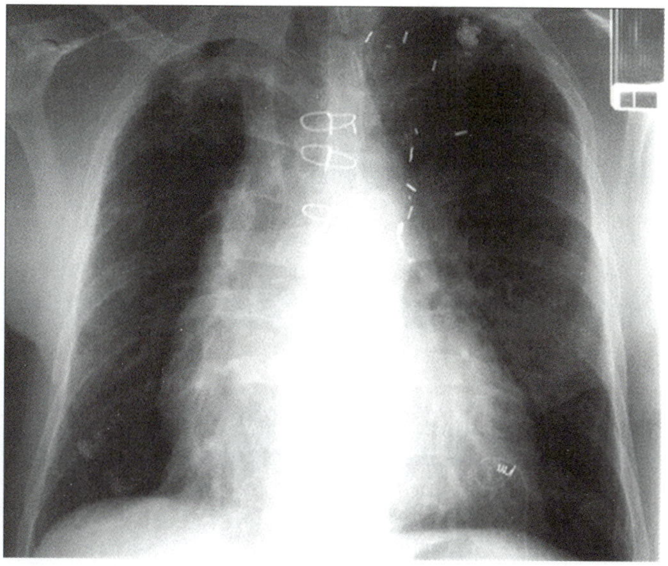

Figure 2 Tricuspid atresia with multiple surgeries in a 43-year-old man

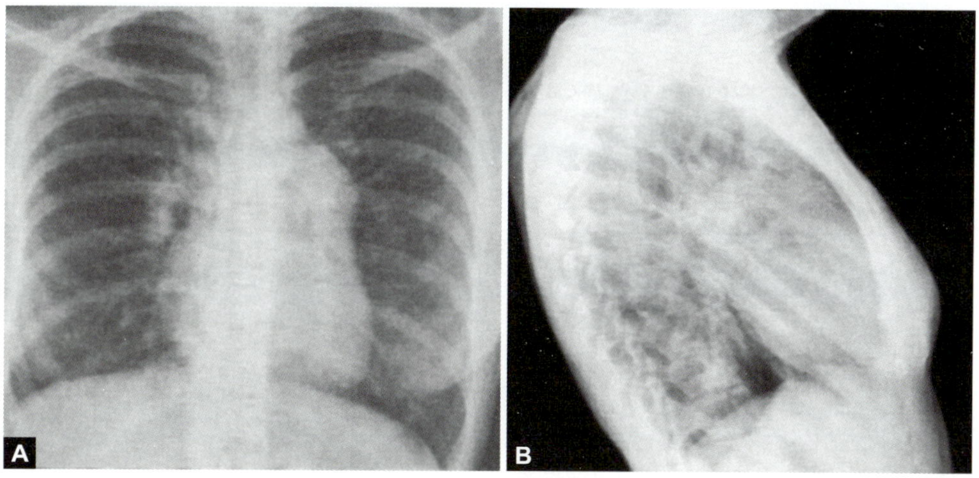

Figures 3A and B Chest film PA and lateral views of a patient with ventricular septal defect with severe pulmonary hypertension Eisenmenger's complex

CHEST X-RAY OF TRICUSPID ATRESIA

- Appearance is variable depending on the amount of pulmonary blood flow.
- Diminished pulmonary blood flow is seen with normal or slightly enlarged cardiac silhouette.
- Concavity in the pulmonic area and decreased pulmonary vascular markings.
- Increased blood flow will be associated with cardiac enlargement and pulmonary congestion (**Fig. 2**).

Shown below is an example of chest X-ray in a patient with tricuspid atresia demonstrating the following features (**Figs 3A and B**).

- Reduced pulmonary blood flow, prominent aortic root (AO) and right atrium (RA)
- The left anterior oblique projection on the right side shows distinctive humped appearance of the anterior cardiac silhouette due to right atrial (RA) enlargement in the absence of a right ventricle.
- The left ventricle (LV) is enlarged.
- A right aortic arch may be observed in some cases.

ECG FINDINGS

ECG findings with TA are very specific (**Fig. 5**):

- Most other cyanotic heart lesions present with increased right-sided forces, i.e. right axis deviation and right ventricular hypertrophy; with the hypoplastic right ventricle of TA, right-sided forces are diminutive or even absent.
- The ECG will show a left and superior axis in nearly 90% of TA with normally related great arteries, and 50% with d-TGA will also be 0 to 90 degrees. The rest should fall in the left inferior quadrant.

CASE PRESENTATION (FIGS 2 TO 7)

A 43-year-old man, born with tricuspid atresia, was palliated in childhood with a Waterston-Cooley shunt (later taken down), a Glenn, a Blalock-Taussig, then a graft from descending aorta to left PA (B-T no longer

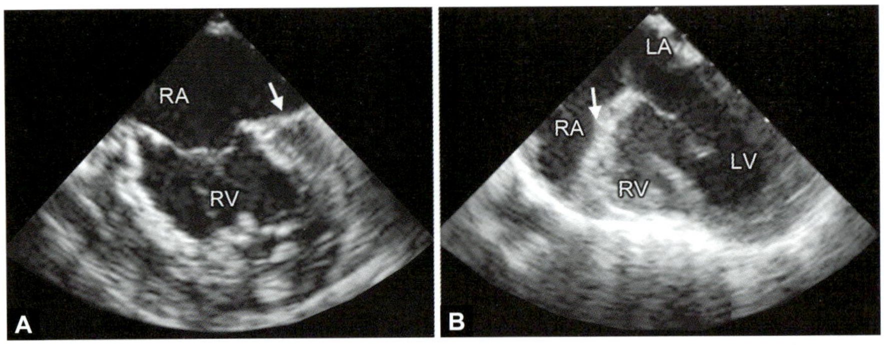

Figures 4A and B Single ventricle physiology. (A) Hypoplastic left heart syndrome. The midesophageal short-axis view shows the mitral atresia (arrow) and hypoplasia of left ventricle (LV); (B) Tricuspid atresia. The midesophageal short-axis view demonstrates the tricuspid atresia (arrow) and hypoplasia of right ventricle (RV). *Abbreviation:* RA, right atrium

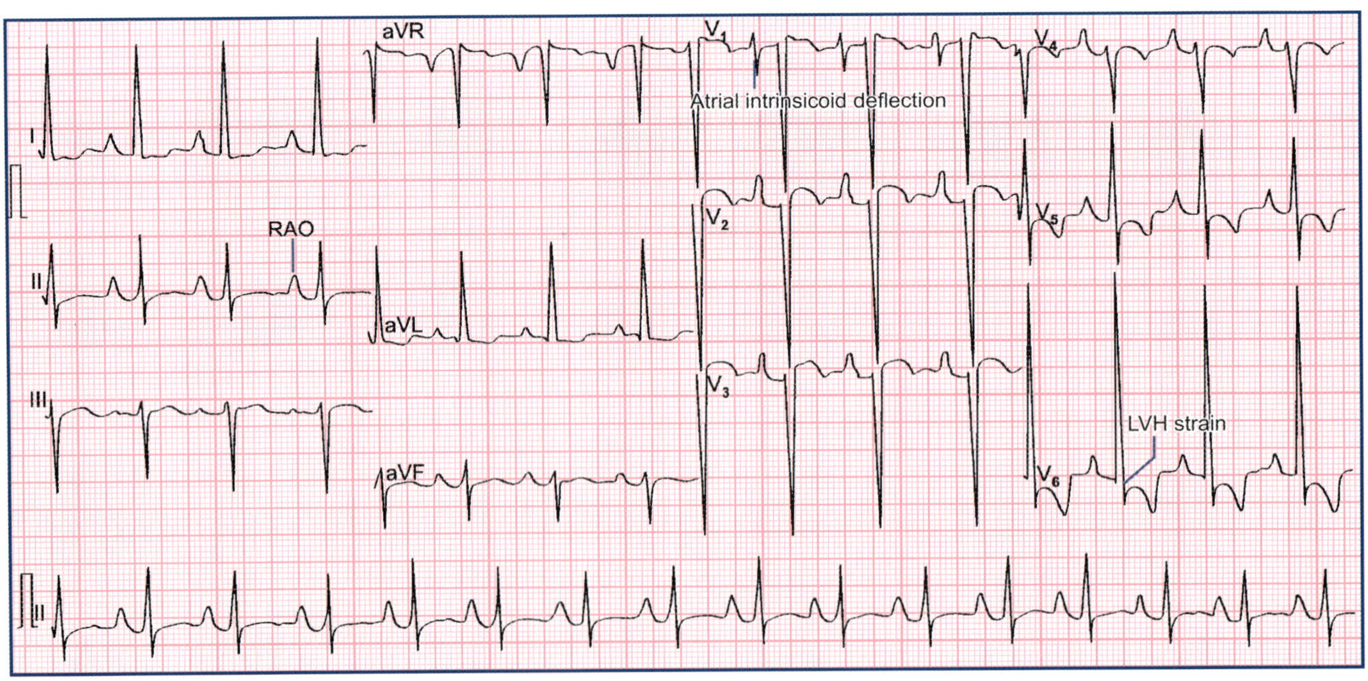

Figure 5 ECG of a patient with tricuspid atresia defect

CHAPTER 24

functional). Hemoptysis required coil embolization of right lung AVMs.

At age 31, the aorta-PA graft was coil embolized in preparation for the Fontan: the PDA was ligated, the VSD closed, the ASD closed, a 6 mm fenestration was created, the RA appendage was connected by graft to the left PA, an opening between the RA and the SVC was slightly enlarged to allow some atrial return to the right lung. Due to cyanosis the ASD was closed with a clamshell occluder 2 months later (see transesophageal echo) (*see* **Figs 3A and B**).

Atrial arrhythmias began at age 25 and were medically treated. Atrial fibrillation recurred 6 years after the Fontan. Sinus rhythm was restored with amiodarone, digoxin, warfarin. An epicardial VVIR pacemaker was placed. VO_2 was 14.5 mL/kg/min at baseline.

TEE CONFIRMS THE DIAGNOSIS OF TRICUSPID ATRESIA

- Ventricular size
- Atrial and ventricular shunts
- Location and function of the AV valves
- Relationships of the great arteries are all well seen with echocardiography.
- Presence of a left SVC and its atrial communication can also be established, which is of importance to the surgical repair.
- The atretic tricuspid valve is represented by dense band of echoes (**Fig. 6**).

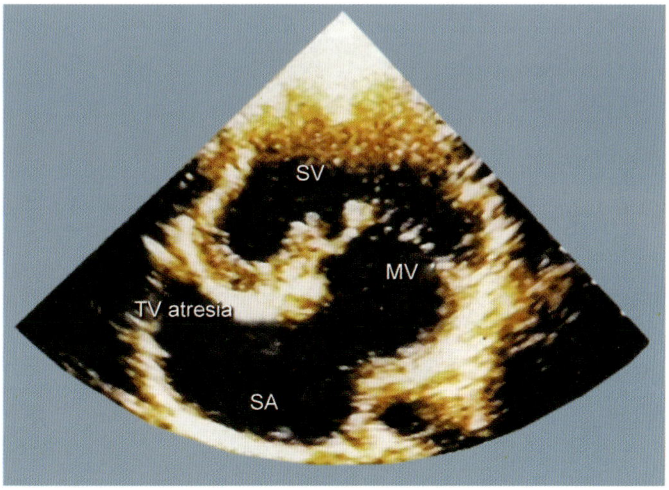

Figure 6 Apical four-chamber view shows dense band of echoes at the site normally occupied by the tricuspid valve and single atrium, as there is no IAS and single ventricle as there is only a small rudimentary septal tissue at the apex

- The 2D echo is not only diagnostic of tricuspid atresia, but is also establishes the position of great arteries, the condition of the interventricular septum and the nature of ASD.
- The ventricular to great arterial connection are best established.
- In ME 4 chamber and RV inflow-outflow view along with CW Doppler study assist in identification of the presence or absence of pulmonic stenosis (**Figs 7A and B**).
- The comparison of the relative sizes of aortic root and pulmonary trunk can also be done. In the common variety of tricuspid atresia identifies a dense band of echoes at the site normally occupied by the tricuspid valve.

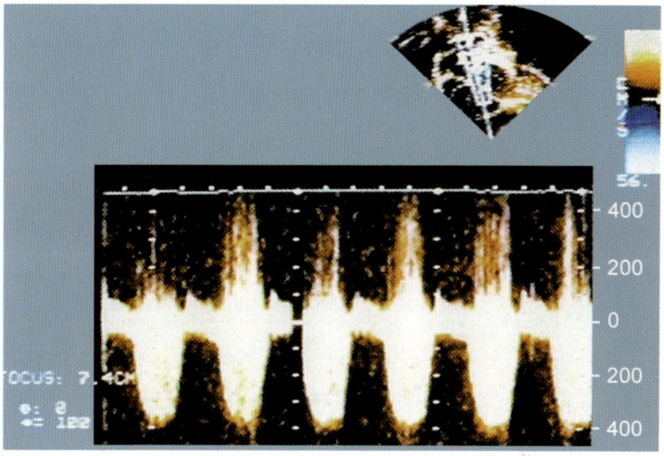

Figure 7A CW Doppler shows associated pulmonary stenosis

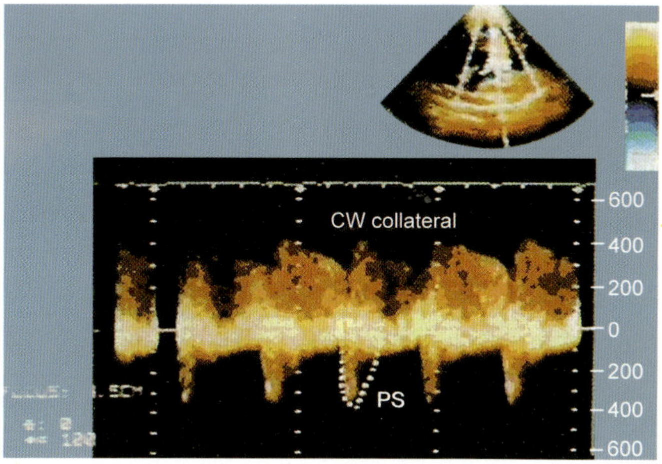

Figure 7B CW Doppler shows continuous signals in associated collaterals

- In tricuspid atresia, the right ventricular cavity is small, and the left ventricular cavity is only moderately enlarged.
- The right atrium is increased in size and the atrial septum bulges towards the left if the inter atrial communication is restrictive.
- When tricuspid atresia occurs with transposition of the great arteries, a large ventricular septal defect is imaged the right ventricular cavity is well developed.
- When pulmonary stenosis is present the echocardiogram identifies the obstruction.

REFERENCES

1. Rao PS. Diagnosis and management of cyanotic congenital heart disease: part I. Indian J Pediatr. 2009; 76:57.
2. Dick M, Fyler DC, Nadas AS. Tricuspid atresia: clinical course in 101 patients. Am J Cardiol. 1975;36:327.
3. Keating P. Tricuspid atresia—profile and outcome. Cardiovasc J S Afr. 2001;12:202.
4. (Cyanotic Heart Disease, Casey Wong MS III) congenital heart disease , Copyright 2001, Yale University School of Medicine.

Chapter 25

Echo Resources

Poonam Malhotra Kapoor, Kalpana Irpachi

Chapter Outline

- Echo Resources
- Societies
- Websites

ECHO RESOURCES

Textbooks

- Deepak K Tempe. Atlas of Trans-oesophageal Echocardiography: An Anesthesiologist's Perspective. Anshan Ltd, CBS, 2005, ISBN: 9781904798231.
- Textbook of TEE by Deepak Tempe, 1st Edition CBS Publishers, 2013.
- Robert M Savage. Perioperative Transesophageal Echocardiography, 2nd Revised edn. Lippincott: Williams and Wilkins; 2010. ISBN: 1605472468.
- David Sidebotham. Practical Perioperative Transesophageal Echocardiography. Butterworth-Heinemann; 2nd edn, 2011; ISBN: 9780702034275.
- Annette Vegas. Real-Time Three-Dimensional Transesophageal Echocardiography. Springer, 2012, ISBN: 9781461406648.
- Poonam Malhotra Kapoor. Review of Cardiac Anesthesia with 2100 MCQs; Jaypee Brothers Medical Publishers, 2013. ISBN: 9789350906590.
- Poonam Malhotra Kapoor. TEE of TV and PV Jaypee Brothers Medical Publishers, 2013 ISBN: 978-9351521297.
- Albert C Perrino, Scott T Reeves. A Practical Approach to Transesophageal Echocardiography, ISBN-10: 1451175604, ISBN-13: 978-1451175608.
- Navin Chandar Nanda, Michael J Domanski. Atlas of Transesophageal Echocardiography Lippincott Williams & Wilkins, 2007, ISBN-10: 0781755034 ISBN-13: 978-0781755030.
- Atul P Kulkarni, Divatia JV, Vijaya P Patil, Gehdoo RP. Objective Anaesthesia Review: A Comprehensive Textbook for the Examinees (2013) ISBN-10: 9350905043 ISBN-13: 978-9350905043.
- Vegas, Annette. Perioperative Two-Dimensional Transesophageal Echocardiography: A Practical Handbook 2011, ISBN-10: 1441999515 ISBN-13: 978-1441999511.
- Fischer, Conrad. Kaplan Medical Internal Medicine Question Book, October 2009, ISBN-10: 1607141264 ISBN-13: 978-1607141266.

- Robert M Savage, Solomon Aronson, Stanton K. Sherman. Comprehensive Textbook of Perioperative Transesophageal Echocardiography, October 2010, ISBN-10: 1605472468 ISBN-13: 978-1605472461.
- Gallagher, Christopher, Sciarra, John C, Ginsberg, Steven. Board Stiff TEE: Transesophageal Echocardiography, second edition April 2013, ISBN-10: 1455738050 ISBN-13: 978-1455738052.
- Gerald Maurer. Transesophageal Echocardiography January 1994, ISBN-10: 0070409889 ISBN-13: 978-0070409880.
- Norbert P De Bruijn, Fiona M. Clements Transesophageal Echocardiography, June 1991, ISBN-10: 0316178160, ISBN-13: 978-0316178167.
- Jose Missri. Transesophageal Echocardiography: Clinical and Intraoperative Applications, November 1992, ISBN-10: 0443088527, ISBN-13: 978-0443088520.

Journals

- Cardiovascular ultrasound (online journal): *http://www.cardiovascularultrasound.com*
- Echo—The journal of The British Society of Echocardiography: *http://wwwbsecho.org*
- Echocardiography—A Journal of Cardiovascular Ultrasound and Allied Techniques: *http://www.blackwell-synergy.com/loi/echo*
- European Heart Journal—Cardiovascular imaging: *http://www.oxfordjounals.org/our_jounals/ehjcimaging*
- The Journal of The American Society of Echocardiography: *http://journal.elsevierhealth.com/periodical/ymje*
- Annals of cardiac anaesthesia TEE tutorials: *http://www.annals.in*
- Journal of the American Society of Echocardiography: *http://www.onlinejase.com*
- Circulation: *http://circ.ahajournals.org*
- National center for biotechnology information: *http://www.ncbi.nlm.nih.gov*
- The Journal of the Society of Anesthesiologists: *http://journals.lww.com/anesthesiology*
- American Society of Echocardiography: *http://www.asecho.org*
- British Journal of Anesthesia: *http://www.bja.oxfordjournals.org*
- Journal of the American Society of Cardiology: *http://www.content.onlinejacc.org*
- The Journal of Thoracic and Cardiovascular Surgery: *http://www.jtcvsonline.org*

Key Guidelines

Key guidance published by the British Society of Echocardiography (BSE) and available from its website (*http://www.bsecho.org*):

- A standard Transthoracic Echocardiogram
- A standard Transesophageal Echocardiogram
- Recommendations for safe practice in sedation during Transesophageal Echocardiography
- Protocol: Mitral Stenosis
- Protocol: Pulmonary Hypertension
- Protocol: Hypertrophic Cardiomyopathy

Posters published by the BSE and British Heart Foundation (details can be obtained from the BSE):

- *Echocardiography:* Guidelines for chamber quantification
- *Echocardiography:* Guidelines for valve quantification

1. Cerqueira MD, Weissman NJ, Dilsizian V, et al. Standardized myocardial segmentation and nomenclature for tomographic imaging of the heart. Circulation. 2002;105:539-42.
2. Douglas PS, Khandheria B, Stainback RF, et al. ACCF/ASE/ACEP/ASNC/SCAI/SCCT/SCMR 2007 appropriateness criteria for transthoracic and transesophageal echocardiography. J Am Call Cardiol. 2007;50:187-204.
3. Douglas PS, Khandheria B, Stainback RF, et al. ACCF/ASE/ACEP/AHA/ASNC/SCAIISCCT/SCMR 2008 appropriateness criteria for stress echo cardiography. J Am Call Cardiol. 2008;51:1127-47.
4. Lancellotti P, Tribouilloy C, Hagendorff A, et al. European Association of Echocardiography recommendations for the assessment of valvular regurgitation. *Part 1:* Aortic and pulmonary regurgitation (native valve disease). Eur J Echocardiogr. 2010;11:223-44.
5. Lancellotti P, Moura L, Pierard LA, et al. European Association of Echocardiography recommendations for the assessment of valvular regurgitation. *Part 2:* Mitral and tricuspid regurgitation (native valve disease). Eur J Echocardiogr. 2010;11:307-32.
6. Lang RM, Bierig M, Devereux RB, et al. Recommendations for Chamber Quantification: A Report from the American Society of Echocardiography's Guidelines and Standards

Committee and the Chamber Quantification Writing Group, developed in conjunction with the European Association of Echocardiography: a branch of the European Society of Cardiology. J Am Sac Echocardiogr. 2005;18:1440-63.

The Task Force on the Management of Valvular Heart Disease of the European Society of Cardiology. Guidelines on the management of valvular heart disease. Eur Heart J. 2007;28:230-68.

SOCIETIES

American Society of Echocardiography

2100 gateway centre boulevard
Suite 310
Morrisville, NC 27560
United states of America
Tel: +9198615574
Fax: +9198829900
Website: *http://www.asecho.org*

British Society of Echocardiography

Doxkland Business centre
10-16 Tiller Road
London E14 8PX
United Kingdom
Tel: 02073455185
Fax: 02073455186
Website: *http://www.bsecho.org*

European Association of Cardiovascular Imaging

European Society of Cardiology
The European Heart House 2035, Route des Colles
BP 179- Les Templiers
06903 Sophia Antipolis
France
Tel:+33.4.92.94.76.00
Fax: +33.4.92.94.76.01
Website: *http://www.escardio.org/communities/EACVI*

Indian Association of Cardiovascular Thoracic Anaesthesiologists (IACTA)

Anaesthesia House, 1st Floor, GCDA Shopping Complex
Panampilly Nagar, Cochin, Kerala, India - 682036
Phone: 0484-4011307, 08129035539
E-mail: *iactasecretariat@gmail.com*
Website: *www.iacta.co.in.*
IACTA Education & Research Cell (IERC, A Subcommittee of IACTA)
Room no - 8, 7th Floor
Cardio-Neuro Centre
AIIMS, New Delhi (India)-110029
Phone: 011-26593858, 09868398103
E-mail: *iactaeduresearch@gmail.com*

WEBSITES

In addition to the websites already listed earlier, the following sites contain material of interest to anyone learning or practicing echocardiography:

- 123sonography: *http://www.123sonography.com*
- Echocardiology.org: *http://www.echocardiology.org*
- e-Echocardiography: *http://e-echocardiography.com*
- Wikiecho: *http://www.wikiecho.com*
- Yahoo! Discussion Group—Cardiovascular Ultrasound: *http://health.groups.yahoo.com/group/echocardiography*
- Yale Atlas of Echocardiography: *http://www.yale.edu/imaging/echo_atlas/contents.*

CHAPTER 25

Index

Page numbers followed by *f* refer to figure and *t* refer to table